Monographien aus dem Gesamtgebiete der Psychiatrie

14

Psychiatry Series

Herausgegeben von
H. Hippius, München · W. Janzarik, Heidelberg
C. Müller, Prilly-Lausanne

The Apallic Syndrome

Edited by
G. Dalle Ore · F. Gerstenbrand
C. H. Lücking · G. Peters · U. H. Peters

With the Editorial Assistance of
E. Rothemund

With 67 Figures

Springer-Verlag
Berlin Heidelberg New York 1977

Professor Dr. G. Peters, Max-Planck-Institut für Psychiatrie,
Kraepelinstr. 2, D-8000 München 40

Professor Dr. G. Dalle Ore, Università di Neurochirurgia di Padova,
I-37100 Verona

Professor Dr. F. Gerstenbrand, Neurologische Universitätsklinik,
Anichstr. 35, A-6020 Innsbruck

Priv.-Doz. Dr. C. H. Lücking, Neurologische Klinik der Technischen
Universität, Möhlstr. 28, D-8000 München 80

Professor Dr. U. H. Peters, Johannes-Gutenberg-Universität Mainz,
Neuropsychiatrische Klinik, Langenbeckstr. 1, D-6500 Mainz

ISBN-13: 978-3-642-81153-1 e-ISBN-13: 978-3-642-81151-7
DOI: 10.1007/978-3-642-81151-7

Library of Congress Cataloging in Publication Data. Main entry under title: The Apallic Syndrome. (Monographien aus dem Gesamtgebiete der Psychiatrie; 14). Includes index. 1. Akinetic mutism. I. Dalle Ore, G., 1924— II. Series. RC394.A43A63. 616.8'5. 77-24951.

Softcover reprint of the hardcover 1st edition 1977

Foreword

The subject of the apallic syndrome is one which has long been familiar to me, although I have not personally studied it as deeply as I would have wished. I became acquainted with this syndrome long before the last war, when my neurosurgical colleague Hugh Cairns (1952), made his pioneer contribution under the term "akinetic mutism". This was an arresting title, but it was one which did not altogether satisfy some of his colleagues, including myself. We found it difficult to suggest an alternative. That is one reason why I welcome the expression "apallic syndrome".

Forensic practice has forced me from time to time to consider rather more deeply this distressing syndrome, and to try and marshal my ideas in a form which would satisfy my colleagues in the legal profession. More than once I have been instructed to make a medicolegal assessment of these unfortunate patients. The points which have concerned my lawyer friends have not been matters of diagnosis, or of morbid anatomy, or of etiology. The factual problem which has been put before me was to make some approximate assessment as to the expectation of life. Vague guess-work is unacceptable in such circumstances. What the lawyers require is a precise and dogmatic answer. How many months, how many years can an apallic victim continue to survive in his state of suspended animation? Much, if not everything, depends of course upon the amount of medical and nursing care which the relatives can command. But what actually is the practical limit of expectation in optimal circumstances? And what complications are there which are responsible for the fatal termination of these patients?

My other question is of a more philosophic character. Many apallic patients cannot be said to be in a state of total unconsciousness. And yet their state of awareness is restricted—usually to a considerable extent. Can it be said, however, that all cognitive processes are necessarily in abeyance? We are familiar with the disarming manner in which some apallic patients appear to fix their gaze upon some person or object around them. Sometimes they seem to follow a moving stimulus with their eyes. Is this a volitional activity? And if so, how much in the way of sense-data is registered at a perceptual level? Or is it merely a reflex phenomenon which takes place far beyond the realm of awareness? And does a purely reflex staring at an object necessarily entail some element of perception, or are barriers of nonregistration set up between the object, the retinal imagine, and the cortex?

In the same way, I would welcome an explanation of those rare instances when the apallic patient breaks silence and ceases, for a moment, to be mute. Every neurologist must have encountered a close relative who has declared with conviction that the patient has suddenly given vent to an utterance. This is difficult to deny, although hard to explain. The vocalization belongs to the category of an "occasional utterance" as described by Hughlings Jackson (1958) in very severe cases of aphasia. The unexpected remark which the apallic patient is alleged to emit is often a phrase or even a sentence and not just an isolated word. Still more odd is the observation that the unexpected utterance is not wholly incongruous in the environmental setting but is disarming, almost startling. Is this phenomenon well authenticated? Or is it merely a figment of mythology, yet another instance of wishful thinking on the part of relatives who are emotionally involved?

One final question concerns those patients, rare no doubt, who make a recovery from a state of apallism. Do such fortunate persons recall anything that has transpired during their protracted illness? Or are these months of convalescence mercifully overlaid by an extended period of amnesia? If not, at what point in convalescence does memory begin?

Lenin once said that a fool can ask more questions in a minute than 12 wise men can answer in an hour. It behooves me, therefore, to make way for those who have had an important experience of this syndrome, with its many theoretical and practical repercussions.

Macdonald Critchley

Preface

The idea for this monograph originated from the desire to take a stand on today's views on this severe cerebral state, as well as to gain a survey of the clinical symptomatology and the morphologic changes, and to consider therapeutic possibilities. Furthermore, an attempt was made to outline the syndromic unity of the apallic syndrome and to compare this syndrome complex with other neurologic and psychiatric disorders which in their clinical symptomatology are similar to the apallic syndrome but so far have not been considered from this aspect. This applies, for example, to cerebral disorders which appear in the course of metabolic brain damage.

Thanks to the many reports and the intensive discussions held during the conference in Verona, it was possible to achieve a fairly good agreement on the clinical symptomatology, morphology, additional examinations, as well as on therapeutic measures to be taken. The literature on the apallic syndrome and analogous neurologic disorders has increased considerably in the last few years. The study of this literature, however, reveals signs of discrepancies in the terminology used. More important, no clear distinction between similar disorders is made, and the syndrome complex described by Kretschmer (1940), specifically the described clinical symptomatology and the course of the disease, as well as Kretschmer's assumed pathophysiologic basic concept of a functional disturbance, has been misunderstood by some authors. For these aforementioned reasons, it was considered best to collect the reports of the conference of Verona in a monograph.

The editors have asked the individual authors to revise their reports in order to take into account recent developments. Therefore, a renewed report on the discussion remarks will be superfluous. The decision to publish the monograph in English is based on the assumption that it will reach a wider distribution, especially since the concept of the apallic syndrome is just beginning to prevail in the Anglo-American countries.

In order to provide a better understanding of the topic and to consider specific problems, additional reports, apart from the program of Verona, were requested by the editorial board. Parts of Kretschmer's original report were included not only for historical reasons but also to demonstrate the classical presentation of this pioneer worker.

It must be particularly pointed out that, although all attempts were made to give a uniform presentation, odd reports were included for various reasons: (1) to inform the reader on the state of regional research and (2) to stress the significance of certain working methods. The editors are of course aware of the fact that this does not completely conform with the basic concept of this monograph.

It is hoped that with this monograph a further clarification of the symptomatology, prognosis, and therapeutic possibilities of this heavily increasing disorder can be brought about, and that it will provide the stimulus for even more intensified research.

The Editors

Contents

IV. Pathophysiology

V. Additional Diagnostic Methods and Investigations

VI. Therapy

List of Contributors

H.J. Avenarius
Medizinische Hochschule, Karl-Wiechert-Allee 9, D 3000 Hannover

A. Benati
Ospedale Civile Maggiore, Dipartimento di Neurochirurgia, I 37100 Verona

B. Bergamasco
Clinica Neurologica dell' Università di Torino, Via Cherasco, I Torino

L. Bergamini
Clinica Neuropsichiatrica dell' Università di Torino, I Torino

A. Berger
I. Chirurgische Universitätsklinik, Alserstr. 4, A 1090 Wien

U. Boeters
Universitäts-Nervenklinik, Zentrum Nervenheilkunde, Niemannsweg 147, D 2300 Kiel

A. Bricolo
Ospedale Civile Maggiore, Dipartimento di Neurochirurgia, I 37100 Verona

G. Dalle Ore
Ospedale Civile Maggiore, Dipartimento di Neurochirurgia, I 37100 Verona

R.A. Dietze
Kinderneurologische Abteilung der Nervenklinik der Humboldt-Universität, DDR Berlin

G. Dolce
Istituto S. Giovanni Battista, Magliana Vecchia 821, I Roma

K.A. Flügel
Universitäts-Nervenklinik mit Poliklinik, Schwabachanlage 10, D 8520 Erlangen

H. Fromm
Neurochirurgische Abteilung am Städtischen Krankenhaus, D 6060 Offenbach/Main

F. Gerstenbrand
Neurologische Unversitätsklinik, Anichstr. 35, A 6020 Innsbruck

N. Grčevič
Department of Neuropathology, Clinical Medical Center Repro, University of Zagreb, YU 41000 Zagreb

B. Heerklotz
Universitäts-Nervenklinik mit Poliklinik, Schwabachanlage 10, D 8520 Erlangen

W.-D. Heiss
Institut für vergleichende Physiologie der Universität Wien, Schwarzspanierstr. 17, A 1090 Wien

L. Infuso
Clinica Neurochirurgia del'Università, Via S. Sforza 35, I Milano

K. Jellinger
Ludwig-Boltzmann-Institut für Klinische Neurobiologie, Wolkersbergenstr. 1, A 1130 Wien

S. Kanowski
Gerontopsychiatrische Abteilung der Freien Universität Berlin, Reichsstr. 15, D 1000 Berlin 19

F. Lackner
Institut für Anaesthesiologie, Spitalgasse 23
A 1090 Wien

G. Lausberg
Neurochirugische Abteilung des Knappschaftskrankenhauses, In der Schornau, D 4630 Bochum-Langendreer 1

C. Lehmann
Städtisches Krankenhaus München-Neuperlach, Anaesthesia-Abteilung und zentrale Intensivbehandlungseinheit, Oskar-Maria-Graf-Ring 51, D 8000 München 83

H.J. Lehmann
Neurologische Klinik der Gesamthochschule Essen, Hufelandstr. 55, D 4300 Essen

G.P. Liebaldt
Universtitäts-Nervenklinik, Neuropathologische Abteilung, Röntgenring 12, D 8700 Würzburg

C.H. Lücking
Neurologische Klinik und Poliklinik der Technischen Universität München, Möhlstr. 28, D 8000 München 80

B. Mamoli
Neurologische Uniersitätsklinik, Lazarettgasse 14, A 1097 Wien

S. Mingrino
Istituto di Neurochirurgia del'Università, I Padua

E. Müllner
II. Medizinische Klinik, Städtisches Krankenhaus Schwabing, D 8000 München 40

K. Pateisky
Neurologische Universitätsklinik, Lazarettgasse 14, A 1097 Wien

G. Peters
Max-Planck-Institut für Psychiatrie, Kraepelinstr. 2, D 8000 München 40

U.H. Peters
Neuro-Psychiatrische Klinik der Johannes-Gutenberg-Universität, Langenbeckstr. 1, D 6500 Mainz

H.P. Preissler
Am Gericht 17, D 3590 Bad Wildungen

R. Rettelbach
FA für Neurologie und Psychiatrie, Dammstr. 1, D 7910 Neu-Ulm

G.F. Rossi
Università Cattolica del Sacro Cuore, Facoltá di Medicina e Chirurgia, Via Della Pineta Sacchetti, 644, I 00168 Roma

E. Rothemund
Max-Planck-Institut für Psychiatrie, Kraepelinstr. 2, D 8000 München 40

M. Salzer
Orthopädisches Krankenhaus Gersthof, Wielemannsgasse, A 1180 Wien

E. Scherzer
Rehabilitationszentrum Meidling, Kündratstr. 37, A 1120 Wien

I. Schleip
Universitäts-Nervenklinik und Poliklinik, Röntgenring 12, D 8700 Würzburg

U. Seifert-Mielke
Bereich der Medizin der Humboldt-Universität, Schumannstr. 20-21, DDR 104 Berlin

E. Sluga
Neurologisches Institut der Universität Wien, Schwarzspanierstr. 17, A 1090 Wien

G. Ule
Institut für Neuropathologie der Universität Heidelberg, Im Neuenheimer Feld 220-221, D 6900 Heidelberg

H.H. Wieck
Universitäts-Nervenklinik mit Poliklinik, Schwabachanlage 10, D 8520 Erlangen

H. Zacherl
A.Ö. Krankenhaus, Hofmeisterstr. 70,
A 2410 Hainburg/NÖ

K. Zhuber
Orthopädisches Krankenhaus Gersthof,
Wielemannsgasse, A 1180 Wien

I. Das apallische Syndrom

Das apallische Syndrom*

E. KRETSCHMER **

Die Beschreibung der psychischen Begleiterscheinungen cerebral-neurologischer Vorgänge bei ausgebreiteten Gehirnerkrankungen, die in erster Linie die Großhirnrinde betreffen, ist an gewissen Stellen noch lückenhaft; statt einer klaren Syndromheraushebung muß man sich dann entweder mit der Aufreihung verzettelter und für sich allein nichtssagender Einzelsymptome begnügen oder man ist gezwungen, benachbarte Syndrombezeichnungen hilfsweise heranzuziehen, die dann den Tatbestand schief und ungenau decken.

Für bestimmte Formen weitgehender Ausschaltung gesamtpsychischer Leistungen, bei gleichzeitigem Erhaltensein der notwendigsten vegetativen Steuerungen des Hirnstamms, haben wir den Begriff der *"hypnoiden Syndrome"*, den wir in seinen schweren Ausprägungen bekanntlich mit dem Ausdruck "Koma", in seinen leichteren Graden als "Somnolenz", "Benommenheit" usw. quantitativ mit einer Reihe von Bezeichnungen abstufen können. Man könnte sie auch als "Bewußtseinsstörungen" im engeren Wortsinn zusammenfassen, wenn der Ausdruck "Bewußtsein" nicht allzu vieldeutig wäre. Ursächlich betrachtet sind der Prototyp dieser Gruppe die pathologisch-physiologischen Störungen, die bei Überschwemmung des Gehirns mit Toxinen eintreten, denen normalphysiologisch die Schlafreaktion auf Ermüdungstoxine entspricht. Wesentlich für alle in die hypnoide Gruppe gehörigen Phänomene ist die in ihnen enthaltene Störung der *Wach-Schlafsteuerung* im Sinne einer herabgesetzten "Helligkeit" des Bewußtseins bis zum Grade tiefer pathologischer Schlafzustände. Wesentlich für den subjektiven Tatbestand ist immer das einfache diffuse Dunkel- und Unscharfwerden des Erlebens mit nachfolgender Erinnerungstrübung bzw. Amnesie. Objektiv ist, wenn dies nicht gezeigt werden kann, mindestens ein zeitweiliges oder angedeutetes Auftreten schläfriger Symptome in der Motorik, hinsichtlich Gesichtsinnervation, Lidsenkung, Gähnen, Atmungstypus, Kopfvasomotorium, sei es mit passivem, ungezieltem, verträumtem Bewegungsspiel (Delir), sei es nur mit Wegsinken der Aufmerksamkeit (Amentia), oder zeitweiliger Desorientierung zu fordern, sofern der Ausdruck "Bewußtseinstrübung" etwas Präzises besagen soll.

Bauen sich in diese diffus quantitative Herabsetzung der psychischen Funktionen partiell sensorische und motorische Reizerscheinungen ein, so entstehen die Syndrome des "Delirs" und des "Dämmerzustandes", die ebenfalls das hypnoide Radikal mit enthalten; während der ebenfalls hierhergehörige "amentielle" Symptomenkomplex, grundsätzlich dem Syndrom der gewöhnlichen schweren Übermüdung ähnelnd, sich von der einfachen Somnolenz hauptsächlich durch die Fluktuationen des Bewußtseins, das Ableiten der Aufmerksamkeit und die dadurch bedingte Ratlosigkeit unterscheidet.

---

* First published: Ztschr. Neurol. Psychiat. **169**, 576-579 (1940).
** Eingegangen am 14. März 1940

Gegen die somnolenten Syndrome oder Bewußtseinsstörungen hebt sich eine andere Gruppe gesamtpsychischer Funktionsminderungen gut ab; das ist die Gruppe der *"Demenz"*. Ihr entsprechen pathologisch-anatomisch eine Reihe von Gehirnprozessen, die zu ausgebreiteten diffusen oder disseminierten Schädigungen der Großhirnrinde führen. Man spricht u.a. nicht von einer akuten Demenz und es gibt auch keine Bilder von akuter Störung der Großhirnrindenfunktion, die vorübergehend und reparabel das psychische Syndrom erzeugen könnten, das man in der allgemeinen chronischen Demenz findet. Die Demenz ist eine Intelligenzstörung, die zuerst die Merkfähigkeit, dann das Altgedächtnis und die Kombinations- und Urteilsfähigkeit fortschreitend in Mitleidenschaft zieht. Steht die Störung der Merkfähigkeit einseitig im Vordergrund, so entsteht der Korsakowsche oder amnestische Symptomkomplex; er ist der einzige dieser Gruppe, der auch in akuten Bildern, z.B. vorübergehend traumatisch vorkommt und insofern eine gewisse Sonderstellung einnimmt. Für die Demenz im engeren Sinn ist charakteristisch, daß sie mit der Wach-Schlafsteuerung nichts zu tun hat, daß sie weder subjektiv noch objektiv somnolente Züge enthält. Ferner, daß sie in reiner Form nicht mit Verlangsamung und Erschwerung der einzelnen seelischen Vollzüge einherzugehen braucht. Unter den einzelnen seelischen Akten werden viele falsche oder minderwertige intellektuelle Vollzüge sein; diese Akte können aber rasch, ungehemmt, selbst flott und mühelos ablaufen, wie etwa bei manchen senil Geschwätzigen oder Paralytikern.

Sind nun mit den verschiedenen Syndromen der somnolenten und der dementen Gruppe die diffusen psychischen Gesamtstörungen der Großhirnrindenfunktion erschöpft? Es gehen in diesen Gruppen nicht auf folgende Bilder: Der Patient liegt wach da mit offenen Augen. Der Blick starrt geradeaus oder gleitet ohne Fixationspunkt verständnislos hin und her. Auch der Versuch, die Aufmerksamkeit hinzulenken, gelingt nicht oder höchstens spurweise; Ansprechen, Anfassen, Vorhalten von Gegenständen erweckt keinen sinnvollen Widerhall; die reflektorischen Flucht- und Abwehrbewegungen können fehlen. Es fehlt manchmal auch das reflektorische Zurückgehen in die Grundstellung, bzw. in die optimale Ruhestellung, mit dem der Gesunde zufällige, nicht mehr gebrauchte, besonders auch unzweckmäßige und unbequeme Körperstellungen automatisch zu beenden pflegt. Infolgedessen können diese Kranken in aktiv oder passiv gewordenen Zufallsstellungen verharren bleiben. Dieses Verhalten kann entweder auf der Unfähigkeit zu sinnvoller Reizerwiderung, oder auf einer primären Antriebsstörung beruhen. Im Gegensatz dazu kann das elementare Irradiieren unverarbeiteter und ungebremster Außenreize enorm gesteigert sein, so daß sensible Reize mit Zuckungen beantwortet werden können. Trotz Wachsein ist der Patient unfähig zu sprechen, zu erkennen, sinnvolle Handlungsformeln erlernter Art durchzuführen. Dagegen sind bestimmte vegetative Elementarfunktionen, wie etwa das Schlucken erhalten. Daneben treten die bekannten frühen Tiefenreflexe, wie Saugreflex, Greifreflex hervor. – Soweit das engere Syndrom, das wir meinen. Es kann mit variablen Begleitsymptomen von anderen Hirnteilen einhergehen, z.B. mit Tonusstörungen, extrapyramidalen Hyperkinesen (Chorea, Athetose, Tremor). Vom Koma unterscheidet es sich durch das Fehlen der *Bewußtseinstrübung* (Wach-Schlafsteuerung), von der Demenz durch die Tatsache, daß letztere eine quantitative *Herabsetzung* der Großhirnleistungen bei in begrenztem Grad noch erhaltener Funktionsfähigkeit bedeutet, während das hier beschriebene Syndrom eine *Blockierung* derselben darstellt, so daß es im Idealfall einer Panagnosie plus Panapraxie gleichkäme. Im übrigen finden wir die Parallelen zu diesen Bildern weniger in landläufigen klinisch psychiatrischen Beschreibungen; sie erinnern dagegen manchmal lebhaft an die von den Gehirnphysiologen geschilderten Verhaltungsweisen des "großhirnlosen Hundes" bzw. der "Enthirnungsstarre", ohne natürlich mit diesen Bildern oder unter sich selbst genau identisch zu sein.[1]

Interessant ist noch die Skala der Vorgänge, mit denen sich das Syndrom einleitet und in die es sich beim Verschwinden wieder auflöst. Es können entweder Erscheinungen aus der apraktisch-aphasischen Reihe den Auftakt und die Schlußfiguren bilden, oder es können sich aus den "exogenen" Gruppen etwa delirante oder amentielle Reihen einlagern.

Beim Übergang von dem schweren cerebralorganischen Bild zur Genesung können sich leicht paranoide Syndrome, etwa in der Form des Beziehungswahns einstellen. Dies sind keine primär gehirnorganischen Zeichen, sondern Sekundärbildungen, die eine beginnende Stellungnahme der wiedererwachenden Persönlichkeit und den ersten Versuch einer Verarbeitung des allmählich wieder herankommenden seelischen Außenmaterials bedeuten. Diese ängstlichen Beziehungs- und Verfolgungsideen spiegeln nichts anderes wider, als das Fluktuieren der Psyche zwischen Verstehen und Nichtverstehen, die diffuse Unsicherheit der Subjekt-Objektrelation. Dies letztere gilt übrigens in gewissem Grad für alle paranoiden Syndrome, gleichgültig, ob die Unsicherheit des Bezugs zwischen Subjekt und Außenwelt wie hier, durch gehirnorganische Funktionsschwankungen, oder, wie in den schizophrenen Randgebieten durch Interferenz zwischen Realwelt und magischer Innenwelt, oder, wie etwa beim sensitiven Beziehungswahn mehr psychisch reaktiv durch die aus der Unsicherheit der Selbstwertlage entspringende Erschütterung der Beziehungen zwischen Ich und Außenwelt bedingt sind.

Das gehirnorganische Syndrom, das wir oben beschrieben haben, soll als *"apallisch"* bezeichnet werden. Der Ausdruck ist absichtlich in derselben Art gebildet, wie die Begriffe "apraktisch", "agnostisch", "aphasisch"; und zwar deshalb, weil das apallische Syndrom zwar keine einfache Addition dieser Zustände darstellt, aber doch folgerichtig dann entstehen muß, wenn durch akutere Krankheitsherde die entsprechenden Rindenfelder gleichzeitig außer Funktion gesetzt werden, was ja nur bei weitausgedehnten Störungen des Palliums in seiner Ganzheitsfunktion denkbar ist. Im Sinne dieser ganzheitlichen Störung der Zusammenarbeit des Palliums in sich, sprechen wir von apallisch. Macht man sich gerade diesen ganzheitlichen Charakter des Syndroms klar, so erhellt auch, daß nicht notwendig jedes einzelne Rindenzentrum isolierte Lokalsymptome geben muß, daß z.B. nicht notwendig Pyramidenbahnstörungen, bzw. Symptome von der motorischen Rindenregion gefunden werden müssen.

Das klinische Vorkommen des Syndroms erstreckt sich weniger auf toxische Störungen, auch nicht auf solche Infektionen, die sich vorwiegend toxisch auswirken. Toxische Störungen gehen vorwiegend mit Bewußtseinstrübung einher; ihre Hauptdomäne sind neben der einfachen Somnolenz die bekannten "exogenen" Syndrome, speziell Delir und Amentia.

Apallische Störungen finden sich dagegen bei panencephalitischen Prozessen[2] mit vorwiegender Großhirnbeteiligung, sodann traumatisch bei Hirnschuß, wenn nach Abklingen der initialen Schockwirkung größere Bereiche beider Großhirnhemisphären ausgeschaltet sind[3]; ferner bei vorwiegend großhirnmäßig ausgebreiteter Lues cerebri, bei disseminierten

[1] Vgl. die Arbeiten von Goltz, Gamper, Scholz, Magnus u.a. Zusammenfassendes darüber bei Kretschmer: Med. Psychologie, 5. Aufl., S. 41f.

[2] Siehe die folgende Arbeit: Conrad u. Dellbrügge: Ein geheilter Fall von Panencephalitis subacuta.

[3] Ein solcher Fall mit schrägsagittalem Durchschuß durch beide Hemisphären soll aus unserer Klinik demnächst veröffentlicht werden.

Erweichungsherden, als vorübergehende Verlaufsphasen schwerer Gehirnarteriosklerosen usw. Es dürfte nicht zufällig sein, daß die Demenz sich mehr auf dem Boden chronisch verlaufender Großhirnzerstörungen entwickelt, die durch Anpassungs- und Ausgleichsvorgänge immer noch eine, wenn auch quantitativ herabgesetzte geistige Gesamtleistung erlauben, während der Blockierungscharakter des apallischen Syndroms mehr der Überwältigung durch akute Gehirnprozesse oder durch schubweise Veränderungen in chronischen Verläufen entspricht. – In schweren Vollausprägungen ist das apallische Syndrom nicht häufig. Doch ist seine klare Heraushebung und Bezeichnung für eine präzise Beschreibung der psychischen Begleitsymptome gehirnorganischer Prozesse unerläßlich.

II. Clinical Problems

1. Clinical Picture and Problems in Terminology

U.H. PETERS and F. GERSTENBRAND

The clinical picture of the apallic syndrome was occasionally described in casuistic studies at the end of the nineteenth century. No special attention was given to the clinical picture, and it was described in a rather incidental way. The first description was probably given by Rosenblath (1899), in which a 15-year-old tightrope walker, after toppling from a high wire, fell immediately into a coma and developed stretch cramps. After 2 weeks the patient became strangely awake and this state did not change until the death of the boy 8 months after the accident. It was not until 1940 when Kretschmer–based on his own clinical observations but without knowledge of the older descriptions–recognized the particular importance of the symptom complex. He called it apallic, since in his opinion the condition occurs as a result of extensive disturbances of the pallium in its entire functioning.

Although identical clinical pictures were later described in other terms which will be discussed below, Kretschmer's term has largely prevailed despite some difficulties[1]. While there are some objections, the authors are very much in favor of retaining the expression apallic syndrome to identify the *clinical* picture. The term is being used extensively and gives some recognition to Kretschmer's original effort. In addition, the term can be easily translated (French: *syndrome apallique*, Italian: *sindrome apallico*, German: *apallisches Syndrom*). However, some misunderstandings have occurred. A misspelling–e.g. "aphalic syndrome"–might suggest a loss of penis; the Italian translation could be retranslated into "syndrome without testicles." These rather remote possibilities for error have not proven to be a serious obstacle to the usage of the term. Furthermore, it should not be used solely in its literal Latin meaning ("derobed") and thus be applied only to diseases that are caused by extensive damage to the cortex.

Philosophical objections of this kind do not often lead to scientific discoveries. It should be emphasized again that, in the authors' opinion, the term applies only to the clinical picture and that the pathogenesis, at this point, has not yet been clearly established–the connection between cortex and brain stem may be interrupted anywhere: e.g. pallium, white substance, midbrain. Furthermore, it is common practice to identify the etiology by adding a special term (for example, traumatic apallic syndrome).

Clinical Picture

As we noted in Kretschmer's original study, the clinical description of the apallic syndrome is based primarily on the report of a case of panencephalitis subacuta (Pette) published in

[1] After Kretschmer the expression "apallic syndrome" was again taken up by a study group in Kiel led by G.E. Störring (see Ule et al., 1961).

1940 by Conrad and Delbrügge, as well as on the case of a brain injury caused by an oblique sagittal shot through both hemispheres. But Kretschmer (1940) pointed out expressly that the same syndrome can be caused by several other diseases such as "lues cerebri concentrated mainly in the cerebrum," disseminated encephalomalacic focus, severe arteriosclerosis of the brain, etc. The "severe full stage" did not often occur.

Kretschmer's clinical description of the condition is so appropriate that we cannot add much to his comments. We will therefore quote the original description from Kretschmer's paper:

> The patient is prostrate, awake, with his eyes open. He either stares straight ahead or his eyes travel back and forth without understanding or being able to focus on anything. Attempts to attract his attention are unsuccessful or only slightly successful. Talking to the the patient, touching him or showing him objects does not result in any sensible response. The reflexive movements of flight and defense are missing. Sometimes even the reflexive return to the basic position, that is, the position of optimum relaxation, is lacking. A normal person usually returns to the basic position from an accidental position or one that is no longer used or necessary for a specific purpose, or is inefficient or uncomfortable.
>
> The patient may therefore be in a position accidentally assumed that can be active or passive. This behavior can be based either on the inability to react sensibly to a stimulus or on the disturbance of a primary impulse. In contrast, the elementary irradiation of undigested and uncurbed outside stimulation may increase enormously. In spite of the fact that the patient is awake he can neither talk, recognize, nor perform sensible patterns of behavior that he had once learned. Certain elementary vegetative functions such as swallowing still exist. In addition, the familiar basic instincts such as sucking and grasping appear. . .
>
> The syndrome differs from the coma in that there is no clouded consciousness (control of sleeping and waking). It differs from the dementia in that the latter results in a quantitative reduction in the function of the cerebrum, whereby the functional capacity is retained to a certain degree. However, the syndrome described here results in a blockage of the functional capacity of the cerebrum, so that in an ideal situation it might equal a panagnosis plus panapraxia.

Important Individual Phenomena:

1. The particular way in which consciousness is disturbed–coma vigile (see below).
2. Suspension of the sleeping and waking rhythm normally regulated by local time. The sleeping and waking phases are regulated instead by normal tiring. We can distinguish between waking and sleeping phases but they are very irregularly distributed over the 24-h day.
3. The lack of emotional reactions.
4. Torso and extremities are in a stretched positon.
5. Slow, pendular movements of the eyes or lack of coordination of the eye movements.
6. Appearance of primitive motor patterns.
7. The integrating systems of the vegetative functions become uninhibited.

We have seen from Kretschmer's (1940) description that the apallic syndrome basically occurs in two different forms (Gerstenbrand, 1967):

1. By an acute process which leads to the loss of the entire cerebral function. This loss may be caused by damage to the cortex, to the brain stem, or to the connecting systems at various levels. It occurs through local processes in the upper brain stem resulting from tumors, circulatory disturbances, or tentorial strangulation. Or it occurs through hypoxidosis of the various etiology, metabolic disturbances of different origin, gas embolism, acute encephalitis, edema of the brain caused by an allergy, brain injury, etc. In these cases the apallic syndrome may be a terminal or transitional syndrome.

2. By a graduated breakdown of the cerebral function which can affect cortex and marrow either separately or simultaneously. The clinical picture of the apallic syndrome caused by

processes of this kind (senile or presenile atrophy of the brain, diffuse sclerotic leukencephalitis, multiple sclerosis, Marchiafava-Binami syndrome, etc.) is terminal.

The development of the apallic syndrome to full stage, caused by graduated processes in the cerebrum, shows phases that can be clinically differentiated. These phases may be regarded as the disintegration of the cerebrum functions to the level of the mesencephalon. During the remission phases we can again differentiate the same kinds of phases as in the graduated disintegration. Reintegration, however, in the remission process, can come to a halt at a certain phase and that phase may remain as a defect syndrome.

Explanations of Terminology

Since a commonly known and recognized expression for the clinical picture of the apallic syndrome was lacking for a long time, the same clinical pictures have been described by various terms. The following is a list of all known terms brought into relation with the clinical picture of the apallic syndrome given above:

1. Coma vigile: The most familiar term is coma vigile, widely used in French literature. In a number of studies this term was the full stage, but the descriptions involved other clinical pictures as well. In the descriptions by Mollaret and Goulon (1959) we recognize rather a sopor. Furthermore, the term coma vigile is really a contradiction in itself, since the familiar connotation of "coma" actually excludes the possibility of being awake. Yet it is this incompatibility of contrasting symptoms in the apallic syndrome—no object content of consciousness and yet being awake—that appear to make the expression so fitting. Since the apallic syndrome includes so much more than only this strange form of changed consciousness, it is not suitable to accept coma vigile as a synonym for the apallic syndrome as a whole. Gerstenbrand (1967) has therefore used coma vigile only to describe the state of consciousness in the apallic syndrome since it is often necessary in a given context to emphasize this side of the entire symptom complex. It is suggested that the use of this term be retained.

2. Parasomnia: This expression was created by Jefferson (1944) to find a better name for that particular type of disturbed consciousness following "normal" brain traumas in which the patient can, for example, react verbally when called but falls immediately back into a kind of sleep. It is important to Jefferson that the patient does not react to stimulation with a response that will assist in analyzing the problem (his definition of consciousness). In accordance with the usual nomenclature, parasomnia can mean a state of clouded consciousness which may extend from slight somnolence to coma, whereas in the apallic syndrome the "skalar" consciousness is still intact. Among the three cases briefly reported by Jefferson, therefore, an apallic syndrome is not present and yet the term parasomnia has been used occasionally to describe the state of consciousness in the apallic syndrome.

A further objection to the usage of the expression parasomnia is the fact that before Jefferson it was used to describe the various forms of troubled sleep (anxiety dreams, somnambulism, spasms when going to sleep).

3. Hypersomnia: Even the old and common term hypersomnia has occasionally been used to identify an apallic syndrome. Façon et al. (1958), employing the term *hypersomnie prolongée*, described a female patient aged 78 whose condition showed, at least occasionally, an apallic syndrome during the 3 years of her illness which occurred after occlusion of the arteria basilaris. French (1952) also talks of hypersomnia in a case which corresponds to an apallic syndrome. The usage of the term hypersomnia does not correspond to the familiar connotation of this expression (Michaelis) and thus should not be applied. The authors, however, might again have wanted to emphasize the particular posttraumatic state of sleep known as parasomnia.

4. Akinetic Mutism: The inhibition of all motor functions, including speech, gesticulation, and facial expressions, is the central symptom of the akinetic mutism, conceptualized and solely based on the phenomena by Cairns et al. (1941). However, according to the description by these authors, the patients can be fully awake and remember everything well. The condition can be entirely functional; patients with akinetic mutism may eventually get up, go to the toilet, and return afterwards to the akinetic mutism (e.g., Case 3, Sutter et al., 1959). A similar situation arose in the first case described by Cairns et al. (1941) of an epidermoid cyst of the third ventricle, in which the akinetic mutism disappeared within a few minutes every time the cyst was drained.

We are dealing, therefore, with a syndrome all on its own which Jefferson (1944) already regarded as being separate from parasomnia. According to him, the difference lies above all in the particular tendency of parasomnia patients to sleep, which does not occur in the akinetic mutism. It is also clear that there is actually no close relation between the akinetic mutism and the apallic syndrome when one looks at their respective full stages. But since apallic patients may for a long time be akinetic and mute, it is not surprising to find the symptoms of the apallic syndrome described in case histories of akinetic mutism. There is one case of an apallic syndrome among the cases of akinetic mutism and occlusion of the A. vertebralis or basilaris described by Cravioto et al. (1960). In one case by Lhermitte et al. (1963) the cause of the apallic syndrome was a thrombosis of the A. basilaris. Vitale (1964) describes the syndrome following an unforeseen event during the stereotactic operation of a patient with Huntington's chorea. The clinical pictures described by Umbach and Riechert (1963) following stereotactic elimination in the basal ganglia also correspond to a large degree to the symptoms of the apallic syndrome. Maspes and Marossero (1957) observed an apallic syndrome when vessels in the area of the thalamus had been damaged. The female patient described by Hermann and Sulat (1959) obviously exhibited the symptoms of the apallic syndrome to some extent. This also seems true of the case described by Grotjahn (1936) more than 30 years ago. Finally, Bruck and Gerstenbrand (1967) were able to show that a case of akinetic mutism caused by high doses of phenotiazine also presented the symptoms of the apallic syndrome.

5. Posttraumatic Encephalopathy: A large number of cases of the traumatic apallic syndrome have been described with this term, for example by Jellinger (1965), Jellinger et al. (1963), Chavany et al. (1955), Trillet (1949, 1961), Dechaume et al. (1962), and others. Osetowska (1964), assuming a morphologic point of view, called the cases of traumatic apallic syndrome *leukoencéphalopathie œdémateuse posttraumatique.* Kramer (1964), on the other hand, uses the expression "progressive posttraumatic encephalopathy" to describe a case which clinically corresponds to the apallic syndrome. The morphologic analysis, however, showed a transition to the *coma dépassée* already described by Mollaret et al. (1959).

6. Decerebration Syndrome or Decerebration Rigidity: We can easily understand why an apallic syndrome is occasionally described by this term (see, for example, Mumenthaler,

1961) since "brain stem spasms" are part of the clinical picture. Kretschmer (1940) showed interest in this question in his original paper and recognized that, although there is a certain similarity between the apallic syndrome and decerebration rigidity, the clinical pictures are not identical. There seems to be a tendency to apply the term decerebration rigidity to the early stages of the central brain syndrome (Sutter et al., 1959) and apallic syndrome to the psychotic changes. Hubach and Poeck (1964), who refer to a traumatic decerebration, demonstrate in a schematic diagram to what extent the development of both partial syndromes can run parallel to or separate from each other. The related expression "decortication" has only rarely been used for cases of the apallic syndrome (Nyström, 1960).

7. Coma Prolongé: The term *coma traumatique prolongé*, which is used frequently in French literature, encompasses more than the apallic syndrome. It can apply to all clinical pictures in which patients survive in a coma for at least 3 weeks (Vigouroux et al., 1964). But many cases of apallic syndrome have been described as *coma prolongé* for lack of a proper term. This fact not only shows up in the synopsis of the remission phases by Vigouroux et al. (1964), which indicates distinct parallels with phases of the traumatic apallic syndrome according to Gerstenbrand (1967), but frequently in case histories we can see that, whenever the *coma traumatique prolongé* is mentioned, an apallic syndrome is actually meant.–Fau (1956), Girard et al. (1963), Le Beau et al. (1958), Leson (1960), Reymond and Fau (1956), Wertheimer and Allegre (1953), Sutter et al. (1959). In the English literature the same expression can be found, translated as "prolonged unconsciousness" (for example, French, 1952). In Russian literature the term "prolonged state of coma" (Ivanoff, 1962; Mägi, 1965 and 1968) is sometimes applied to the apallic syndrome.

8. Posttraumatic Catatonia: This expression has occasionally been used as a synonym for the apallic syndrome (for example, Jellinger et al., 1963). Sutter et al. (1959), however, wanted to create a general term for all traumatic brain damage which is followed by catatonic stupor. Of the four cases described, only the first can be considered to be an apallic syndrome. The authors even deduce the therapeutic consequences of the treatment from the expression (see Case 3 involving a posttraumatic twilight state). Since heterogeneous clinical pictures were mentioned under this term in the original study, we fear that further use of the term posttraumatic catatonia might lead to misunderstanding.

9. Stupeur Hypertonique Posttraumatique: Fischgold and Mathis (1959) have used this term to describe a clinical picture corresponding to apallic syndrome.

10. Lucid Stupor is used by Ajuriaguerra et al. (1953) to describe a clinical picture corresponding to the apallic syndrome caused in their case by a tumor in the mesodiencephalic area.

11. Severe Dementia Following Brain Injury. In pathologic-anatomic casuistics Sabina Strich (1956) describes typical apallic syndromes as "severe dementia following head injury." These two terms are synonymous to that extent. The author did not go into details of clinical symptomatology in her later papers. Apparently her term has not been used elsewhere.

12. Démence Progressive avec Cachexie: This is the term used by Gruner (1965) for the clinical picture of a traumatic apallic syndrome which corresponds largely to the classical description.

13. Vita Reducta was introduced by Masshoff (1963a and b) and Neuhaus (1963) and is sometimes discussed in connection with the apallic syndrome. According to the definition, it is clinically related to a "deep coma, or rather a state which follows a deep coma"

(Kubicki, 1963, 1965). Schliack (1963), Schliack and Kubicki (1964) have already pointed out that the clinical picture of the vita reducta may change to an apallic syndrome. The symptoms of the vita reducta, which may briefly be described as complete loss of reflexes, poor muscle tone, and breakdown of the vegetative functions (Kubicki, 1965), show no parallels to the apallic syndrome.

This collection of the numerous terms which have hitherto been used makes visible again the usefulness of the term "apallic syndrome". But also from clinical, pathophysiologic, and therapeutic points of view this appears most useful as long as the view is not anatomic but clinical, the apallic syndrome being a total but functional interruption of the cerebral functions.

2. The Symptomatology of the Apallic Syndrome

F. GERSTENBRAND

Introduction

From the type of motivating disease and the course of the first observed cases of an apallic syndrome described by Kretschmer (1940), the conclusion can be drawn that the concept "apallic" was conceived by its creator as a term denoting a functional disturbance of the cerebrum and was not intended to describe the existing brain damage as a morphologic substrate. Thus in the apallic syndrome a functional dynamism exists and in some cases remission is possible.

The apallic syndrome can develop in two different ways:

1. Following an acute process of the brain which affects the total cerebrum or which interrupts the ascending and descending pathways by a local lesion in the midbrain region, or a combination of both. The latter constitutes the most severe acute brain damage. To this group belong cerebral hypoxydosis of different origins (strangulation, obstruction of the trachea, anesthesia accidents, cardiac arrest, heart operation, etc.); brain edema caused by allergic reaction, etc.; diffuse encephalitis; gas embolism; metabolic disturbances (hepatic coma, uremic coma, etc.); prolonged insulin shock; exogenous intoxication (carbon monoxide, mercury poisoning, etc.); and brain injury as well as processes of the midbrain region such as tumors, circulatory disturbances (upper basilar syndrome), and subarachnoidal hemorrhage with tamponade of the basal cisterns and incidents after stereotactic operations. In the majority of events mentioned in this group the diffuse brain edema is the cause of a mass movement in the supratentorial cavity followed by tentorial herniation and secondary lesion of the oral brain stem. In this form of apallic syndrome a remission is possible, but the full syndrome can remain until the death of the patient without the slightest tendency towards remission.

2. A diffuse progressive process of the cerebrum affecting the cortex, or the white matter, or both together. Neurologic diseases which can cause an apallic syndrome in this manner are, for example, senile or presenile brain atrophy, diffuse brain sclerosis, subacute sclerotic leukencephalitis, the severest forms of multiple sclerosis and the Marchiafava-Bignami syndrome. The apallic syndrome occurring in a progressive process of the cerebrum is an irreparable end-state.

In accordance with the above description, the apallic syndrome develops in certain stages. In the acute processes of the brain an initial stage is obligatory, showing the different phases of the acute midbrain syndrome, in rare cases the acute bulbar brain syndrome, followed by a transient stage.

In the remission stage several phases of the reintegration of the higher brain functions are to be found. In an apallic syndrome, as a consequence of a diffuse progressive process of the brain, the same phases as in the remission stage occur in a particular sequence, according to the disintegration of the higher brain functions, but only in reverse.

The symptomatology of the apallic syndrome in all its stages can be divided into the symptom categories of the disturbance of consciousness (activity and content of consciousness) and vigilance; the reaction to external stimulation; the emotional reaction; the optomotor function; the motor function of the face, throat, and body; the body posture; the primitive motor patterns; and the autonomic functions.

The Symptomatology of the Full Stage

The symptomatology of the full stage of the apallic syndrome is as follows:

1. Coma vigile with sleep-awake regulation controlled by exhaustion. The patient is awake but has no conscious activity nor any conscious capacity. The apallic patient lies with eyes open, not noticing events around him (Fig. 1). He can neither focus nor follow optically. The threatening reflex cannot be evoked, but the blinking reflex is present. This awake state becomes independent of time and is interrupted by periods of sleep, which are characterized by their depth. During the awake state the autonomic functions are in a sympathetic tonus, during the sleep periods in a parasympathetic tonus.

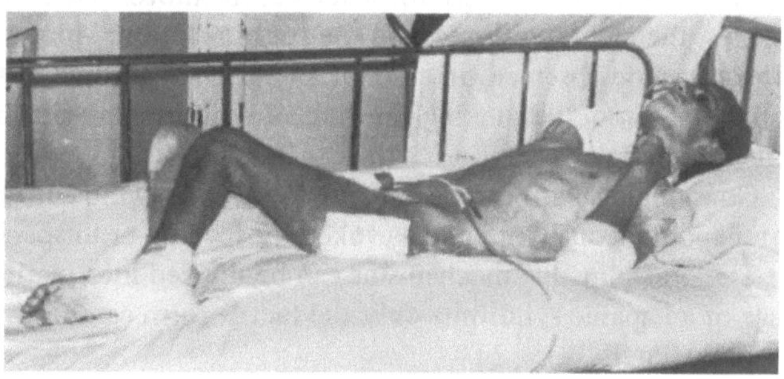

Fig. 1. Traumatic apallic syndrome, full stage (Patient A.D., age 17 years, male, 7 months after accident). Coma vigile, flexion position of extremities with contractions of main joints, signs of marasmus, decubital ulcers

2. The patient shows no reaction to external stimulation. Pain stimuli cause, after a period of latency, mass movements of the extremities corresponding to the holokinetic movements of the newborn (Lesny, 1965), accompanied by a stress reaction (enlarging of the pupils, increase in breathing and pulse rate as well as increase in blood pressure).

3. Emotional reactions are not present.

4. The eyes are in a divergent position and are of different size; convergent reaction is not evocable. Eye movements are slow and saccadic and are mostly evoked by vestibular stimuli. The oculocephalic reflexes (doll-head phenomena) are diminished; the vestibulo-ocular reflex (cold calorization) shows a tonic reaction. Size of the pupils varies according to the autonomic tonus. The light reaction is diminished and tonic; the pain reaction (ciliospinal reflex) is slightly positive.

5. The tonus of the masseter muscle is increased, especially in apallic cases after brain hypoxia; the masseter reflex is also increased. There is a significant amimia. Swallowing movements occur only as automatisms together with chewing automatism and are considerably slowed.

6. The posture of the extremities shows a slight flexion in the elbow and knee joints, an adduction of upper and lower extremities, a fist position, and a plantar flexion in the foot angle. The trunk is extended (Fig. 1). In some cases the flexed position is seen; in other cases a stretch position of the legs can be observed. Sometimes the posture of the asymmetric tonic neck reflex with deviation of the head to one side and a stretched position of the chin extremities and flexion of the other side can be observed. In young children with an apallic syndrome an abduction posture of the upper extremities is possible. The muscle tonus of the extremities and the trunk is increased and shows signs of spasticity and of rigidity ("rigido-spasticity": Narabayashi, 1962). There is a hyperreflexia of all tendon reflexes. However, in some cases the tendon reflexes are diminished because of contraction of the joints, periarticular ossification, as well as a highly increased muscle tonus. The pyramidal signs can be evoked. In some cases the escape reflex can be evoked in the lower extremities, in rare cases overlapping onto the other side or from the legs to the arms. The escape reflex is always accompanied by sympathetic reaction corresponding to a stress reaction.

7. Primitive motor patterns. The primitive motor patterns have a pathognomonic value in the apallic syndrome. These motor actions can be divided into different groups, according to their functional basis, for instance, the motor patterns of the oral sense, the grasping reflexes, the mental reflexes, and the fright reaction. Moreover, the position and posture reflexes can be observed. In cases of an apallic syndrome of the primitive motor patterns of the oral sense, the sucking-chewing automatism appears; in others only the sucking component appears.

Gnashing of teeth can be an equivalent of chewing automatism. This motor pattern may occur spontaneously or can be evoked by specific or unspecific stimulations.

The oral adjusting mechanisms can be divided into tactile and optic forms. In the full stage of an apallic syndrome only the tactile form can be elicited; this is accomplished by perioral stimuli.

Sometimes the tactile adjusting oral mechanisms are followed by sucking movements, similar to the lick-sucking, and by the bulldog reflex. During a sustained bulldog reflex the lick-sucking can continue. In rare cases the tactile adjusting oral mechanisms are followed by magnet reaction.

The snout reflex can be elicited in most cases of apallic syndrome.

In single cases the motor pattern of breast searching can be observed. This motor pattern occurs particularly in cases of progressive brain damage or after a diffuse encephalitis.

In some cases an intensive yawning is observed. The yawning motion may be repeated several times. It is similar to the yawning of the brain-damaged newborn.

The grasping reflexes are divided into the phasic and the tonic grasping reflexes (Wieser, 1957). The tonic grasping, which is evoked by proprioceptive flexion of the fingers, can be followed by a flexion of the elbow joint and by an adduction of the whole arm. An intensive tonic grasping reflex enables one to pull the patient up. It is possible to intensify the motor patterns of the oral sense by the grasping reflexes. In rare cases the Chodzko reflex can be elicited.

The so-called mental reflexes–mental because of the contraction of the mental muscles–first described by Marinesco and Radovici (1920) are obligatory in the apallic syndrome. Different types are known, the most common being the palmomental reflex, elicited by scratching the palm with a blunt object. Not only the homolateral mental muscle is contracted but also the reflexogenous zones often spread to the whole arm, sometimes to the trapezius muscle. The pollicomental reflex can be elicited by intensive scratching of the top of the pollux. Other types belonging to the mental reflex group are the cygomatico-, mento-, labio-, and corneomental reflexes, as well as some others.

The same pathophysiologic basis as in the mental reflex group can be observed in the Babkin reflex, elicited by simultaneous intensive pressure of both palms, followed by an opening of the mouth sometimes combined with an attenuated stretch position of the trunk. This motor pattern can be found in every premature baby and in cases of an anencephalus. Very rarely is the Lesný reflex, the one-sided Babkin reflex, observed.

Of the group of fright reflexes, the glabellar reflex, the head retraction, and the total-fright reflex are most often observed.

In some cases climbing movements of the legs–also called tread movements–appear. The Galant reflex is also very seldom observed. (After scratching of the lateral trunk the homolateral hip moves towards the stimulated side.)

From the position and posture reflexes the asymmetric and symmetric tonic neck reflexes are elicited in nearly every case in a more or less intensive form. Sometimes the posture reflexes can be found from one extremity to the other, or at the head. These reflexes usually occur latently. It must be pointed out that these reflexes are of great importance for early physiotherapy in the so-called method of tonus-regulating reflex therapy.

The support reaction can be found only in some cases and nearly always as support reaction in the flexion position. These reflexes can also be used in early physiotherapy.

8. The disinhibition of the autonomic functions has a distinct influence on the condition as well as on the further course of an apallic patient. As mentioned above, during the awake state all signs of a sympathetic tonus regulation may be found shifting over after the entrance of the sleeping period in a parasympathetic regulation level. The period of the predominance of the sympathetic tonus regulation has a tendency towards chronification of an emergency reaction. This tendency towards a sympathetic tonus regulation state may explain the necessity for hypercaloric nutrition in apallic patients. In connection with this regulation of the autonomic system, complications such as marasmus, bedsores, and so on may be observed.

In the course of autonomic dysregulation the incontinence of bladder and rectum must be cited. Of special importance is the diminishing resistance to infections of various kinds. Most cases have a cystitis. The overaction of some glands producing hypersalivation, ointment face, and sweating yield parallels a Parkinson symptomatology which is enforced by the presence of akinesia and amimia. Therefore, Parkinson symptomatology was found to be a part of the apallic syndrome (Gerstenbrand, 1967).

As already mentioned in the introductory remarks, the apallic syndrome can develop in two different ways. In both ways, in the apallic syndrome occurring (1) after a severe acute brain lesion, as well as (2) in a progressive process of the cerebrum, a fixed course towards a syndrome can be determined. In the apallic syndrome, as an end state of a progressive process of the cerebrum, the full state appears after a decrease of the higher brain functions, corresponding to the distintegration of the cerebral function (Jackson, 1958). The course of disintegration of the higher brain functions is directly comparable to the reintegration of the brain activity during the remission stage of an apallic syndrome resulting in severe brain damage.

In cases of an apallic syndrome following an acute brain damage, of different etiology, an initial stage and a transition stage appear before the full stage. The initial stage and the transition stage are described in Chapter 3.

The Remission Stage

During the remission stage of an apallic syndrome due to acute damage of the brain, reintegration of the higher brain functions appears, together with a decrease in activity of the primitive motor patterns which become integrated into the increasing voluntary movements, and a normalization of the disinhibited autonomic functions. During the course of the remission, considered from the functional point of view, two periods may be differentiated: (1) the stage of establishing contact with the surroundings, coupled with an increased mental awareness, as well as with a reintegration of the turning-towards movements (*Zuwendungsmotorik*), and (2) the second stage during which the remaining disinhibition symptoms disappear and voluntary motor as well as higher brain functions reappear.

The clinical course of the remission stage can be divided into several phases. The beginning of the remission is indicated by the emergence of primitive emotional reactions in response to pain stimulus, corresponding to a primitive alarm reaction and accompanied by an emergency reaction. Moreover, a change in the sleep-awake rhythm influenced by day-night regulation, as well as a disappearance of the chewing-sucking automatism can be observed. These first signs of remission can occur either after several days of a lasting full stage or after some months. The duration of this phase can vary from several days to several months or may become a final one.

In the further course of remission optical fixation occurs (Fig. 2). The patient turns towards objects brought into his visual field. At the same time a differentiation of the emotional reaction can be observed. Besides the primitive alarm reactions during nursing care

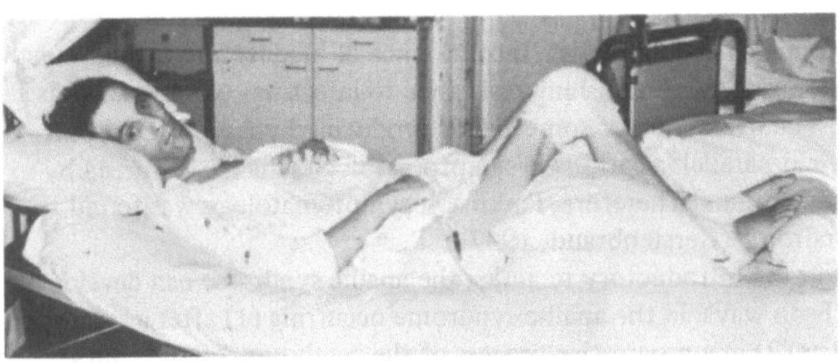

Fig. 2. Traumatic apallic syndrome, remission stage, second phase (Patient A.Z., age 29 years, male, 10 months after accident). Optic fixation, turning towards, voluntary movements

and injections, displeasure reactions are elicited. The change in the sleep-awake regulation progresses. This development parallels a progressive disappearance of the coma vigile. This phase may also last for a varying length of time but can be the end stage of the remission.

During the progression of the remission the apallic patient shows optic following together with deviation of the eyes, later of the head, with initial convergence reaction of the bulbi and diminishing of the divergent position of the eyeballs, as well as grasping of objects put in front of him. The emotions show positive effects with slight signs of recognition of special persons and the first signs of a smiling reaction (Fig. 3). The first voluntary movements occur, usually in the fingers. At the end of this phase the patient responds to very simple orders (opening of the mouth, closing of the eyes, etc.). In this phase the latest symptoms of superimposed focal lesions of the cerebrum and sometimes of the cerebellum may be found (hemiparesis, etc.).

The following phase is marked by the symptomatology of the Klüver-Bücy-Terzian-Dalle Ore syndrome. The main symptoms are grasping and bringing to the mouth every object in the surroundings, followed by biting and swallowing (Fig. 4); change in the

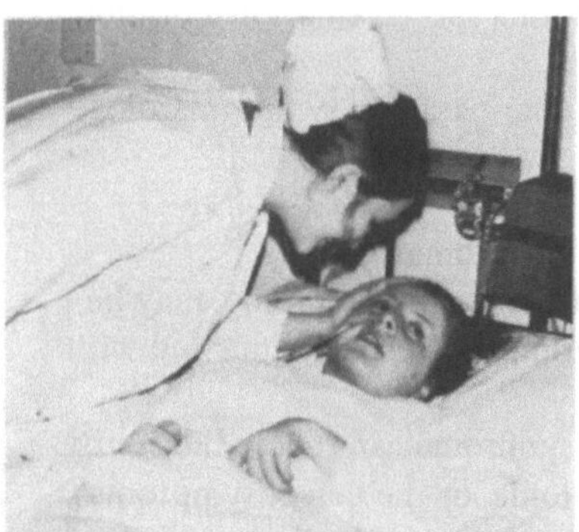

Fig. 3

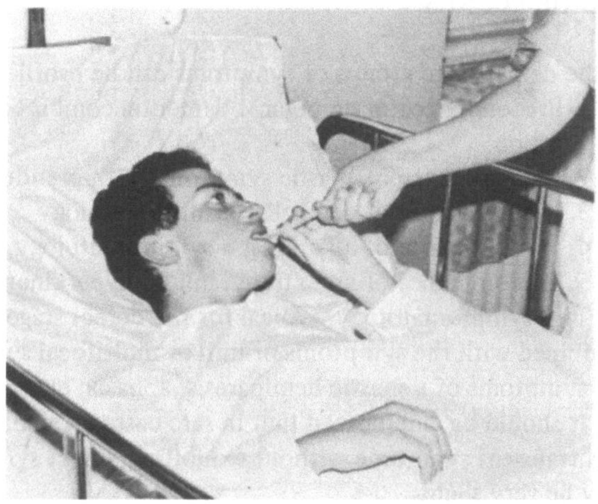

Fig. 4

Fig. 3. Traumatic apallic syndrome, remission stage, beginning Klüver-Bucy phase (Patient A.X., age 12 years, female, 10 months after accident). Adulation reaction (*Schmeichelreaktion*)

Fig. 4. Traumatic apallic syndrome, remission stage, Klüver-Bucy phase (Patient N.D., age 20 years, male, 20 days after accident). Shown object grasped immediately and put into mouth, followed by sucking and biting movements

emotional reactions to positive effects; establishment of an euphoric mood; hypersexuality with hetero- and homosexual tendencies and lack of shame reactions during masturbation; and lack of fear reactions sometimes accompanied by the appearance of rage reactions, bulimia, and by a lack of memory. The primitive motor patterns show a further differentiation and some disappear (Babkin reflex, Chodzko reflex, posture reflexes, etc.). The voluntary movements show a progressive development; muscle tonus is only slightly increased. Hyperreflexia and pyramidal signs are to be found in many cases. Symptoms of parkinsonism can be observed in some patients. In this stage coma vigile has disappeared.

The symptomatology described above is completely different from that of the apallic syndrome and could be explained by the rising of the functional niveau to the higher level of the disinhibited limbic system. It must be emphasized that in a number of cases only a partial symptomatology of the Klüver-Bucy-Terzian-Dalle Ore syndrome can be observed in this remission phase.

During remission the symptomatology of a Korsakoff syndrome occurs. In the meantime, having started in the first phase, the redevelopment of speech and other higher brain functions has progressed and voluntary movements have been normalized. Significant signs of emotional lability can be found. In some cases psychotic decompensation may appear during this phase. The symptoms of a local brain lesion can now be clearly determined. In rare cases this phase can last up to 1 year.

During further recovery the phase of psychoorganic syndrome occurs followed by a defect stage.

The Defect Stage

In the defect stage groups of symptoms can be profiled:

1. Predominance of an organic dementia combined with a special emotional disinhibition.
2. Predominance of spastic symptoms with pseudobulbar-paralytic symptomatology
3. Predominance of cerebellar symptomatology
4. Predominance of a Parkinson symptomatology
5. Predominance of an extrapyramidal hyperkinetic symptomatology

This symptomatology, typical for the defect stage of the apallic syndrome, may be combined with the symptoms of uni- or multifocal superimposed brain lesions and with the symptoms of a spastic hemiparesis, aphasia, etc.

It should be emphasized that in rare cases an apallic syndrome can follow the course of a transient syndrome without exhibiting defect symptoms, or the defect symptoms may be very slight.

The exitus of an apallic patient after acute brain damage may be caused by an irreversible breakdown of the circulatory system, or by a renewed secondary midbrain syndrome followed by a bulbar brain syndrome. Death of the apallic patients in the former group usually occurs during the full stage, or during the early period of the remission stage. After entry into the Klüver-Bucy-Terzian-Dalle Ore phase the prognosis for survival is favorable.

The Apallic Syndrome as a Sequel to a Diffuse Progressive Brain Process

In the progressive cerebral processes followed by an apallic syndrome as a final state, the apallic symptomatology develops correspondingly to the disintegration of the higher brain functions involving the remission stage, but in reverse. It can be presumed that, due to progress in intensive care treatment, the number of apallic patients of this etiology will increase, especially those cases with metabolic brain damage.

The clinical course of the progressive loss of brain function to the apallic level is described in Chapter 5. In order to give a rough idea of the course of development, it should be mentioned that during the first period of the clinical course psychiatric symptoms predominate. These symptoms can occur either in the different forms of the exogenic reaction types as described by Bonhoeffer (1910) in a sequence of different pictures, or with the psychoorganic syndrome according to E. Bleuler (1969). In most cases a Korsakow symptomatology appears followed by a Klüver-Bucy-Terzian-Dalle Ore syndrome as has been described, for example, by Pilleri (1961a). The further course to the full stage corresponds on the whole to the first period of the remission.

The full stage of an apallic syndrome as a sequel to a progressive process of the cerebrum shows for the most part the same symptomatology as an apallic syndrome after acute brain damage without local symptoms of a brain stem lesion.

Conclusions

The full stage of an apallic syndrome, independent of its etiology, is remarkably uniform and may be explained by a restriction of the brain functions to the mesodiencephalic level. The remission of an apallic syndrome, as well as the disintegration of the brain functions to an apallic syndrome, show in their development a systematic sequence. A difference is found, however, in the remission course caused by superimposed brain lesions. While in cases with a progressive brain process the apallic syndrome is a final state, the full stage of an apallic syndrome caused by an acute brain lesion can be reversible to a defect stage, in some cases without clinical symptoms as a transient syndrome without defect (*defektfreies Durchgangssyndrom*).

3. The Transition Stage from Midbrain Syndrome to Traumatic Apallic Syndrome

H.J. AVENARIUS and F. GERSTENBRAND

In those cases of apallic syndrome which occur after acute brain injury, an acute midbrain syndrome is observed as a preliminary stage. This syndrome, caused by tentorial strangulation, develops into the complete stage in three phases. It is characterized clinically by increased curtailment of consciousness to a comatose state, release of the motor functions of the midbrain with increased stretching of the extremities and trunk, and finally, by accompanying stretch synergisms in the complete state of the syndrome, as well as a release of the vegetative systems of the midbrain (with hyperpnea, trachycardia, hypertonia, and hyperthermia (Gerstenbrand, 1967). If intracranial pressure persists, a strangulation in the foramen occipitale magnum can develop and thereby an acute syndrome of the medulla oblongata (bulbar brain syndrome) can occur, which develops after subsidence of the symptoms of midbrain damage (McNeal and Plum, 1962; Müller, 1965). When the strangulation pressure decreases, a development from the bulbar brain syndrome to the midbrain syndrome is possible only if the bulbar brain symptoms have not existed longer than about 30 min. The acute midbrain syndrome can revert back through the same phases which are to be observed in the development of the complete state of the disease. The acute bulbar brain syndrome, however, can also develop into a irreversible loss of brain function, a condition which corresponds clinically to the death of the brain.

With patients who show an apallic syndrome after acute injury to the cerebrum following hypoxia or diffuse encephalitis, the phaselike development to a acute midbrain syndrome is generally not evident, nor is the complete state of the disease well defined. The same holds true for the apallic syndrome patients with exogenous or endogenous poisoning, such as mercury or insulin poisoning. In these cases the otherwise clearly defined acute midbrain symptoms are changed by local injury in the region of the brain stem.

If the acute midbrain symptoms do not decrease directly, a subsidence of the symptoms sets in after a few days, and the complete stage of an apallic syndrome develops after 10-20 days. This phase–the observation of which is of great importance for the prognosis of acute midbrain syndrome in serious brain injury–is termed the "transition stage" (Gerstenbrand, 1967). Individual phases of the transition stage are derived from the chief symptom, disturbance of consciousness. The further symptom categories, such as the release of the motor system and vegetative functions, can be assigned to the characteristic state of consciousness in each case. The development of the transition stage to the apallic syndrome can best be exemplified by discussing the recovery after a secondary acute midbrain syndrome following head injury. Corresponding to the disturbance of consciousness existing in the transition stage, we have termed the three definable stages as follows: (1) *coma prolongé* (Fau, 1956; Vigourous et al., 1964), (2) *parasomnia* (Jefferson, 1944), and (3) *akinetic mutism* (Cairns et al., 1941; Cairns, 1952). In Figure 1, the development of the individual phases is graphically represented by means of the cardinal symptoms present.

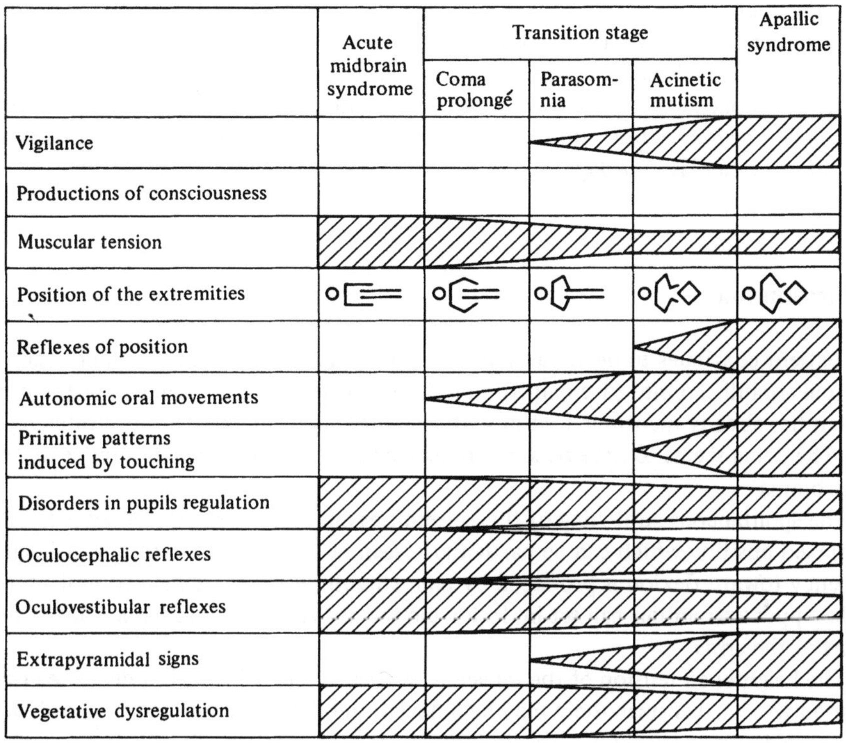

Fig. 1. Development from acute midbrain syndrome to apallic syndrome. Graphic representation of cardinal symptoms

1. Coma Prolongé

Although deep unconsciousness continues (*coma prolongé*) and the patient shows no reaction to external stimuli, the spontaneous stretching spasms subside generally after 3-5 days, and in this phase are only actuated by pain stimuli, initially in pronounced form, but later to a lesser degree. The extremities are stretched out and the patient's trunk and neck are also extended. At the end of this stage, however, a flexed position of the arms begins to set in, which can then be intensified by stimulation. The heightened tension of the body muscular system is considerably increased; coordinated movements of any kind are lacking. The tendon reflexes are increased; Babinski reflexes are generally more easily actuated than in the acute midbrain syndrome.

After the Babinski examination, an increased tendency to stretch the extremities is sometimes observed. The eyeballs are divergent but no longer in a fixed position. The oculocephalic reflexes are only slightly actuated; the vestibuloocular reflex shows an initial reaction to heightened tension. The reaction to light of the somewhat less than medium-wide pupils is retarded and sluggish; the ciliospinal reflex is clearly accentuated. The vegetative functions tend to be equilibrated.

In the course of this stage spontaneous chewing mechanisms set in. At the beginning, these exist only in a few chewing movements, whereby the lips are slightly open, but sometimes they remain closed too, so that the movements are carried out only by the lower jaw. Poeck and Hubach (1963) interpret these movement lapses as a primitive type of oral mechanism–not one connected with the environment, but an organized one nonetheless.

This stage can last 3-7 days, before changing into the "parasomnia" stage.

2. Parasomnia

The patient continues to be unconscious, lies with closed eyes, and shows no reaction to external stimuli. To intensive pain stimuli, however, the mass movements of the upper extremities already mentioned set in with a simultaneous increase in the stretching of the legs. The coma seems to have become superficial and resembles a state similar to sleep (parasomnia).

The spontaneous stretching of the extremities changes, in an intensified manner, into the flexed position which can be particularly seen in the upper extremities. A heightened tendency toward flexion is produced by pain stimuli. With severe pain stimuli an extension of the upper extremities can set in, following the above-mentioned tendencies to mass movements of the arms.

The heightened tension of the muscular system is still evident, but decreases further in its intensity. At this stage there may be a deviation of the eyeballs and the head, accompanied by the holding of the asymmetrically hypertensive neck reflex. The tendon reflexes are enhanced; the pyramidal signs are actuated. The divergence of the eyeballs has further diminished and remains variable; the eyeballs roll slightly. The oculocephalic reflex is actuated; the vestibuloocular reflex shows a hypertensive reaction. The vegetative reactions demonstrate a further stabilization; the sympathetic reaction state is not so strongly pronounced; with pain stimuli, however, an emergency reaction is produced. The automatic chewing actions appear at this stage in augmented form; they are spontaneous or actuated by external stimuli, such as the introduction of a nasal probe, etc. At the end of this stage the lip-closing and snout reflex can be demonstrated, and the bulldog reflex is slightly present. Hypertensive clutching is present in a number of cases. The parasomnia stage can also last 3-5 days.

3. Akinetic Mutism

At this stage patients open their eyes, initially for short periods of time, later for more extended periods. However, the blinking and menacing reflexes are not present.

During those periods of time when the patient has his eyes open, an increased tendency to vegetative stimulis response exists. The vegetative hypertension is shifted to the sympathetic tense state. In the following periods of a condition resembling sleep, a parasympathetic state of hypertension predominates. In his posture the patient shows a slight flexing tendency; also present in the legs, while the arms demonstrate a clear bending posture. The pronounced flexing of the upper and also the lower extremities presents a bad prognostic sign. The above-mentioned tendency to asymmetric, hypertensive neck reflex can increase. After pain stimuli, mass movements of the arms and, to a lesser degree, also of the legs, latently appear. With intensive pain stimuli, an increase in the flexing and stretching posture of the extremities follows. The muscle reflexes are intensified, the hypertension of the muscular system is heightened, and the pyramidal signs can be actuated, resulting occasionally in a flexing movement and a flight reflex in the legs. The eyeballs of the patient are in a position of divergence, spontaneous horizontal movements occur. The oculocephalic reflexes are actuated, the vestibuloocular reflex is heightened tonically. The medium-wide pupils show a lively reaction to light, the ciliospinal reflex is clearly evident. The vegetative functions have been stabilized but still remain displaced in the sympathetic tonic condition.

Primitive motor patterns show a further differentiation. Tactile oral adjustment mechanisms are carried out which are generally followed by spontaneous automatic chewing movements. Lip-closing and snout reflexes, as well as the bulldog reflex, are clearly apparent at this stage. The asymmetric tonic neck reflex is generally evident. Sporadically Babkin reflex can be actuated; seldom can a Chotzko reflex be demonstrated. The mental reflexes and the glabellar reflexes are present in almost all cases.

The third phase of the transition stage is in most cases curtailed compared with the other two, and lasts 2-5 days. It follows the overall picture of the apallic syndrome.

Compared with this phaselike development in cases with a traumatic apallic syndrome or after tentorial strangulation from a supratentorial increase in volume of different etiology, the symptoms in the transition stage after hypoxic damage and also after poisonings are generally less well definable. This can be explained particularly by the intruding symptoms conditioned by the brain stem.

In the time lapse of the transition stage, prognostic inferences can be made from various long pauses of the individual intermediary phases. A pause in the first two sections, over a period of 5 days each, is to be interpreted prognostically as an unfavorable sign; generally a temporal extension of the *coma prolongé* stage over 7 days appears particularly unfavorable. Thus the intensification of hypertension and/or the presence of permanent stretch synergisms remains the most important factor, together with the disturbance of consciousness, for an unfavorable prognosis.

With exact registration of the development of symptoms in the transition stage, an orientation in the sphere of transition between the acute midbrain syndrome and the apallic syndrome is possible.

4. Surgery of Traumatic Apallic Syndrome

G. DALLE ORE

Severe cerebral traumatic disease evolves toward apallic syndrome through an acute stage characterized by a midbrain syndrome, a transition stage with remission of the most severe symptomatology, and a chronic stage with the complete picture of apallic syndrome.

The cerebroanatomic lesions of apallic syndrome usually form during the acute stage. They are either in partial remittance or stabilized during the apallic syndrome stage.

A. Acute Stage

The acute stage is characterized by a midbrain syndrome very often caused by an uncal herniation which progressively compresses and finally tightly constricts the brain stem.

A valuable prophylactic measure for preventing herniation is the immediate removal of an intracranial hematoma and/or any lacerocontusive foci.

If uncal herniation has been stabilized for a long period of time and is far advanced, the simple removal of the hematoma is no longer sufficient, and tentorial decompression to free the brain stem becomes necessary.

Reduction of the herniated uncus may be sufficient to decompress the brain stem and to obtain proper circulation of the cerebrospinal fluid in the basal cisterns. In most cases, however, it is necessary to excise the uncus and the adjacent temporal lobe, as reported by Vincent et al. (1936). In the most severe cases an incision of the tentorium just posterior to the superior border of the petrous bone will eliminate the constriction.

Extensive bone decompression, up to complete hemicraniectomies, can sometimes be added to the above surgical procedure. This allows better control over intracranial pressure and cerebral edema in the postoperative period.

Other chapters in this book discuss the importance and usefulness of reanimation and especially of early mechanical hyperventilation during the acute stage.

B. Transition Stage

During the transition stage it is sometimes possible to obtain through surgery an earlier regression of some symptoms and a consequent decrease of irreversible neurologic impairment.

Hemorrhage into the subarachnoid spaces occurs often in severe head injuries. This may lead to impairment of the CSF reabsorption (Zander, 1969). to the onset of hydrocephalus, and to changes in the cerebral metabolism.

The introduction of atrioventricular shunts and the demonstrated usefulness of these derivations in hypertensive hydrocephalus as well as in normotensive hydrocephalus (Ojemann et al., 1969; Salmon, 1971) has led to the use of this operation in head injuries with protracted courses. After the patient has overcome the acute stage, this operation can, in some cases, speed recovery and limit functional damage.

The author's experience is limited to a few cases. Therefore, definite surgical indications cannot be provided. This type of surgery certainly does not appear curative. However, given exact indications, it can eliminate one of the many factors responsible for the severe traumatic neurologic syndromes and contribute to a more complete recovery.

Hassler (1969a and b) proposed stimulating the unspecific projection system into the forebrain, assuming that apallic syndrome can be at least partially due to a blockage of the unspecific projection system. This stimulation can be performed with stereotactically implanted flexible bipolar electrodes. The operation was performed on two patients with apallic syndrome by stimulating simultaneously the lamella pallidi interna and the base of the contralateral VA several times daily for a period of 3 weeks. Both patients experienced electroencephalographic arousal and modest clinical improvement.

Even though the results of the operation were positive, it is not believed to have any practical application. At present it is easier to obtain stimulation with pharmacologic means, by using neuromodulators and especially L-dopa.

C. Chronic Stage

During the chronic stage the apallic syndrome may appear either as a transitory condition which will eventually evolve toward a more favorable neurologic situation or—more rarely—as a fully stabilized clinical situation.

Apallic syndromes which had been fully stabilized for over 2 years were seen in the author's department until 1967. Ten of these cases were especially followed and studied clinically. All patients died within 6 years from the time of the head injury, without any change in their clinical pictures. In the years that followed no such cases were observed. Patients who survived the acute stage had temporary apallic syndromes, even though many experienced very severe psychoorganic deficiencies. This may be due to more accurate early surgical and reanimatory care during the acute stage.

In the fully stabilized stage of apallic syndrome there are no surgical possibilities.

Figure 1 refers to a patient who died of pulmonary complications while in an apallic syndrome which had been stabilized for 6 years. The cerebral cortex is reduced to a slight atrophic layer, the structures of the basal ganglia and especially of the thalamus and pallidus have practically disappeared. The corpus callosum appears as a thin plate between the two hemispheres. Only the bulbar and the mesencephalic structures, which were partially retained, allowed this patient to survive in the completely stabilized stage of apallic syndrome.

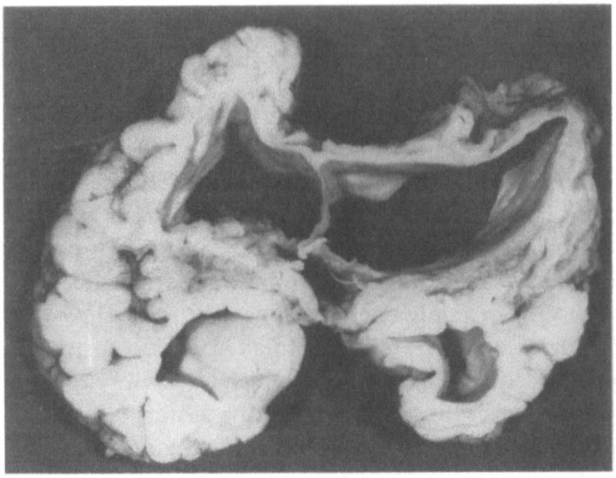

Fig. 1. Patient died after 6 years of fully stabilized apallic syndrome

This post-mortem study confirms that it is impossible to act surgically to improve the functional conditions of a practically destroyed brain.

In conclusion the surgical problems connected with apallic syndromes are primarily concentrated on the acute stage of head injury, when all efforts must be directed toward avoiding the spread of the primary cerebral lesions. Improvement of surgical and reanimatory techniques have largely increased the possibilities of preventing the onset of apallic syndromes. In the chronic or apallic stage of head injuries, surgery has no chance of success.

5. The Apallic Syndrome in Metabolic Disorders of the Brain

F. GERSTENBRAND, H.J. AVENARIUS, and H.P. PREISSLER

Introduction

Cerebral symptoms caused by insufficiency of brain metabolism in endogenous and exogenous metabolic disorders have been known for a long time (Frerichs, 1860). Pentschew mentions in his article (1958) that Jackson in 1882 already understood such neurologic pictures as a "stepwise disintegration of the cerebral integration efficiency." Nevertheless, the nonspecific term "metabolic encephalopathy" is widely used, as in the subtile presentations describing cerebral symptoms occurring in metabolic disorders in diseases of the liver (Summerskill et al., 1956; Penin, 1967), of the kidney (Tyler, 1968; Prill, 1969), in diabetes mellitus (Pentschew 1958; Levine, 1969), as well as in cases of anoxia (Strauss, 1931; Weinberger et al., 1940). Numerous other publications report disorders in serum electrolytes (Riecker, 1967), intra- and postoperative casualties (Gerstenbrand et al., 1968), as well as intoxications with narcotics (Victor and Adams, 1962), psychopharmaca (Corcoran et al., 1949; Bruck and Gerstenbrand, 1967), methanol (Plum and Posner, 1966), ethanol (Kieser, 1957), cyanide (Butenuth, 1970), paraldehyde (McDougall and Wyttie, 1932), water (Swanson and Iseri, 1958), carbon monoxide (Mumenthaler, 1961), and carbon dioxide (Sieker and Hickam, 1956). The above-listed references are limited to the given topic; severe brain damage in connection with metabolic disorders in the widest sense are reported.

The various authors describe similar psychopathologic transitory syndromes of the acute exogenous reaction type, without comprehension of the pathophysiologic connection between damage and respective central nervous reaction patterns. The published neurologic reports range from a slight reduction of the cortical level with varying disorders of consciousness and cortical dropout, to severe and partly irreversible damage of the brain and brain stem.

Comparison of clinical and experimental parameters with pathophysiologic analysis until a few years ago showed little unity and apparently divergent results (Erbslöh, 1958; Hoff and Jellinger, 1967; Jakob, 1964; Müting, 1962; Zysno et al., 1966; and many more). A few authors (Gerstenbrand et al., 1969; Tyler, 1970) have only recently started to re-emphasize the functional connections of the integration output of the central nervous system by pointing out similarities between the various neurologic findings in the development of the comatose syndromes on the one hand and the phylogenetic or ontogenetic stage of maturity of the central nervous system on the other.

At the same time it was possible to work out a uniform pathophysiologic concept of the comagenesis by using differentiating experimental and clinical tests to evaluate the brain metabolism. The energy requirement of the brain for the synthesis of the so-called energy-rich phosphates, which maintain the active intraextracellular exchange of potassium and sodium ions as a prerequisite for the excitability of the cells, is mainly supplied by the aerobic catabolism of glucose (Fazekas and Bessman, 1953; Gottstein, 1966; Sherlock, 1957; Tyler, 1968; Zysno et al., 1966). Two types of disturbances of energy metabolism can be discussed. First, a reduction of the substrate and/or oxygen may arise, caused by a deficiency involving the whole metabolism, or insufficient blood circulation of the brain (for both, the possibility of a limited compensation is given), and secondly, either a disturbance of the utilization of the substrate through a decrease in enzyme activity, a change in the acid-base balance (pH) and electrolytes, or the presence of nonmetabolized toxic substances may be the cause. A disturbance of acid-base balance may be evident at the blood-brain barrier (Fishman and Raskin, 1967; Freeman et al., 1962), as well as intracellularly (Fazekas and Bessman, 1953; Schenker et al., 1967; Sokoleff, 1971). In some comatose conditions differences in the chemical composition of serum and spinal fluid were observed, with a change in the normal distribution of the individual chemical substances (Agrest et al., 1962; Cowle et al., 1962; Müting, 1962; Plum, 1971; and others).

In extreme glucose deficiency the brain cells are capable of catabolizing, within limits, substrates such as amino acids and lipoproteins. This emergency oxidation of the cells' own substances occurs, according to Sokoleff (1971), in comatose cases which are irreversible even after sufficient supply of glucose. Since histopathologic examinations are primarily impossible in processes like this, discrepancies between clinical and pathologic reports may arise.

Finally, it is of significance (Erbslöh, 1958; Hoagland et al., 1939; Weinberger, 1940) that the energy turnover is less in ontogenetic older parts of the central nervous system and subsequently not as sensitive to glucose or oxygen deficiency.

The desire for a more distinctive clinical syndromatology of comatose states (Gerstenbrand et al., 1969; Jouvet and Dechaume, 1960; Polli, 1971) to avoid the nondistinctive term of encephalopathy is therefore not only justified, but also necessary for a more exact diagnostic and prognostic evaluation of the individual cases. In accordance with other reports (e.g., Conomy and Swash, 1968; Mumenthaler, 1961; Engerth and Winkler, 1933), it was found that daily intensive neurologic examinations are essential.

The literature reports that, especially with hepatic coma and hypoglycemic coma, lesional changes in the brain stem appear, upon analysis of the reports, to be regarded as an acute midbrain syndrome (Sherlock, 1957; Swanson and Iseri, 1958), rarely also as an apallic syndrome (Conomy and Swash, 1968; Cravioto et al., 1960) or bulbar-brain syndrome (Ziegler et al., 1965; Sieker and Hickam, 1956). In fact, with sufficient neurologic examinations of the patients, single phases are distinguishable in the transient phases in the development of the cerebral coma symptomatology. These phases are of changing and varying duration; a phase may be omitted or may overlap into the next, persist in any one stage, and also occur partly in reverse order or be remittent.

Approximately 160 patients were observed with a severe comatose course of different etiology. Four of these cases may serve as examples here.

Case Histories

Case 1. Hepatic coma (R.R., age 52, female): At the age of 48, after years of alcohol abuse, decompensated cirrhosis of the liver, and diabetes mellitus, the patient was hospitalized because of recurrence of ascites and prodromata of coma.

Two weeks later she was rehospitalized because of ascites and confusion in the morning, unexpected vomiting and within 30 min unconsciousness as well as a flexed/stretched position of the limbs accompanied by flex/stretch cramps of the extremities, as well as further symptoms of an acute midbrain syndrome of the third phase (Gerstenbrand and Lücking, 1970). After 30 min, there was spontaneous remission of midbrain symptomatology to a psychoorganic syndrome. On the following days, she presented symptoms of a diffuse brain damage with ever-increasing reflexes, frontal lobe signs, and slight-to-moderate dementia, corresponding to the state prior to the midbrain syndromatology. There was improvement of the pathologic findings of the liver by constant therapy with spirolactone, potassium, and Rocmalin treatment.

Eight days later, without external cause, renewed unconsciousness occurred within a few minutes, simultaneously with a stretch position of all extremities, as well as all signs of an acute midbrain syndrome in the full state. The stretch cramps subsided after 10 min, but, continuing increase of tonus, hyperreflexia, and pyramidal signs accompanied by simultaneous appearance of primitive motor patterns (spontaneous chewing automatism, oral and grasping patterns, mental reflexes, postural reflexes), as well as coma vigile, were seen. The position of the bulbi was divergent and the extremities were in the flex/stretch position. After 12 h, there was optic fixation and optic following, as well as primitive emotional reactions. This was followed 24 h later by the acute state symptoms of a Klüver-Bucy syndrome with simultaneous increase in voluntary movements. Twelve hours later, there was a transition to a Korsakoff syndrome followed by the development of a psychoorganic syndrome to the previous state of a diffuse cerebral lesion. After 8 weeks and intensive treatment of the liver, the patient was released from the hospital.

A few days later, she was rehospitalized with a fracture of the pubic bone caused by a fall in a state of confusion. Upon admission, she showed symptoms of a paranoid hallucinatory picture with intensive motor unrest, and also marked neurologic disorders exhibited by hyperreflexia, pyramidal signs, slight increase in tonus, as well as primitive motor patterns, primarily oral and grasping ones. With intensive treatment of the liver, remission into a neurasthenic state of the exogenous reaction type (Bonhoeffer, 1910) and transition into the previous state of cerebral defect, she was released from the hospital after several weeks of treatment.

Two days later she was readmitted to the hospital with suddenly appearing flashes of consciousness and strong motor unrest with mass and roll movements. Within 3 h an acute midbrain syndrome in the full state developed, lasting only 3 h, followed by subsidence of the stretch cramps and development of coma vigile. After approximately 6 h, the full state of an apallic syndrome with all characteristic symptoms appeared. After 20 h, there was sudden renewed stretch position of all extremities with stretch synergism and coma, and disappearance of the primitive motor patterns. After 6 h the stretch cramps subsided with simultaneous onset of gasping-breathing and finally breathing with only base-of-mouth movements. Within the next hour breathing was arrested, posture was atonic, reflexes were absent, and the pupils wide and without reaction. Twenty minutes later, cardiac standstill and death.

Neuropathologic findings (Neurologisches Institut, Vienna): Older walnut-sized hemorrhage of the white matter with perifocal necrotic edema parietooccipital dextra, slight diffuse brain atrophy (pre-aging glial and axonal dystrophy, as in chronic liver damage, no signs of acute brain edema with herniation).

Summary: The 52-year-old female patient, a chronic alcoholic, developed several times an acute midbrain syndrome, which transformed itself into an apallic syndrome. Remission followed through a Klüver-Bucy syndrome, as well as a Korsakoff symptomatology, into a psychoorganic syndrome to a defect state which existed previous to the acute incident. In between, an exogenous psychosis developed, in the course of which the patient fell, breaking her pubic bone. Death resulted during an apallic syndrome when a renewed acute midbrain syndrome developed, followed by a bulbar brain syndrome. Autopsy showed diffuse cerebral damage, but, without signs of an acute midbrain or bulbar brain herniation.

Case 2. Uremic coma (T.K., age 61, female): After repeated hospitalization because of shrinking nephropathy and high blood pressure, the patient was rehospitalized because of unrest and depression, anxiety, lack of drive, disturbed concentration, pain sensation, reduction of the higher brain functions accompanied by neurologic symptoms such as hyperreflexia, slight increase in tonus, slight amimia and akinesia, flapping tremor, slight cerebellar symptoms, slight primitive motor patterns, as well as the symptoms of a polyneuropathy. Twenty-four hours after admission, she exhibited severe motor restlessness and fear, marked paranoid ideas, and optic and acoustic hallucinations. At the same time there was moderate intensification of the neurologic symptomatology, with slight pyramidal signs and a marked reduced convergence reaction of the bulbi as well as increased amimia and akinesia. In the course of 36 h, the restlessness subsided, as did the paranoid thoughts, but hallucinations continued, together with increased confusion with Korsakoff symptoms and a moderate increase in the neurologic symptomatology. After 12 h, she was comatose, and showed undirected movements of defense. Within the next 4 h lower extremities were in the stretch position, the arms were flexed, there was marked increase in muscle tonus, hyperreflexia, on both sides a positive Babinski sign, further divergent position of the bulbi with sluggish reaction to light and moderately marked primitive patterns (oral reflexes, tonic grasping, asymmetric tonic neck reflex).

Within the following 12 h coma vigile occurred with typical sleep-awake rhythm, lack of emotional reaction, divergent position of the bulbi, moderately marked oculocephalic reflexes, medium-wide, left somewhat smaller, pupils with delayed reaction to light, positive reaction to pain, flex/stretch position of the extremities with increased tonus, hyperreflexia, pyramidal signs on both sides, mass movements to intensified pain stimulation, primitive motor patterns (chewing automatism, oral reflexes, tonic and phasic grasping, asymmetric tonic neck reflex of both sides), as well as moderate amimia, a tendency to tachycardia, and other signs of autonomic disinhibition.

For 30 h there was no change. Then the coma vigile disappeared, the legs assumed the stretch position with undirected mass movements of the arms upon pain stimulation, and there was beginning disinhibition of the autonomic functions. Two hours later there was coma, flexed position of the arms, stretched position of the legs, and divergent position of the bulbi. One hour later the acute midbrain syndrome with all typical symptoms appeared, especially stretch cramps. After 3 h without change gasping-breathing began with a simultaneous decrease in muscular hypertonus, as well as hyperreflexia, and finally, atonic posture of the upper extremities while the legs were in a stretched position. The pupils were dilated with only a moderate reaction to light, and there was increased divergent position of the bulbi. This state continued for over 24 h, followed by atonic posture of body and limbs, areflexia, disappearance of pyramidal signs, marked divergence of the fixed bulbi, dilated pupils, no reaction to light, slight dyspnea, drop in temperature to 36°C, and bradycardia. Death after 1 h was caused by cardiac arrest. There was continuous increase in BUN and creatinine unchanged by therapy during the comatose state.

EEG (at the stage of the beginning of the bulbar brain syndrome): diffuse general changes, without side signs or focus.

Neuropathologic findings (Pathologisch-Anatomisches Institut, Vienna): Brain edema with slight basal pressure signs, recent damage of the white matter.

Summary: In this 61-year-old female patient suffering from shrinking nephropathy and high blood pressure, during an exogenous type of reaction according to Bonhoeffer (1910), a hyperemotional weakness state appeared first, which finally developed into a paranoid hallucinatory state and later into a marked psychoorganic syndrome with symptoms of severe diffuse cerebral damage. Upon intensification, an apallic syndrome in the full state developed, from which an acute midbrain syndrome evolved, finally progressing to the transitory phase of an acute bulbar brain syndrome which was shortly followed by the death of the patient. The neuropathologic findings showed brain edema with slight signs of herniation.

Case 3. Diabetic coma, hyperglycemia, uremic coma with diabetic nephropathy (Kimmelstiel-Wilson) (M.L., age 72, female): Diabetes with insulin therapy for over 20 years, for 3 years increased BUN. The patient was admitted because of decompensation of carbohydrate metabolism and pneumonia with a "comatose state." Upon pain stimulation, she exhibited undirected defense movements with latency, flexion tendency of the arms, flex/stretch position of the legs, increased muscular tonus, hyperreflexia, decreased Achilles tendon reflex, slight pyramidal signs, divergent position of the bulbi, oculocephalic reflex slightly releasable, moderately dilated pupils with decreased reaction to light, and slight reaction to pain, primitive motor patterns partly releasable (grasping reflexes, oral pattern, asymmetric tonic neck reflex, slight chewing automatism), coma vigile, slightly increased somewhat deeper rhythmic breathing, tachycardia, BP 100/70; blood-sugar 944 mg%, no ketone bodies in the urine, and acidosis. Within 24 h metabolism was balanced with normal blood sugar and acid-base balance. Twelve hours after commencement of therapy there was a passing intensification of the primitive motor patterns, especially of the chewing automatism, disappearing coma vigile, optic fixation, afterwards optic following, beginning of undirected spontaneous mass movements, increase in the grasping reflexes with tendency to grasp objects, sound reply upon calling; 24 h after admission, turning-toward, as well as performing simple tasks, remains of a stretch position of the lower extremities with slight increased tonus of the arms and legs, slight divergent position of the bulbi upon limited convergence, directed voluntary movements, slight primitive motor patterns of the oral sense and of grasping. Six hours later the psychoorganic syndrome, with increase in orientation was observed, with slight neurologic symptomatology with hyperreflexia, slight increase in muscle tone, as well as slight cerebral reduction signs, and further symptoms of polyneuropathy.

After another 7 h there was rapid development of motor restlessness and fear, followed 2 h later by acoustic and optic hallucinations, simultaneous increase in the neurologic symptomatology with hyperreflexia, and slight tonus increase, oral and grasping reflexes. After 1 h the hallucinations subsided, but anxiety, depression, and severe restlessness continued. The neurologic symptomatology decreased.

Three days after admission there was a rapid decrease in diuresis, finally polyuria, an increase in BUN to 124 mg%, creatinine to 2.6 mg%, and potassium to 6.3 mVal/1, followed 1 day later by increased motor restlessness, logorrhea, and increased Korsakoff symptomatology. There was a simultaneous increase in the primitive motor patterns, hyperreflexia and slight pyramidal signs. After 12 h symptoms of a Klüver-Bucy syndrome with further intensification of the neurologic symptoms appeared: marked flapping tremor, myoclonia on the face as well as the upper and lower extremities. On the 6th day of treatment there was marked limitation of consciousness with a decreased reaction to external stimuli, slight divergent position of the bulbi, flexed position of the upper extremities and a flex/stretch position of the lower extremities, increase in muscular tone and reflexes, and pyramidal signs. After 8 h the patient exhibited coma vigile, lack of emotional reaction to pain stimulation, latent onset of undirected mass movements, flex/stretch position of the extremities with increase of tonus, hyperreflexia and pyramidal signs, marked primitive motor patterns, including the tonic asymmetric and symmetric neck reflexes, and marked autonomic overexcitability. Twelve hours later there was rapid development of coma with stretch position and stretch synergism of all extremities. The bulbi were divergent, with decreased reaction to light, tachycardia, tachypnea, as well as all symptoms of an acute midbrain syndrome. After 4 h the full state of a bulbar brain syndrome appeared; 15 min later the patient died of cardiac failure.

Summary: In this 72-year-old female patient coma developed with hyperglycemia with all symptoms of an apallic syndrome, which on admission showed the remaining symptoms of an acute midbrain syndrome. After normalization of blood sugar and of the acid-base balance, remission began. Still in the phase of a psychoorganic syndrome, an exogenous type of reaction started which developed increasingly into a state of hallucination. After renewed remission a Korsakoff syndrome developed, followed by a Klüver-Bucy symptomatology and again an apallic syndrome. During this time a disturbance of kidney function developed, with a severe increase in BUN and creatinine as well as potassium. The apallic syndrome developed into a renewed acute midbrain syndrome and finally into a bulbar brain syndrome ending in the patient's death.

Case 4. Hypoxic coma (K.B., age 11 months, female); (cf. Amann et al., 1971): During an examination of the mouth with a spatula because of laryngitis sudden heart and breathing arrest occurred, followed 5 min later by setting in of the heart's action, and after 15 min spontaneous breathing. Within 2 days heart arrest occurred 2 more times. Upon admission the patient was in acute midbrain syndrome with coma, showed divergent position of the bulbi, and stretch cramps of all extremities. Because of repeated heart arrest, thoracotomy and manual heart massage was done, but cardiac arrest occurred again. After stabilization of the heart's function, the acute midbrain syndrome continued. Three hours later the arms were abducted. On each of the following 2 days there was heart and breathing arrest. On the 3rd day after the incident, there developed myoclonia of the eyes and face, as well as of the arms and legs in the posture pattern as described previously. On the 8th day symptoms appeared of a transitory stage into the apallic syndrome with increasing primitive motor patterns, primarily of the chewing automatism, with simultaneous decrease in the myoclonia. Three weeks after onset of the disease, the patient exhibited the full state of an apallic syndrome with coma vigile, typical sleep-awake rhythm, lack of emotional reactions, flex/stretch position of the extremities, marked primitive motor patterns, including the Babinski sign, as well as severe autonomic lability. Five weeks after the start of the disease with unchanged neurologic state, a pontine crying pattern developed. Death was caused by irreversible failure of the circulatory system, 57 days after onset of the disease.

EEG (16 days after heart arrest): Extremely flat curves with slight theta and beta activity, no noticeable side difference.

Neuropathologic findings: Extreme form of postanoxic encephalopathy with extensive necrosis of the cerebral cortex, symmetric necrosis of almost all central gray matter, diffuse total atrophy of the cerebellar cortex and symmetric focal necrosis in the mesencephalon and pontine tegmentum. Secondary embolic-metastatic focal encephalitis was also found.

Summary: In this 11-month-old girl cardiac and respiratory arrest set in during an examination of the pharynx. After reanimation an acute midbrain syndrome developed, which changed only after 8 days into the transitory stage to an apallic syndrome and finally into the full state of this syndrome. The apallic symptomatology was maintained without noticeable changes until death, 57 days after the acute incident. Besides the characteristic midbrain symptoms, rhythmic myoclonia of the face and extremities developed which could not be observed in the full state of the apallic syndrome. During the course of the apallic symptomatology a pontine crying pattern developed. In this case, massive hypoxic damage to almost all gray matter and also edematic damage to the white matter occurred. Further, a diffuse total atrophy of the cerebellar cortex and of the nucleus dendatus, as well as of the lower oliva, developed. At the end of the course of the disease a metastatic focal encephalitis existed.

Discussion

Actual knowlege of cerebral metabolic disorders in coma of various genesis allows the following hypothesis:

The cerebrum shows a decreasing sensitivity towards an impaired energy supply, conditioned through its phylogenetic functional planes (Richardson et al., 1959). The supply and utilization of glucose, essential for the functions of the central nervous system, depend in comatose states upon the respective damage. If the energy turnover is lowered to such an extent that the output for a central functional level is insufficient, the cerebral integration output will be reduced to the phylogenetic older functional plane still sufficient for energy supply, whereby the rostrally situated parts of the brain then cease to function (Fazekas and Bessman, 1953; Gottstein, 1966; Tyler, 1970; and others). This process was termed a functional cerebral disintegration independent of its etiology.

Biochemical parameters or the encephalogram (Conomy and Swash, 1968; Polli, 1971; Tyler, 1968; Kitani, 1959; Penin, 1967; Parsons-Smith et al., 1957; and many others) are only a rough aid in the therapeutic and prognostic evaluation. Strict neurologic and psychiatric observations during the whole course are important in differentiating certain functional syndromes which may be brought into relation to the central disintegration levels. Not every step can be observed in the individual case; however, the course of various hepatogenic, hypoglycemic and other forms of coma, as well as postoperative hypoxemic complications, show that the various disintegration levels may be present in all comatose states.

Several authors (Erbslöh, 1958; Prill, 1969; Stefenelli, 1962) have pointed out that the clinical course is subject to the acuity of the decompensation process. Depending upon whether the brain has enough time for a relative adaptation, the acute and subacute courses (electroencephalographic; Penin, 1967) may be differentiated.

In the development of the coma syndrome, the variable acute midbrain syndrome (Cases 1-4) dominates with a characteristic disorder of consciousness, a flexed-stretched position of the extremities and the trunk, which may be intensified by pain stimuli, increased muscle tone, increased reflex action, positive pyramidal signs, disorder of the optomotor system and autonomic disinhibition. With an intermittent bulbar brain syndrome (muscle atonia, loss of reflexes, light-rigid mydriasis, disintegration of autonomic functions), this picture, if it persists, may lead to death. Other cases may go into remission shortly after direct cessation of the midbrain symptomatology—very rarely, however, with a brief previously occurring bulbar brain or apallic syndrome. The severity of the functional disintegration depends upon how acute the comatose state appeared (Case 4). If the comatose state can be controlled therapeutically, late damage may often result. In contrast to the reports of Plum and Posner (1966), personally observed cases show neurologically complete remission, even after an acute midbrain syndrome in its full state, caused by metabolic disorders as well as traumatic events. In lethal cases, especially in younger patients who die during one of the acute phases, the brain shows conditioned basal pressure signs or even transtentorial or foraminal herniation (Case 2). A causal connection between herniation and clinical course, however, cannot be established, since the actual intracerebral metabolic or other disorders causing local changes (Weinstein, 1947) cannot be differentiated clinically in the individual case.

In contrast to this, the subacute "coma forms" in their various central disintegration phases are more easily distinguishable. This is shown in our second case, where it was possible to analyze some symptomatologically different disintegration phases, namely, a neurasthenic phase (Penin, 1967) showing cortical disintegration with loss of vitality; pain sensation; irritated, anxious, depressive disposition; an exogenous paranoid-hallucinatory phase; a phase of a Korsakoff syndrome followed by an apallic syndrome which was interrupted by different phases of the acute midbrain syndrome (Gerstenbrand and Lücking, 1970). This was followed by a transient prephase of the bulbar brain syndrome and the full picture of a bulbar brain syndrome, which soon after led to death.

Effective therapy of the basic metabolic disorder will favor a stepwise reintegration of the higher central function levels in the remission course of the apallic syndrome with an increasing stabilization of the energy balance. Here, too, the various phases may be omitted in individual cases or may not be noticed because of their short duration. The explanation for the nonappearance or short duration of the individual transitory phases may lie in the condition of the patient (e.g., age, varying degree of disturbance of the various central structures, local vascular disorders, previous cerebral damage, rate of metabolic restabilization).

The remission as well as the disintegrating course corresponds for the most part to the course of the apallic syndrome of traumatic genesis. Clinical details are given in Chapter 2. Particular attention is given to the Klüver-Bucy phase (Case 1) which shows in disintegration as well as in remission hypersexuality, lack of shame reaction, complex primitive motor patterns with oral priority, lack of object identification, a manic-depressive mood and sometimes bulimia. The Korsakoff syndrome, with massive amnestic disorders, disturbed sense of time, logorrhea, euphoria, and rapid tiring combined with a disappearance of the primitive motor patterns and improvement of the spontaneous voluntary movements, is well known as a transitory phase in the development and remission of comas of various etiology. A defective state marked by organic dementia, affective disinhibition and/or persisting extrapyramidal, spastic or cerebral symptoms, appears in a certain percentage of the cases in the apallic syndrome with metabolic or hypoxic or traumatic genesis.

Through the indicated analysis and the symptomatologic classification of a coma syndrome of various etiology, a deeper understanding of the cerebral functions may be gained. Adequate consideration of the patient's age, duration and severity of the central disintegration, and the acuity of the dominating functional disorder allows a faster and more reliable prediction of the effectiveness of modern therapy. Furthermore, a better prognosis of individual cases can now be made than was previously possible from laboratory tests or electroencephalographic reports. However, many questions remain, such as the manner and exact location of the damage causing the coma and its pathophysiologic pattern. Improved routine laboratory tests on the spinal fluid, for example, may further assist the clinician to supplement the neurologic reports and possibly aid in the commencement of additional therapeutic measures on the central energy metabolism—as an aid in the analysis of individual factors outside the acute metabolic disorder requiring therapeutic attention. Finally, the analysis of function as well as brain morphology and ontogenesis of the primitive motor patterns will prove useful.

It should also be mentioned that chronic central cerebral damages caused by endogenous or exogenous disorders of metabolism may possibly lead to an apallic syndrome. These disorders are, for example—besides the causes already mentioned—diabetes mellitus and chronic alcoholism, hyperthyroidism, chronic lead and mercury intoxication, and usually congenital disorders of lipoid or amino acid metabolism in children. The clinical symptomatology of the apallic syndrome caused by these diseases has, as far as we know, not been described, with the exception of mercury poisoning.

Summary

The central nervous structures show a varying degree in rate of energy turnover, depending upon their phylogenetic age. The disturbances in oxygen utilization in comatose states of various genesis is the most important and last step in cerebral metabolic disorders, whereby a stepwise progressive disintegration of the cerebrum occurs with a uniform central remission pattern, independent of the coma etiology, in the levels of the cortex, limbic system, midbrain, and lower brain stem. Four characteristic cases serve as examples of these reaction patterns and the development of the apallic syndrome. Laboratory tests and the electroencephalogram are only a rough aid in evaluating therapeutic measures and prognosis in the individual coma cases, but they may be significantly supplemented by keen neurologic observations.

6. Apallic Syndrome Following Protracted Hypoglycemia

G.P. LIEBALDT and I. SCHLEIP

A rarer form of the apallic syndrome is considered in the case reported below. Severe hypoglycemia, precipitated in this case by an islet-cell adenoma of the pancreas, produced the clinical manifestations of cerebral cortical failure with apallic syndrome. The pathologic changes were widespread cortical necrosis in the neocortical region of the cerebrum, leaving the brain stem and the phylogeneticallyolder cerebral cortex with the allocortex largely spared. The distribution of the changes, nonidentical to those produced in the CNS cerebral anoxia, but peculiar to a lack of glucose, is of special interest. This particular distribution of changes should be considered neurohistologically and in the light of its phyloontogenetic localization, as well as biochemically with regard to the metabolic requirements, and clinically with regard to the neuropathology of wakefulness and consciousness.

Case History (Dr. I. Schleip): Patient E.Pf., female, born 1930 (Neurological Clinic of the University of Würzburg): The patient had always been healthy apart from childhood complaints. She was of pyknic build, with no history of familial diseases or endocrine abnormalities. At the end of 1962, 9 months before her first admission to the hospital, she complained of morning fatigue, a tendency to perspire, paresthesia in the limbs, air hunger and anxiety, followed by confusion and sometimes loss of consciousness. These attacks lasted 15-30 min. In the hours following she complained of impairment of physical ability and concentration and blurred vision. She had had menstrual irregularities since the development of these attacks. There was a gradual intensification in the degree and frequency of these morning attacks, and in August 1963, she was admitted to the Neurological Clinic in Würzburg for protracted disturbance of consciousness following an attack.

Neurologic Findings (on the day of admission): Cranial nerves N.A.D., muscle tone of limbs greater on left side than on right, increase in muscle reflexes, more on left side than on right, bilateral signs of pyramidal tract involvement.

EEG: Marked focal signs over right hemisphere, maximal in the parietal region. Focal signs also present over left occipital region.

A complete medical examination was carried out for suspected spontaneous hypoglycemia due to an islet-cell tumor of the pancreas, and the suspected diagnosis of hyperinsulinism was confirmed.

A few days after admission there was ocular paralysis with upward deviation together with generalized tetanic spasms and trismuslike hypertonia of the jaw musculature, followed by repeated chewing movements of the lower jaw. The tetanic spasms faded 15 days before death, at the same time as the automatic choreiform movements, which were more pronounced on the right. The abnormality of consciousness finally took the form of coma vigile, with no response to optic, acoustic, and tactile stimuli, and absence of any movements of expression and spontaneous mimicry. The blink reflex was present and the corneal and pupillary reflexes were intact. The tetany was aggravated by nursing procedures and was accompanied by groaning. There was no disturbance of circulatory or respiratory function, although increasing cachexia developed. The patient died December 18, 1964, of circulatory failure following pneumonia, 16 months after admission.

Clinical Diagnosis: Brain damage of the apallic syndrome type, with protracted hypoglycemia. Encephalitis?

Post-mortem Findings

Examination of Body (performed December 19, 1964 at the Pathological Institute, University of Würzburg, Director: Prof. H.W. Altmann): Islet-cell adenoma of the pancreas, the size of a cherry, histologically composed of beta cells. Diffuse moderate fatty infiltration of the liver, slight fatty infiltration of the midtubular portion of the kidneys. Cause of death: bronchopneumonia.

Examination of Brain (Dr. G.P. Liebaldt, Department of Neuropathology, Neurological Clinic and Policlinic, Würzburg):

Macroscopic Findings: Brain weight: 1250 g, fixed in formaldehyde. The consistency of the brain appeared to be generally reduced. Whitish clouding of the leptomeninges over the convexity, especially in the region of the borders of the pallium. Thickening and adhesions of the cisternal connective tissue in the basal cisternal region. Basal arteries normal, soft-walled. Cerebral convolutions reduced in the region of the frontal pole back to the junction with the gyri recti, and as far as the orbital convolutions.

Frontal Sections: The ventricular system was slightly and symmetrically dilated in the middle sections. The ventricular wall was smooth. The brain substance contained more fluid than normally. The medullary layer of the right temporal lobe showed disintegration of the status spongiosus or status lacunaris type. There was extensive necrosis of the cerebral cortex (Fig. 1a). The orbital cortex and the cerebellum (Fig. 1b), and the allocortical portions of the cerebral cortex (Fig. 1a) were for the most part spared. Apart from patchy

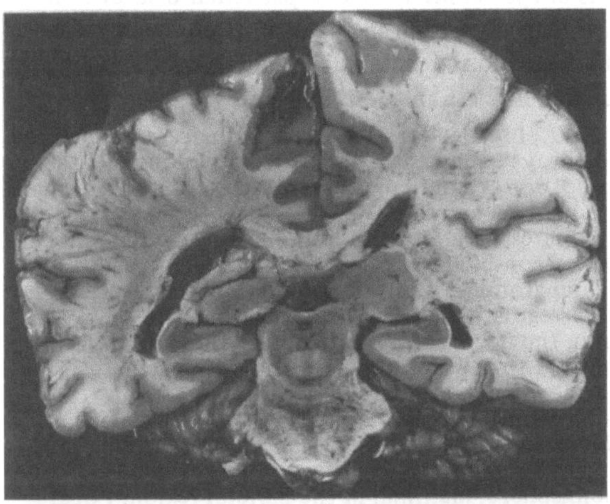

Fig. 1a

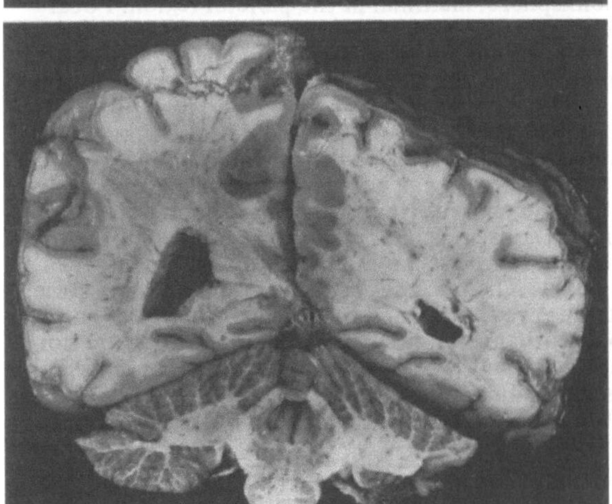

Fig. 1b

distributed areas of hyperemia, there were no focal pathologic changes in the other regions of the brain.

Histologic Findings

There was severe lipoid degeneration throughout the neocortical cerebral cortical regions, with fine- to medium-sized deposits of fat in ganglia and glial cells. In the white matter there was degeneration of the medullary sheath and spotty fat deposits in the cellular elements. There was total necrosis of the second to sixth cortical layers in the frontal–and especially in the temporal–cortex, and a greater number of "fatty glia" in the molecular layer (Fig. 2c). Diffuse disappearance of ganglion cells characterized in cortical areas, show-

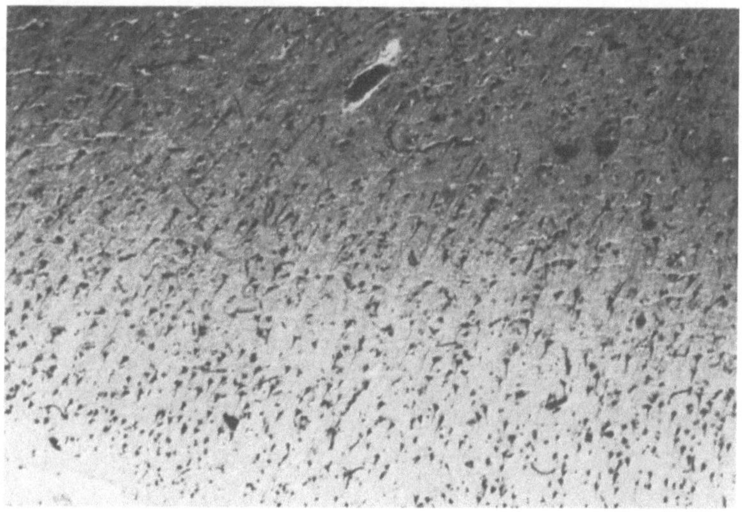

Fig. 2a

ing necrobiotic change, together with atrophic ganglion cells showing pronounced pyknotic alterations without marked glial reaction. There was moderately marked recent status spongiosus in the granular layer of the hippocampus, and moderately distributed atrophy of ganglion cells in the pyramidal cell layers. Only a small amount of neuronal degeneration was found in the area striata, and the craniolateral portions of the occipital lobes showed extensive necrosis of the deeper cortical layers. No pronounced increase in glial fibers could be seen in the necrotic areas with the use of Holzer's glial fiber stain. There was severe atrophy of ganglion cells in the caudate nucleus, the putamen, and the thalamic nuclei. In the central diencephalic gray matter, the ganglion cell components were generally normal, as in the indusium griseum and in the reticular formation of the subthalamic region. There were fresh focal clear areas in the medullary layer. Central myelinolysis was observed in the oral pons with scattered disappearance of ganglion cells in the pontine nuclei. The cerebellar cortex was extraordinarily well preserved. Even the dentate nucleus of the cerebellum showed only very scattered ganglion cell atrophy. More pronounced lipofuscin deposition occurred in the ganglion cells near the vagal nucleus in the medullar oblongata. The spinal cord (cervical cord) showed partly atrophic, partly primarily irritated ganglion cells in the anterior horn region, together with diffuse ganglionic degeneration. Irregular degeneration of the medullary sheath was determined in one of the peripheral nerves examined.

Histologic Assessment

High-grade parenchymatous damage with widespread atrophy of the ganglion cells (Fig. 2a) was seen in the frontal and parietooccipital cerebral cortex, interspersed in places with extensive necrobiosis (Fig. 2b), going as far as total necrosis of the cortex (Fig. 2c) and of the

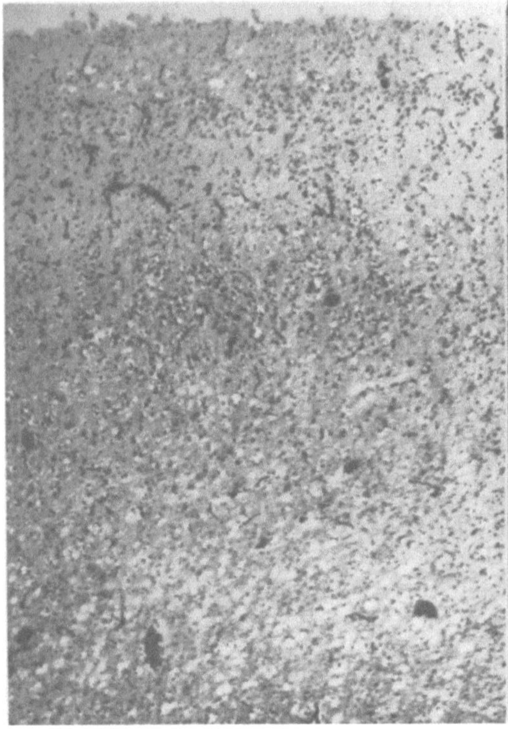

Fig. 2b

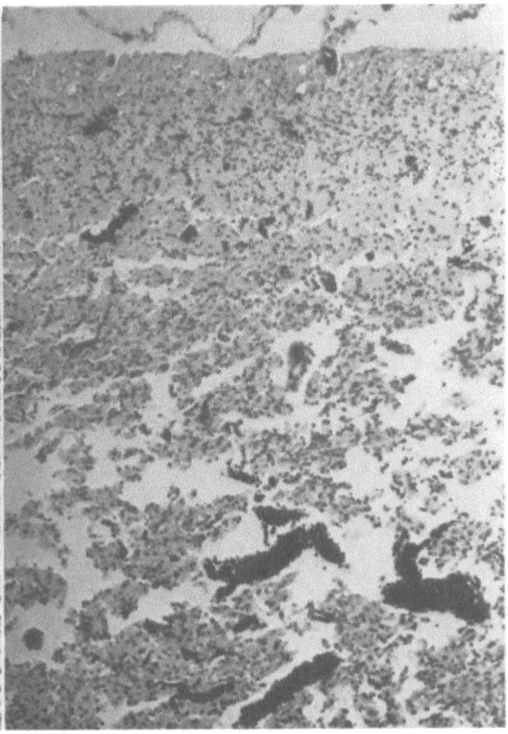

Fig. 2c

underlying subcortical medullary layer in the temporooccipital region. In addition, atrophy of ganglion cells with diffuse necrosis of ganglion cells was found in the neostriatum (putamen and caudate nucleus) and in the medial and lateral thalamic nuclear areas associated with the neocortex. Surprisingly few pathologic changes were found as compared with the cerebrum) in the cerebellum, the cerebellar nuclei, and the brain stem (paired and unpaired brain stem and allocortical regions of the cerebrum).

Discussion of Changes and Comments

When we come to the question of chemistry in the formal pathogenesis of the changes described here, we must bear in mind Opitz's statement (Opitz, 1952), that "the amount of energy turnover necessary for the reversible maintenance of structure and hence also of recovery, may be regarded as a thermodynamic criterion for the differentiation of structure. In view of the very short recuperation time of central nervous structures, it is presumed that the structure turnover in the brain is very high." According to C.G. Schmidt (1956), brain tissue possesses "only very small reserves of carbohydrate, so that any interference with the supply of glucose through the bloodstream will imperil brain metabolism and energy release."

Because of its low level, the glycogen content of the brain does not exert any noteworthy compensatory effect. It was determined that the hypoxia-sensitive regions and cell types of the CNS were not at all affected. Neither the hypoxia-sensitive Purkinje cells nor the granular layer of the cerebellum, nor the dentate nucleus of the cerebellum, were definitely involved in the damage described here. Even the damage to the hippocampal formations was marginal as compared with the changes, which extended as far as total necrosis, in the neocortical cerebral cortex. The histologic findings generally show that the brain stem regions—and of these, particularly the phylogenetically older structures as well as the allocortical cerebral cortex—and the nuclear regions were clearly the least affected. Thus the main weight of the findings in our case falls preferentially in the phylogenetically younger cortical regions, and with decreasing intensity in the associated neocortical nuclear areas (neostriatum). The smallest changes were seen in the allocortical paleo- and archicortex and in the brain stem, i.e., in the phylogenetically old, central lobular structures.

In the authors' opinion, these findings are significant in view of the clinically impressive apallic syndrome. There is indeed some degree of overlap, but in view of the difference in distribution of damage due to hypoxia and to hypoglycemia, some evidence is obtained concerning the various biochemical architectonics of the CNS. Naturally, in the case of hypoglycemia, endogenous pathogenetic influences are acting on a complicated system of energy metabolism (cellular respiration and assimilation), which cannot fail to affect structure. It is striking that in our case the type of damage is not uniform, even within the neocortical region. In one region we have severe and universal atrophy of ganglion cells in the cortical layers, and in other sections we see the appearance of necrobiosis or total necrosis of the cortical layers (Fig. 2c). This stepwise gradation of severity of the tissue damage in the neocortical layers appears to indicate a varying intensity in the energy processes in these areas. With the close interrelationship and interaction of intermediate metabolism as regards the assimilatory and dissimilatory processes, which in the CNS—with a respiratory quotient of about unity—corresponds to a generous provision of energy and hence a great deal of carbohydrate breakdown, it is understandable that the cortical areas requiring most energy are first and most severely damaged. In cases of hypoglycemia there is a reduction in glucose supply to the CNS in the presence of a normal oxygen supply. The reduced glucose supply means that the cells of the CNS undergo a corresponding reduction in possible carbohydrate breakdown on which, as we know, the CNS is especially dependent, so that a reduction in available glucose inevitably leads to a corresponding reduction in the energy processes, and so to atrophy of the ganglion cells.

Since the atrophic process was only very slight in the allocortex and brain stem areas in this case, the conclusion follows that these areas clearly possess a relatively lower assimilatory level as compared with the cerebral cortical areas and their associated nuclear regions (the neostriatum and the neothalamus). The evidently smaller structure metabolism of the cellular cerebellar elements is also striking. Cellular respiration is also a contributory factor in the maintenance of structure and thus facilitation of function, in addition to the assimilatory level. Here it is of interest that, according to E. Albert (1952), the central lobular ganglia have a lower O_2 consumption than the neocortical cerebral areas and their nuclear regions (caudate nucleus and putamen), thus confirming the phyloontogenetic relationship of the neocerebral regions to the neocortical cortex. Since the energy turnover for the reversible maintenance of structure is of considerable magnitude in the brain and is normally almost exclusively covered by carbohydrates, glucose lack is expressed as a process going beyound atrophy, via a compensatory oxidative utilization of the structural elements of the cell, inasmuch as cellular respiration remains intact.

Although the frontal cortex showed high-grade atrophy of ganglion cells in our case, there was no tendency to necrobiosis and necrosis of the cortical layers, as was clearly present in the parieto-occipital and—particularly—in the temporal cortical regions. Thus, brain structures of different location are involved in these different expressions of vulnerability, and these characteristically affect the clinical picture.

On the basis of an analysis of brain stem tumors, especially of the mid- and hindbrain regions, and a comparison of the clinical symptomatology of wakefulness and consciousness, Orthner (1969) concluded that disturbances of wakefulness appear preponderantly in cases of damage to the areas of the mid- and hindbrain in the neighborhood of the ventricles. Processes in brain areas lying further caudally from the third ventricle and the aqueduct, however, may indirectly affect wakefulness, either as a result of a generalized increase in intracerebral pressure, or as a result of displacement of tissue, which may cause strangulation of the brain around the ventricles in the tentorial gap or interfere with the blood supply. However, as our investigations of the apallic syndrome have shown, it is primarily the cerebral cortex which is concerned with the maintenance of consciousness. Undifferentiated, nonconscious wakefulness, on the other hand, appears to be localized in the brain stem. Wakefulness is thus translated into consciousness in the cerebral cortex. Both factors, consciousness and wakefulness, as is clearly shown in our case, are associated with phylogenetically different structures. On the basis of biochemical individuality, wakefulness and consciousness can evidently be separately interfered with. Which phylogenetically special, biochemical, structural characteristics are involved?

If we now consider the known chemoarchitectonics of the brain stem as compared with those of the neocerebral end-brain, the increase in content of "trace elements" in the brain stem immediately strikes us. The hippocampus, for example, has in some areas a relatively high zinc content, while in the midbrain, especially in the globus pallidus, the substantia nigra and the red nucleus are rich in iron, and the cerebellum shows an increased copper content. According to E. Albert (1952), the brain stem ganglia have a lower O_2 consumption than the neostriatum and the neocortical cerebral cortex, and are thus less sensitive to oxygen lack. The high iron content of the midbrain and hindbrain indicates that the respiratory enzyme content of these brain stem structures is higher. Thus, the substantia nigra has a marked cytochrome absorption spectrum. At the same time, these brain stem ganglia also contain considerable lactoflavin. The low O_2 consumption of these nuclear regions is clearly due, therefore, to the fact that even a small amount of available oxygen can be better utilized, thanks to the high concentration of respiratory enzymes (utilization), than is the case in the neocortical cerebral cortex (cortex and neostriatum).

To what extent the less generous capillary circulation of the brain stem nuclei (see Table in 3rd Mosbach Colloquium, 1952) is involved, as compared with that of the neocortical cerebral regions, either directly or indirectly in the phyloontogenetic development, together with the physiologic increase in respiratory enzymes and the iron enrichment described here, is another question. In addition to the phylogenetically determined differences, there are evidently also biochemical differences between the neocortical cerebral and cerebellar cortices, as the different vulnerability to glucose lack of the individual cortical areas shows. These different responses to glucose lack are, however, so obvious in the authors' case that further investigation seems to offer great promise.

Summary

It can thus be said that severe hypoglycemia, induced in this case by a pancreatic beta-cell adenoma, produced a special distribution of changes in the CNS, which involved preferentially the phylogenetically younger neocortical cerebral cortex and its associated neocortical nuclei, whereas the brain stem and the allocortical, phylogenetically older, cerebral and cerebellar cortical components were largely spared, and hence did not correspond to the schema of sensitivity to anoxia. With the help of reliable data from the literature, an explanation of this distribution of changes was sought on the basis of phylogenetically determined biochemical characteristics, and a concept of vulnerability of brain structures offered, in a special sense. From the viewpoint of phylogenetic brain localization this confirms certain earlier assumptions and neuropathologic localization analyses, in which "wakefulness" is associated with the anterior and middle brain stem (Orthner, 1969), while the differentiation of wakefulness to wake-"consciousness" is the property of the neocortical cerebral cortex (pallium). The apallic syndrome in its true sense thus exclusively involves the neocortical cerebral cortex via its neocortical associated nuclei, which, as the present case clearly shows, can be *biochemically* damaged in isolation by protracted hypoglycemia. The underlying phyloontogenetically determined biochemical conditions are discussed in the light of the distribution of changes in the CNS. The physiologically lower energy turnover rate in the phylogenetically older brain stem structures as compared with the neocerebral brain structures led, in our case with glucose lack (with different degrees in the various brain regions), via a reduction in energetic processes to atrophy of the ganglion cells and, in the neocerebral regions, where turnover is intensive, to necrobiosis and/or necrosis by structural breakdown. This may perhaps explain the particular distribution of CNS changes which developed in our case as a result of glucose lack—a distribution which in some ways markedly differs from that due to anoxia.

7. Apallic Syndrome in the Metabolic Diseases

L. INFUSO

Several authors have studied the neuropsychic changes referred to as "comatose conditions" which are present during different stages of metabolic diseases of various origin (hepatic, renal, diabetic, respiratory, hormonal, etc.) (Engel et al., 1944; Adams and Foley, 1953; Sherlock, 1957, 1960; Rossi, 1962). These researchers, as well as several other authors who undertook the study of coma of various origins, found it necessary to classify the neuropsychic changes with different criteria according to the degree of severity: primarily clinical (Rowbotham, 1945; Mollaret and Goulon, 1959; Bozza-Marrubini and Rossanda, 1961), clinical and electroencephalographic (Loeb and Rosadini, 1957; Rossi, 1962; Bergamini and Inghirami, 1962), primarily electroencephalographic (Fischgold and Mathis, 1959) and neurophysiologic (Jouvet, 1964).

It is easily understandable how such diverse concepts, as well as the adoption of different terminologies according to the degree of severity of the coma, have caused serious difficulties in the evaluation and comparison of the various classifications, even if each one of these, with its advantages and limitations, is very useful in the particular aspect of the problem which its authors wanted to emphasize. Being aware of the problem and carefully examining the material on hand, it was decided that in order to classify neuropsychic symptoms of dismetabolic patients in a less haphazard way, this was possible only by working out a new quantitative evaluation of the degree of neuropsychic involvement on the basis of a special diagrammatic examination (Infuso et al., 1967), including a list of 13 groups of functional parameters which have been described according to the percentage of involvement.

With this classification an attempt was made to obtain greater uniformity and precision in the evaluation of the clinical picture, as well as the possibility of quantification of the examination, within a fixed ranged of scores. By this method the various cases could be compared, their evolution in time could be followed, and finally, the degree of neuropsychic changes with the impairment of other factors (biochemical, humoral, electroencephalographic, etc.) could be more closely correlated. At the time the results of previous research on 80 cases of metabolic comas were reported, some of the most significant findings revealed by the data had already been summarized.

The author would like to especially emphasize characteristics of the neuropsychic changes found in the groups of patients, stressing the most common and constant characteristic of metabolic diseases. In the large majority of cases of hepatic, diabetic, and uremic patients, the examination revealed either an initial neuropsychic involvement or a more or less deep comatose state. A sharp and often very rapid fluctuation of neuropsychic conditions, which in some cases improved up to complete recovery, but more often deteriorated severly and sometimes irreversibly, (even within a few hours) was noted either spontaneously or, more often, after therapy.

Thus, it is believed that such instability with frequent fluctuations in the severity of involvement should be considered one of the peculiarities of metabolic coma.

Comparing metabolic neuopsychic disorders with the apallic syndrome, the following observations can be made:

1. Apallic syndrome should be considered a neuropsychic picture with progressive acute, subacute, or chronic development, caused primarily by cerebral lesions (traumatic, neoplastic, vascular, etc.), which at times are focal. Various stages of evolution are more or less clearly recognizable in the course of the disease. Some may be due to the involvement of structures located at different functional levels (cortical, subcortical, midbrain, bulbar), accompanied by a complex clinical picture.

Further, the apallic syndrome, because of its prevalent lesional etiology, often presents an irreversible evolution (about 50% of cases, according to Gerstenbrand, 1967), even though there is the possibility of functional recovery, either partial or delayed.

2. Metabolic coma appears to be a neuropsychic syndrome due to functional disorders involving the entire body, and to biochemical malfunctions that affect the entire brain in a diffuse if not homogeneous way. There is a complete unforeseeable course, with typical *poussées*, often disassociated from the evolution of the metabolic disease per se, with morbid episodes which are at times interspaced by long intervals of neuropsychic well-being.

The instability and the possibility of complete remission of the neuropsychic symptomatology thus appear conditioned by the reversibility—at least during the early stages—of the diffuse cerebral changes, without specific characteristics in the various metabolic diseases.

The above observations lead us to believe that, even though it is not easy to compare apallic syndrome and metabolic coma from an etiopathologic, anatomic-functional, and symptomatic point of view, it is possible that during the course of a metabolic disease clinical pictures may occur which, even if temporary, may be comparable to some stages of the apallic syndrome.

8. Apallic Syndrome Due to Pharmacotoxic Effects

S. KANOWSKI

Since the introduction of psychopharmacologic therapy it is known that severe psychic and neurologic side effects are found during treatment with neuroleptic and antidepressant drugs. At first, disturbances of the extrapyramidal motor system were observed, such as paroxysmal dyskinesias, a Parkinson-like picture with tremor and akinesia. Finally, persisting extrapyramidal motor disorders were described, mostly in the form of choreiform permanent hyperkinesia (Degkwitz and Luxemburger, 1965; Delay et al., 1957; Haase, 1954; Hartmann and Hippius, 1959; Uhrbrand and Faurbye, 1960). Ayd (1961) stated that nearly 40% of persons submitted to neuroleptic treatment developed such neurologic side effects. Later focal neurologic disturbances during the course of psychopharmacologic therapy were reported in case material (Helmchen and Hippius, 1962). Finally, in 1967, Bruck and Gerstenbrand described the psychopharmacotoxic apallic syndrome, in 1968 Grahmann and Reimer psycopharmacotoxic encephalopathy and in 1969 Boeters and Grahmann the development of a pharmacotoxic dementia. It should be added that purely psychopathologic deficiencies of the acute exogenous reaction types—for example, delirious and amential forms or Korsakoff-like pictures and the *Durchgangssyndrome* (Wieck, 1962)—are known (Helmchen and Hippius, 1962).

In 1967 Bruck and Gerstenbrand stated that nearly a third of the schizophrenic process psychoses treated with Mayeptil developed into a typical apallic syndrome under treatment. Mayeptil (thioproperazine) is a piperazinyl-substituted phenothiazine derivative, as its chemical structure shows. It has a strong extrapyramidal motoric and generally activating effect and was introduced into psychopharmacotherapy by Delay et al. in 1959. Those patients who developed an apallic syndrome under treatment were on a high average dose, although varying according to the individual. There was a fixed temporal correlation in the manifestation of the apallic syndrome, insofar as the apallic syndrome occurred during the third period of neuroleptic treatment (Flügel, 1954; Selbach, 1961). This is just the time after the usual appearance of a pharmacogenic parkinsonoid syndrome. Reviewing all that is known about somatic side effects of psychopharmacologic treatment, the authors believe that the apallic syndrome is the most severe form of the undesirable effects of neuroleptic therapy.

Upon first impression, the clinical picture could be described as an akinetic mutism (Cairns et al., 1941), but after detailed examination it can be distinguished from this syndrome by accessory symptoms and can clearly be recognized as a true apallic syndrome. In all essential details it corresponds to the rather frequent traumatic apallic syndrome (Gerstenbrand, 1967). A description of the clinical picture can be found in Chapter 2.

As Bruck and Gerstenbrand (1967) have stated, the apallic syndrome diminished and disappeared without exception within 2-6 weeks. The psychic functions were restored after having passed intermediately through a Korsakoff-like state.

Further information on apallic syndromes due to psychopharmacotoxic effects have not yet been published. In reviewing his cases from the beginning of psychopharmacologic therapy, the author discovered that no previous single incident of this kind existed, although Mayeptil was used from 1958 until 1960 as a test preparation in our clinic, but only in a small number of cases. Altogether, only 12 women between 19 and 62 years old (four schizophrenics, four paranoid-hallucinatory psychoses, two depressive psychoses, one atypical cyclic psychosis, and one primitive reaction with abnormal personality) were treated during the above-mentioned period with this drug. Two women showed clear symptoms of cerebral atrophy. The individual dosage of Mayeptil varied between 5 and 130 mg/day; more than half the patients received doses of 80 mg/day or more. In most cases the drug was discontinued between the 7th and 12th day of treatment. Due to side effects, only one patient was under medication longer than 40 days. According to the treatment scheme of Delay and Deniker (1961), the dosage was increased by 10 mg/day. Nearly all patients developed considerable side effects in the form of motor impulse increases, severe akathisia, tremor, and sleeplessness (Kryspin-Exner, 1963). Frequently, paroxysmal dyskinetic syndromes were seen with this drug. There was no doubt that Mayeptil had a good antipsychotic effect. None of our patients developed signs of an apallic syndrome. Only a 53-year-old woman developed psychomotoric stereotypes and a 62-year-old woman showed a transient akinetic catatonic picture.

The absence of apallic syndromes in our population could be explained by the short duration of treatment and the small number of patients treated, so that the expected frequency to be for apallic syndromes may not differ very much from zero. Besides the report of Bruck and Gerstenbrand (1967) and incidents during narcosis, we know of no drug which in the range of therapeutic doses caused the manifestation of such serious neuropsychic disorders.

As far as incidents of narcosis are concerned, they are not due to the direct influence of the narcotic drug. Secondary mechanisms leading to severe hypoxidosis–e.g., cardiac arrests–are the determining pathogenetic factors. Under toxic doses, on the contrary, the apallic syndrome is not unknown as a prefinal or transitional stage during pharmacotherapy. However, in those cases the apallic syndrome is not a question of effects of specific classes of medicaments. All chemical substances which are able to affect particularly the cerebral metabolism in a direct or indirect way can also produce an apallic syndrome (e.g., in carbon monoxide or opiate intoxications). A strongly marked coma vigile in a 47-year-old female patient during a serious lithium intoxication was observed. This patient had been treated with lithium for 2 years because of a severe manic-depressive illness, despite the fact, that she suffered from a cardiac insufficiency due to a myocardial infarction. Therefore, she had been under intermittent digitalis therapy since 1962.

During lithium therapy the lithium serum concentration varied between 0.7 and 1.1 mVal/1 serum within the therapeutic range. For an unknown reason she suddenly developed cardiac failure, and clinical treatment was necessary. Under antiedemic therapy the lithium serum concentration suddenly rose to 1.56 mVal/1 serum and 6 days later to 3.75 mVal/1 serum. During this period the patient passed through a Korsakoff-like state to a severe coma vigile, which was accompanied by the typical neurologic signs of lithium intoxication (Koufen and Consbruck, 1972; Schou, 1969): severe muscular weakness, muscular fasciculations, and severe intentional tremor. Furthermore, there was a delayed response to pain and a grasp reflex more noticeable in the right hand. The patient did not show any spontaneous reactions. Her eyes were open without fixing upon any object. She responded to orders very slowly with delay. She remained in passively produced attitudes. This clinical picture continued for the next 3 days. During this time the lithium serum concentration fell to 0.5 mVal/1 while forced diuresis and hemodialysis were performed. At this point the patient recovered rapidly. Afterwards she had a vague remembrance of the intoxication and no remaining symptoms persisted. The development of the intoxication was paralleled by severe electroencephalographic changes in the form of a general slowing and intermittent nonrhythmic activities. The electroencephalographic changes were normalized 4 weeks after the patient had fully recovered from the intoxication.

Other neuropsychic syndromes which may develop under psychopharmacotherapy and which have already been mentioned above include, besides the frequent pharmacogenic *dysphoric-depressive states, Durchgangssyndrome*, and typical *delirious forms.* For the latter we found a relative frequency of 5.8% in our population (Helmchen, 1961); patients with an amnestic-anoetic syndrome who were under psychopharmacologic therapy were seen repeatedly (Girke et al., 1971).

These syndromes bear a close resemblance to the apallic syndrome. They could be observed under neuroleptic therapy with medium and high doses and showed in most cases in addition a characteristic predominantly motor aphasia. General changes could be observed in the EEG, running parallel to the intensity of the clinical picture. These changes were paroxysmal dysrhythmias, general slowing, and focal disturbances in the dominant hemisphere. From the clinical point of view there is a striking resemblance to Alzheimer's disease.

Intermittent catatonic syndromes, partly of the febrile type preceded by depressive syndromes could also be observed under neuroleptic therapy (Mucha, 1966; Riser et al., 1958). Here it may be difficult to discriminate a pharmacogenic reaction and the manifestation of a catatonic syndrome from a schizophrenic process. In accordance with Boeters and Grahmann (1969), we saw in some patients who were under psychopharmacotherapy a persisting organic brain syndrome following an acute exogenic reaction type. Helmchen (1961) has suggested that this organic brain syndrome is precipitated out of latency by psychopharmacotherapy (Girke et al., 1971).

Regarding the neuropsychiatric side effects of psychopharmacotherapy as described above, the following three main questions can be asked:

1. What are the neurophysiolgic structures responsible for the different neuropsychic disorders provoked by psychopharmacotherapy?
2. Do any correlations exist between the different forms of these syndromes?
3. What are the determining factors responsible for individual forms of decompensation under psychopharmacotherapy?

Question 1: As far as we know, neuroleptic and antidepressant drugs affect mainly parts of the brain stem to varying extents. The spectrum of their desired and undesired effects with influence on vegetative, motor, and psychic functions can be summed up by the *Hirnstamm-Trias* of Reichardt (1944) or the *hirnlokales Psychosyndrom* of Bleuler (1969). The electroencephalographic changes under psychopharmacotherapy, extending from paroxysmal dysrhythmias and abnormal rhythms to provocation of SW complexes, as well as changes in vigilance, support the hypothesis that these drugs act at the brain stem level (Bente, 1964; Helmchen and Künkel, 1964). Therefore, the author agrees with Gerstenbrand (1967), who carefully proved that the pharmacotoxic apallic syndrome is most likely a functional decerebration which results from the interruption of the activating reticular brain stem system.

Question 2: The author believes that a relationship exists between the apallic syndrome and the amnestic-anoetic syndrome on the one hand, and the akinetic-abulic syndrome and the catatonic one on the other hand (Liebaldt and Scheller, 1971; Girke et al., 1971). This is supported firstly by Gerstenbrand (1967), who observed that the traumatic apallic syndrome frequently disappears after having passed an amnestic-anoetic (Korsakoff-like) interval, and secondly by the fact that the traumatic apallic syndrome may be preceded by an akinetic-mutistic phase. Furthermore, the pharmacogenic delirious states are also to be considered as consequences of functional disturbances in the brain stem area. As Helmchen (1961) pointed out, this is proven by close temporal relationships between the psychic symptoms and the manifestation of extrapyramidal motor and vegetative signs. The provocation of delirious syndromes by the combination of psychopharmaceutic preparations and other drugs affecting the brain stem system—e.g., antiparkinsonian drugs—gives further support to this assumption. Finally, in some cases of delirious decompensation under psychopharmacotherapy, atrophic processes in the area of the brain stem ganglias could be demonstrated by pneumencephalography. Similar reflections are valid for the catatonic *Durchgangs-Syndrom* and for the pharmacotoxic encephalopathies and dementias as described by Boeters and Grahmann (1969) and Grahmann and Reimer (1968).

Question 3: Individual cerebral dispositions, the quality of the specific drug, or the interactions of different drugs in the case of combined treatment, as well as the absolute level and gradient of the dose regimen, are the important factors in deciding whether neuropsychic disturbances develop under psychopharmacotherapy and what kind of syndrome will be produced individually. These factors play a definite role in the provocation of extrapyramidal motor, delirious, and amnestic disturbances (Ayd, 1961; Helmchen, 1961; Myrianthopolous et al., 1962). There is nothing so far in the literature connecting them to the apallic syndrome. However, since two-thirds of patients treated with Mayeptil in the Vienna clinic did not develop any apallic syndrome, individual factors in those patients developing this therapeutic complication must be taken into account.

Not much is known about the biochemical interactions between psychopharmacologic drugs and cerebral substrates. It seems, however, that psychopharmaceuticals may have a direct effect upon ganglia cells by interfering with their metabolism, or an indirect effect by changing their membrane permeability or by decreasing cerebral blood flow (Himwich, 1960; Quadbeck and Sachsse, 1961). The latter may be responsible for the provocation of focal neurologic attacks. Whether or not the biochemically induced changes remain at the therapeutic level and do not cause pharmacogenic neuropsychic disturbances up to the apallic syndrome is probably determined by preexisting, often latent cerebral defects which cannot be established by routine clinical investigation.

Summary: The pharmacotoxic apallic syndrome under psychopharmacotherapy in therapeutic doses, as far as we know, has only been seen during treatment with Mayeptil. This therapeutic complication may be the result of a functional blocking of the activating impulses coming up through the reticular formation in the brain stem. A relationship exists between the apallic syndrome and other neuropsychic disturbances provoked by psychopharmacotherapy. This view is supported by taking into account the transition from one picture to another, the determining factors of the individual reaction, and the cerebral structures which are probably responsible for this kind of neuropsychic decompensation under pharmacotherapy. For those syndromes not only characterized by focal attacks, specific systems of the brain stem—perhaps different for each of the clinical pictures—must be assumed to be the locus of the pharmacogenically induced functional disturbances (Liebaldt and Scheller, 1971).

9. Courses of Protracted States of Coma*

H.H. WIECK, R. RETTELBACH, B. HEERKLOTZ, and K.A. FLÜGEL

Introduction

The following study is an investigation of the semeiologic position of protracted stages of coma within the *Funktionspsychosen* (functional psychoses). Apart from numerous single case observations made possible by a hospital that is concerned with the admission of patients with *severe cerebral disorders* of various origin, the syndrome analysis presented here is based upon 100 cases of severe cerebral contusion and 141 cases of hypnotic intoxications, the courses of which have been studied systematically.

In 1956 we divided the *körperlich begründbare Psychosen*, defined by Kurt Schneider (1967) (i.e., organic psychoses) into irreversible and reversible syndromes (Wieck, 1956). In order to have a simple term at our disposal, the reversible syndromes were called *Funktionspsychosen* (Wieck, 1967/1).

Function Psychoses

Severity of Functional Psychosis: In progressive general disturbance of brain function, the functional psychosis begins with the *mild* transit syndrome (*Durchgangs-Syndrom*) and develops via the moderate and severe transit syndromes and via clouding of consciousness into the state of unconsciousness.

The severity of the psychosis may be determined by observing the clinical picture. A greater degree of accuracy can be achieved with the aid of psychopathometric techniques (Böcker, 1961; Böcker and Kinzel, 1969). Suitable for this purpose are syndrome tests (Böcker, 1961; Böcker and Kinzel, 1969; Wieck and Stäcker, 1964), which not only deal with disturbances of individual psychic functions but also determine the degree of severity of the syndrome as a whole.

The term "transit syndrome" has continued to gain ground in the past few years. Gerstenbrand (1967) describes in the course of remission of apallic syndromes transit syndromes that are free of defects or lead to a mild degree of deficiency. The term transit syndrome, however, is not always used to describe the state between the normal condition and the clouding of consciousness. Because the functional psychosis must pass through this state, the term "transit" syndrome was originally chosen. Thus, an unconscious person is *not* in

* This paper does not correspond in its main parts with the terminology used elsewhere in this book. The editors, however, feel that it contains many interesting aspects and thus have chosen to include it.

a state of transit syndrome. Some authors occasionally also call transitory disorders in endogenous psychosis transit syndromes. The term is used here in the sense of exclusively reversible syndromes of organic psychoses.

The *semeiology of the clinical picture* is influenced to a great extent, but not exclusively, by the degree of the basic disturbance. Thus, the severe transit syndrome usually appears as an amnestic-confabulatory syndrome or Korsakoff's psychosis. Behind the picture of a "chronic brain syndrome" often a moderate or severe transit syndrome is hidden.

Relation to the Underlying Pathologic Process: In exogenous intoxications—especially those caused by barbiturates—the course of the disorders of cerebral function can be followed precisely, because the process determining syndrome dynamics can be determined quantitatively by means of the barbiturate blood level, as has been shown in previous studies (Penin, 1970; Peters, 1970; Rix, 1967; Tönnis et al., 1968).

With the decrease in the barbiturate blood level, which is demonstrated in the lower diagram of Figure 1, the disturbances of individual psychic functions also decline, as the

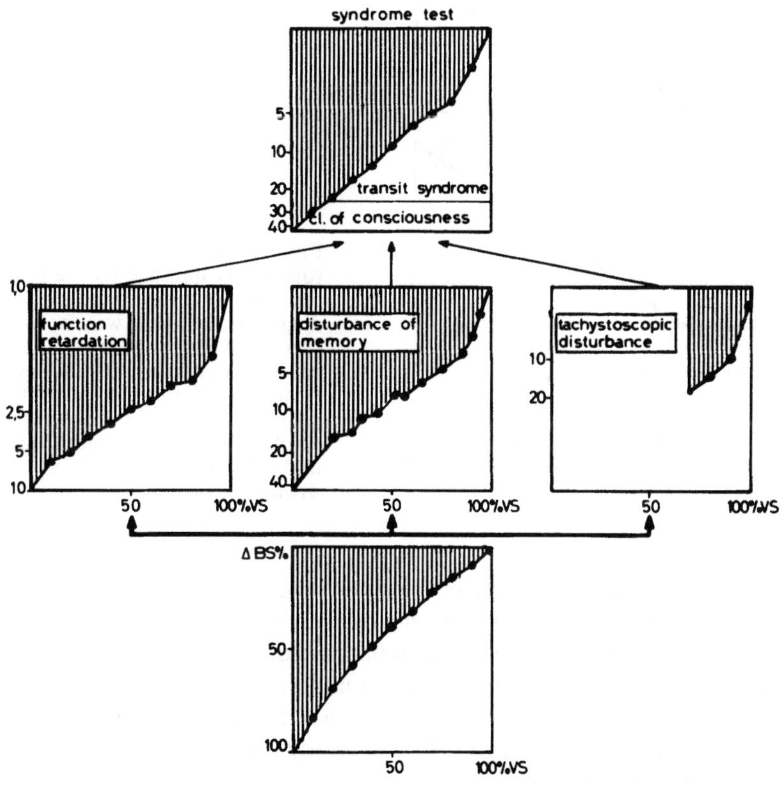

Fig. 1. Functional psychoses in barbiturate intoxication. Mean value of 23 cases. Similar courses in 118 other cases. Abscissa: Based on 100 standardized courses (100% VS) from begin of clouding of consciousness up to the end of the transit syndrome in decreasing barbiturate intoxications. Ordinate of upper and middle diagram: Logarithmic partial results of syndrome test. Ordinate of lower diagram: difference of barbiturate blood level in percent (Δ BS %). Lower diagram: course of barbiturate blood level (indication of syndrome dynamics). Middle diagram: course of test results concerning some individual psychic functions. Upper diagram: course of total syndrome

middle diagram illustrates. Due to the uniformity of the course, the term "homogeneous syndrome dynamics" (*homogene Syndromdynamik*) is applied. There is a significant correlation between the severity of functional psychosis and the somatic process determining the syndrome genesis (Wieck et al., 1962).

In the case of singular events–such as traumatic brain lesions, acute cerebral hypoxidosis, or acute inflammatory processes–the cerebral process determining syndrome genesis cannot yet be traced quantitatively. Its severity must be deduced from the clinical appearance with its resulting difficulties. In brain contusion the primary etiologic somatic process lasts only a fraction of a second. The pressure wave passing through the brain tissue, however, leaves behind a residue of the disturbance, which after a certain period of latency (recovery latency) gradually disappears (recovery time).

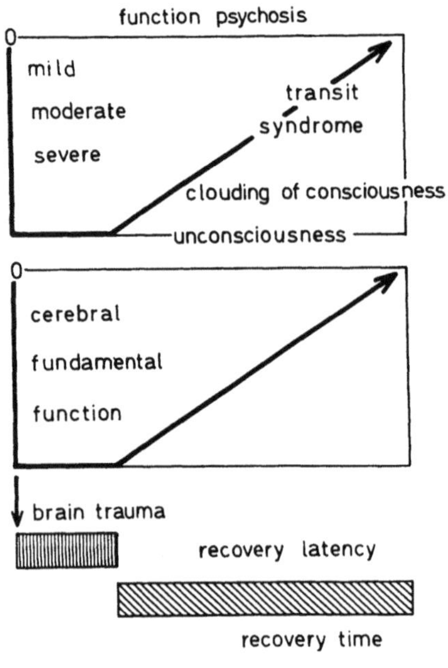

Fig. 2. Functional psychoses after brain contusion. By damage to the brain an immediate blockage of fundamental function (lower diagram), in other words, unconsciousness (upper diagram) results. Latter diagram indicates recovery latency. Recovery time extends from end of unconsciousness to the complete passing away of functional psychoses. It extends over stages of clouding of consciousness and of severe, moderate and mild transit syndromes

In these cases the severity of the lesion manifests itself–if it is to be determined by clinical means–in the duration of the recovery latency and recovery time. Recovery latency is indicated by the duration of unconsciousness. Those cases in which unconsciousness has lasted for 2 days or more are considered the most severe forms of brain damage (Frowein et al., 1968). This was the case in 426 out of 1802 patients with traumatic brain lesions. Of these 426 patients, 294 (i.e., nearly 70%) died. Of the 132 surviving patients 100 were reinvestigated.

Neuropsychiatric Symptoms of Comatose States

Unconsciousness in the Course of Functional Psychosis and Sleep: With the state of unconsciousness, the functional psychosis has reached its extreme end. There is no "deep"

unconsciousness, for a patient cannot be more than just unconscious. There are, however, various stages of sleep depth. As sleep and pathologic sleepiness are basically different from functional psychosis in respect to syndrome genesis (Wieck, 1956, 1967/2), it is not correct to transfer the concept of depth, which is valid for sleep, to consciousness.

Neurologic Symptoms of Coma: When the underlying cerebral process proceeds above unconsciousness, it causes the level of cerebrosomatic reactions to deteriorate (Frowein, 1963). The activity of reflexes and the central regulations are especially restricted and finally disappear.

While functional psychoses from the mild transit syndrome up to unconsciousness are purely psychiatric syndromes, coma must be regarded as a neuropsychiatric phenomenon, in which unconsciousness is combined with the neurologic symptoms of coma. In spite of this combination both types of syndromes—psychoses and neurologic symptoms—should be strictly separated. This separation should also be applied when single symptoms are checked. Since the patient is unconscious, he can no longer demonstrate any emotional reactions. It is, therefore, unnecessary to particularly accentuate the loss of emotional functions in coma, as is sometimes done.

Grade of Severity of Coma: Thus, the quantitative estimation of the state of coma can only be carried out in terms of neurologic criteria. A number of investigations are available to gain useful dimensions (Infuso, 1970; Lücking, 1970a). Our team of co-workers has been concerned with the quantitative determination of the borderline state between clouding of consciousness and unconsciousness. This state is called "borderline syndrome" (Rix, 1967).

Underlying Pathologic Process: The neurologic symptoms of coma after traumatic brain lesions are most frequently caused by complications (Hassler et al., 1969b; Peters, 1970). These complications must be discriminated from the remaining traces of the disturbance which is directly caused by damage to the brain. The pathodynamics of complications are independent and have to be especially taken into account during the recovery phase. Moreover, it must be taken into consideration that the neurologic symptoms of coma differ from the neurologic signs, which in cerebral lesions are caused by *local* peculiarities, such as hemiparesis, which is due to a corresponding cortical contusion focus. These are *supplementary* neurologic symptoms, which can also exist together with milder degrees of functional psychosis.

Apallic Syndrome

Disappearance of Neurologic Symptoms of Coma: Frequently, the neurologic symptoms of coma, which are expressions of a *reduction* of reflex activity and central regulatory functions, disappear without intermediate states.

Symptoms of the Full Apallic Syndrome: In the *apallic state* some neurologic functions recover, which is in contrast to that type of coma which is determined only by a reduction of functions. The patient remains unconscious. However, all other signs of the full apallic syndrome, which Gerstenbrand (1967) has described, are clearly neurologic criteria, especially those concerning reflex activity, motor system, and sleep-waking cycle. To these may be added, for instance, the reflectory primitive movements, the postural abnormalities, and the primitive motor automatisms. The clinical picture is mainly characterized by the functioning of the sleep-waking system (Gerstenbrand, 1967; Kretschmer, 1940). This functioning can, however, manifest itself only in the form of external appearance, such as keeping the eyes open and coordinated eye movements. Furthermore, an arousal effect can be demonstrated in EEG and behavior (Hassler, 1970). The impression of "wakefulness" (coma vigile) should, however, not blind one to the fact that the patient is unconscious. Thus, it is meaningless to speak of a "particular" type of unconsciousness, as is sometimes the case (Peters, 1970). The allegory of the "stage" of consciousness, as Jaspers (1959) expressed it, cannot explain the situation. For if one is in accord with this allegory, it must also follow that in unconsiousness, with the disappearance of its content the stage itself also disappears.

Recovery from the Apallic Syndrome: The recovery latency is very variable in respect to the diverse individual cerebral functions. For instance, the sleep-waking system obviously has a shorter latency than the "fundamental function," the disturbance of which causes functional psychosis (Wieck, 1967a, b). Only in this way can coma vigile result. When the underlying cerebral process improves, the barrier of unconsciousness is overcome.

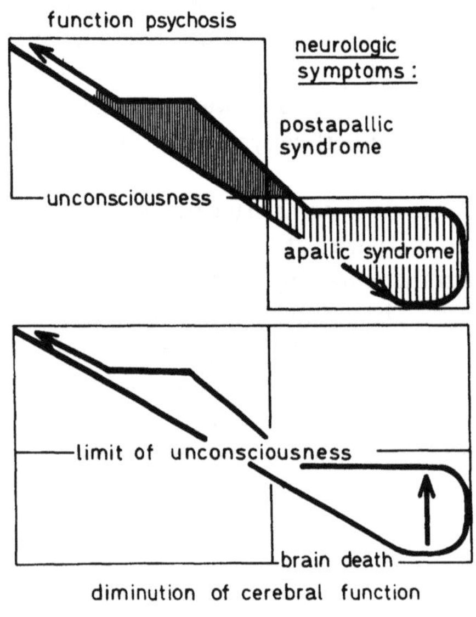

Fig. 3. Apallic symptoms. In protracted states of coma, recovery latency of some neurologic functions is reached (arrow pointing upwards in lower diagram). This resulting in apallic syndrome (upper diagram). In the course of recovery the postapallic syndrome develops and accompanies the involution of functional psychoses

The patient is then no longer unconscious, but has severe clouding of consciousness. In this phase, in addition to neurologic improvement, psychiatric recovery, which manifests itself in regressions of functional psychosis, is initiated. The states of remission following the apallic syndrome have been given different terms (Gerstenbrand, 1967). Whether one should speak of "apallic" or of "postapallic" syndrome is a matter of choice. It is, however, important to note that the neurologic symptoms are responsible for the particular appearance of the clinical picture.

The functional psychosis, on the other hand, passes through the same states as in every other kind of cerebral process. Long before attention was given to the full picture of apallic syndrome, the various modes of action in functional psychosis were observed, and not only the variations of semeiotic appearance but especially the quantitative reduction were investigated (Böcker, 1961; Böcker and Kinzel, 1969; Frowein et al., 1968; Kinzel, 1971; Rix, 1967; Wieck, 1967b; Wieck, in press; Wieck et al., 1962; Wieck and Stäcker, 1964). If patients with postapallic functional psychosis are tested, gradual improvement can be recognized in the psychopathometric results. Clouding of consciousness is followed by the severe transit syndrome, which gradually changes to moderate and mild forms. The recovery time, which continues until functional psychosis has disappeared, lasts, according to the experiences of numerous authors, generally up to 2 years. In about 10% of the observed cases the recovery time required 3 years and occasionally even 4 years (Frowein et al., 1968).

The semeiotic appearance of the clinical picture, in spite of homogeneous syndrome dynamics, varies to quite an extent. An example is the transit syndrome with depressive or paranoid character (Wieck, 1967b). Which factors are responsible for the semeiotic features cannot be determined with certainty. The underlying pathologic process was often blamed. Therefore, the question arises whether the recovery from traumatic apallic syndrome shows any clinical peculiarities that cannot be applied to the neurologic symptoms, including aphasia, apraxia, and agnosia. It is remarkable that in the postapallic state disturbances of drive prevail, so that aspontaneity characterizes the clinical picture, as many authors have pointed out and the authors' experiences have confirmed.

Syndromes of Psychic Deficiency

Brain Death: The underlying cerebral process may lead to the loss of all cerebral functions resulting in brain death, as the lower diagram of Figure 4 illustrates.

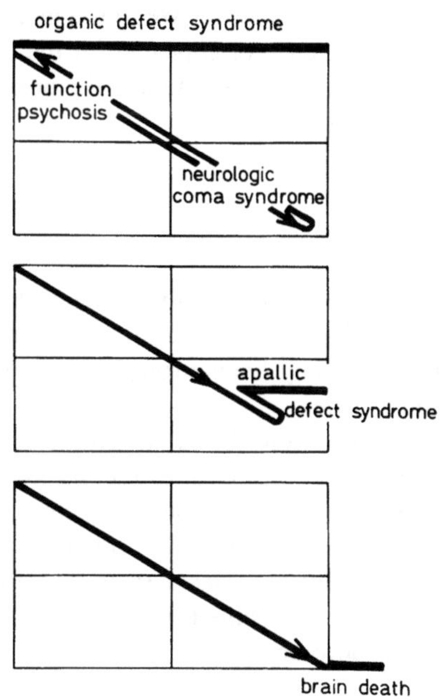

Fig. 4. Defect syndrome and brain death

Apallic Defect Syndrome: This occurs when the brain stem regains the functions which determine the clinical symptoms, but the fundamental function remains irreversibly damaged. The dimension of mentality is thereby lost altogether. The patient is, therefore, not only an unconscious but also without any psychic functions (middle diagram of Fig. 4).

From the beginning the apallic defect syndrome must be distinguished from brain death (Penin, 1970).

Organic Defect Syndrome in the Psychic Field: Only when the functional psychosis has completely passed the organic defect syndrome can be accurately determined. A psychopathometric defect test has been developed by Kinzel (1971). In the foreground are alterations of personality, since intellectual deterioration is not as apparent. A predominant feature of the organic personality alterations has been the previously observed loss of initiative (Wieck, 1956), a fact early investigators have repeatedly stressed. The loss of initiative can be seen in defect syndromes of *different* origin. It is by no means specific for the postapallic defect syndrome.

Of 100 patients with traumatic brain lesions we were able to study 38 psychopathometrically with the defect test (Frowein et al., 1968; Kinzel, 1971). As expected, a high degree of correlation was found between the severity of organic defect and the degree of inability to work. Two patients had no alterations in personality and were able to perform their work. On the other hand, 11 persons with very severe personality defects were either completely or almost completely incapable of working. Moreover, it was obvious that the duration of unconsciousness significantly correlated with the severity of the personality defect. There were some special peculiarities with respect to age. The older the patients, the more severe was the defect syndrome, when persons with equal duration of unconsciousness were compared. Our investigations show that the therapeutic management in the initial stage of brain lesion is prognostically important (Frowein, 1963; Frowein et al., 1968; Tönnis et al., 1968). Apart from the psychic defect syndrome, the neurologic permanent symptoms must also be considered. We found neurologic defects in 39 patients, while in 21 patients epilepsy worsened or appeared for the first time. In these cases paroxysmal functional psychoses, which may simulate the organic personality defect, must be taken into account.

Summary

The semeiotic position of protracted states of coma in their relationship to functional psychoses has been investigated. In coma the patient is unconscious. The clinical appearance is determined by the neurologic symptoms. This is also true in the full apallic syndrome and in coma vigile.

Recovery from the full apallic syndrome takes place via the various degrees of functional psychosis, i.e., via clouding of consciousness, severe, moderate, and finally, mild transit syndrome. In this respect, the postapallic type does not differ from other functional psychoses. However, the remission of postapallic functional psychosis extends over a long period of time. Furthermore, special semeiotic types of appearance must be considered. Apart from the basically reversible functional psychoses, attention must be drawn to the irreversible defect syndromes.

10. Apallic Syndrome in Diseases of the Cerebral White Matter

H.J. LEHMANN

Apallic syndromes after acute cerebral lesions, e.g., severe cerebral trauma and acute cerebral anoxia, are well-known conditions that have been much discussed in recent years. In acute cerebral anoxia there is primarily some damage to the cerebral cortex (Ingvar and Brun, 1972). Due to this general lesion, an apallic syndrome–in the literal sense, a "demantling" of the brain–develops. In the traumatic apallic syndrome, the compression of the midbrain with its consequences, besides edema of the white matter, contributes materially to the development of the apallic syndrome. Such clinical pictures, occurring dramatically after acute lesions of the cerebral cortex or parts of the brain stem, have diverted attention from the fact that a disconnection of the primarily intact cerebral cortex from the primarily intact brain stem structures may also lead to similar conditions.

Destruction or functional blockage of the subcortical myelin layer is found above all in the final stages of so-called demyelinating diseases. Frequently, the cortico-subcortical connection is anatomically still maintained. The axis cylinders of the nerve fibers are preserved, but the fibers become functionally inefficient because proper impulse conduction is no longer possible owing to loss of the myelin sheath. Disconnection of the cerebral cortex from the brain stem is a known result in diseases of the white matter, for example, in the diffuse form of multiple sclerosis (Ule et al., 1965), in metachromatic leukodystrophy (Grahmann et al., 1969), and in subacute sclerosing leukencephalitis (Lehmann and Ule, 1964).

The blockage in cerebral white matter diseases often starts insidiously and can be demonstrated only experimentally at first (Lehmann and Gloeckner, 1972). Increasing disturbances in the association systems characterize the progression. With advancing disease frequent focal disturbances develop, as well as disturbances of recognition and action with initially still satisfactory affective resonance (Ule et al., 1965). With increasing paralysis a progressive indifference and a loss of drive develops, leading finally to an apallic syndrome. Similar events were reported in leukodystrophy by van Bogaert and Scholz (1932) and others. They occurred in patients who came from families with a history of metachromatic leukodystrophy and who were under the author's observation during the later stages of the disease (Grahmann et al., 1969). The events in this disease leading to an apallic syndrome were also described by Born and Binder (1962).

In the hereditary-degenerative diseases of the myelin sheaths the decerebration rigidity–usually more marked in apallic syndromes–is often less obvious. In leukodystrophy this is particularly striking in adults, less so in children and adolescents. This is because the demyelination in a protracted course also affects the peripheral nerve fibers and especially the posterior roots. As in posterior column diseases, spastic toe signs may be present, but increased proprioceptive reflex and increased tonus are absent.

In inflammatory diseases of the cerebral white matter, on the other hand, the decerebration rigidity becomes obvious early. Observations by the author of apallic syndromes in the final stage of subacute sclerosing encephalitis (see also Rabe et al., 1971), as well as in the diffuse form of multiple sclerosis (Ule et al., 1965), increased tonus in the extremities occurred even before the development of the actual apallic syndrome.

The clinical courses of demyelinating diseases ending in an apallic syndrome have a common onset with indefinite focal disturbances and an increasing loss of cerebral functions down to the level of the midbrain, parallel to progressive white matter destruction. The final stage corresponds to the well-known picture of the apallic syndrome, with an inability to recognize and to act, absence of affective resonance, decerebration rigidity in cases with intact peripheral innervation, and appearance of primitive motor manifestations in the form of so-called early deep reflexes and aimless general movements. There are coarse oscillations of the bulbi; the sleep-and-waking rhythm is automatized and independent of the time of day. Autonomous disturbances of central origin with hyperthermia and profuse sweating are regularly present.

In the apallic syndrome the primary lesion may be localized in different structures, such as the cerebral cortex, cerebral white matter, or oral brain stem. The clinical syndrome results from a lesion in the same functional system on different organization levels. For a number of inflammatory and degenerative cerebral demyelinating diseases, the apallic syndrome is, in a way, the common final stretch which is reached when the pallium is functionally completely disconnected from the brain stem structures by destruction of the subcortical white matter.

11. Psychopathology of the Apallic Syndrome

U.H. PETERS

It seems only natural that there should be a psychopathologic side to the apallic syndrome. However, studies published on this aspect of the subject are scarce.

Full Stage of the Apallic Syndrome

The psychopathologic side of the full stage of the apallic syndrome is rather inconspicuous. The problems center on concepts of consciousness, and it is in this respect that the apallic syndrome (or more specifically, the coma vigile in the apallic syndrome) offers a fascinating ground for discussion. Bailey (1955), for example, in his study on the importance of the brain stem and cortex in the generation of consciousness, illustrates his findings with a single case, an apallic syndrome. What is particularly revealing in Bailey's study is that at that time he did not recognize the apallic syndrome as being a separate clinical entity. It is obvious that his attention was directly stimulated by the clinical picture of the apallic syndrome which he called akinetic mutism and which was caused by an operation on the thyroid gland. According to Bailey's description, it is mainly the cortex which is responsible for the generation consciousness. However, as in the case of a radio or television tube which can only function when heated, in order to be able to generate object content in consciousness the cortex needs the warming and wakening stimuli of the reticular activating system. Bailey then introduced this metaphor: man's consciousness without cortex leads an existence as meager as the shadows in Hades; i.e., consciousness exists but in the form of shapes without life.

Noetic object content of consciousness, however, is not the only concern. During the coma vigile emotions cannot be stirred. This is a very important point, since we know from the psychopathology of severe somatopsychic disturbances that an emotional response can be established relatively easily. The first appearance of emotions may also indicate the end of a coma vigile.

One of the basic concepts of consciousness which is part of the metaphor of the shadows in Hades has to be rectified because of knowledge gained during study of the apallic syndrome. It is the concept that consciousness is only characterized by its object content. One may object to the observations made on the apallic syndrome, as they can only apply in a limited way to the theory of consciousness since the patients cannot report anything experienced while in that state. As for the evaluation of consciousness in cases of clouded consciousness, sopor, coma, and twilight state, only objective observations are possible. When the apallic patient is in the coma vigile, unable to focus on an object, exhibiting no intellectual or emotional activity, but having definite waking and sleeping periods, the following conclusion seems to be justified: an alert and bright consciousness does in fact exist, and as there can be maximum alertness, it is possible to say "graduated" consciousness is intact. It is not, however, filled and animated by object content. This condition may be illustrated by means of the *Bewußtseinsbühne* (theatrical stage of consciousness), an image which has already been used by Jaspers (1959), and later by Weber and Jung (1940). In the state of coma vigile the stage of consciousness is brightly lit, the curtain is open, but the stage as well as the auditorium are empty and there is no sign of life backstage. This comparison can be used also for the different remission phases: the first movement in the props or the appearance of an actor on stage may be likened to the moment when for the first time consciousness is animated by object content and the coma vigile ends.

A further fundamental observation should be made at this point. In another section of this book is a description of how the development of the apallic syndrome may come to a halt in any of its phases. However, this applies not only to the phases but also to the separate psychopathologic phenomena. Remission (or further development) of a single phenomenon may stop at any moment, whereas the remission of another phenomenon may still go on. In addition, each pathologic phenomenon may, during the process of remission, disappear completely or leave some kind of defect.

The phenomenon of consciousness devoid of object content can still be observed in the late and even the latest phases of development. Also noticeable in the late phases is the fact that again and again the patients can sit motionless for long periods of time, as if in deep thought, and yet during those periods do not experience any object content in consciousness. Since this state is closely connected with impulse, a more detailed example will be given below. Even with patients who have seemingly fully recovered, one occasionally hears reports from relatives that many years after the apallic syndrome the patient (often a child) will "stare in front of him" or "daydream for hours on end." If asked, the patient will always say that he had "not been dreaming of anything" or "had not been thinking about anything."

Remission Phases

The psychopathologic aspects of the apallic syndrome offer a much more varied picture than the coma vigile, making the introduction of definite outlines considerably more difficult. This is also apparent in previous attempts to study this problem. While the author was a member of the hospital staff in Kiel, he began studying the psychopathology of the apallic syndrome in the remission phases in 1959 when Döhner and Ule first drew attention to the problems. Some of the first cases have already been followed for 13 years. There are a few studies in which observations have been recorded on the same patients. Besides Döhner and Ule, the following are taking part in these studies: Störring, Lehmann, Laux, Hauss, Boeters, Bues and Bredow. However, a larger and really complete study on the apallic syndrome has yet to appear. In 1961 Döhner announced the attempt at a psychopathologic analysis which has not yet materialized, as is also the case with the psychiatric investigation announced by Sauter in 1965. Even though Gerstenbrand (1967) has included many psychiatric investigations in his monograph, there is practically no work in existence, with the exception of a study on impulses by Boeters (1969), which deals exclusively with psychopathologic problems.

The question arises whether all those attempts to describe psychologically a remission or a "terminal syndrome" have not failed because of an inherent problem within the subject itself. When visiting another psychiatric hospital, one can almost always spot a patient who either has or has had an apallic syndrome. It appears that there is something like a "syndrome of the remission phases" that can be described as psychopathologic and which the author prefers to term "postapallic syndrome." Yet in trying to more accurately define the syndrome its outlines become more and more indistinguishable. Whenever one draws up a concept which includes all previous observations, and a new case arrives at the hospital with which one would like to prove the idea, a completely new aspect appears. Following is a description of some psychopathologic aspects of the postapallic syndrome, but allowances will have to be made for the fact that there are no definite boundaries; however, certain outlines can be drawn that are worth pursuing. One point must be given special emphasis: the pictures as they appear in the remission phases of the apallic syndrome are not identical to the common posttraumatic pictures or those caused by organic brain disease, although the individual phenomena are all familiar from the psychopathology of somatopsychic diseases. The expression "organic dementia" has been used occasionally in the literature, but it does not exactly describe the situation. Finally, the expression "anoëtic syndrome" (Duensing, 1949) is sometimes used to describe the psychopathologic remission phases—for example, by Hubach and Poeck (1964) and occasionally in the study group in Kiel by Ule et al. (1965). But there are technical and linguistic-etymologic objections to this usage. The anoëtic syndrome has only certain similarities with the clinical picture following the apallic syndrome and is not at all identical to it—a fact already pointed out by Duensing in 1949. In addition, this expression leads to the faulty assumption that only the intellectual powers are disturbed. The expression "anoëtic" is used, furthermore, in French psychiatry with two different meanings which were not recognized by Duensing. In that context, anoëtic means lack of understanding of object content, that is, a state in which the world is perceived by the senses but cannot be understood. In spite of certain similarities, this description does not apply to the coma vigile, nor to the later remission phases of the apallic syndrome.

Impulsion

One common disturbance seems to appear almost regularly in all patients: disturbance of impulses. It is referred to as "aspontaneity" and "lack of initiative" in one of the earliest descriptions of the late apallic syndrome by Möllmann (1940), which of course was not recognized as such at that time. In almost all casuistic reports of a later date, disturbances of impulsion are mentioned in a few words such as "aspontaneous" or "without interest." Boeters (1969) defined the problem clearly and noted three degrees of severity:

1. *Severe defect* in which spontaneous impulse and response to outside stimulation are severely disturbed.

2. *Medium defect* in which self-impulsion has been lost but outside impulsion has been retained. Response to outside stimulation might possibly be excessive.

3. *Slight defect* in which impulse and spontaneity are diminished.

Furthermore, Boeters showed that in the early remission phases the diencephalic disturbances of impulsion play a larger part, whereas in the later phases it is the frontal disturbances which make the greater contribution.

Following is an example of a medium defect (loss of self-impulsion, excessive response to outside stimulation):

Two years after the accident, a female patient is hardly different from the other patients; she laughs, jokes, and immediately answers every question. It even seems as if she were totally at the mercy of all outside stimulation, since she reacts to everything. In the examination room she still answers every question promptly. But when left to herself without any questions, in other words, without outside stimulation, she will just sit there—motionless. She will take no notice of the doctor writing at his desk, nor of her surroundings. The unprejudiced observer might think that she is absorbed in her own thoughts, perhaps daydreaming, because that would be the behavior of a healthy person in a similar situation or position. But it is more likely that the patient's imagination is void and that no emotions are present. Even after the patient has been allowed to wait for quite a while, she will not show any signs of impatience or boredom. If she is asked "What have you been thinking all that time? " she will quickly answer, "Nothing." It is obvious that her train of thought has not been interrupted. The phase of recalling, known in healthy persons, is also missing. This example also gives proof of the familiar psychiatric assumption of how much the process of thinking (not in its object content) depends on impulsion. As soon as the general impulse ceases, the specific impulse for thinking will also disappear and consciousness can become completely devoid of object content, if consciousness can at all be evaluated.

This "apallic relapse" can be observed quite often during the late phases many years after the initial full stage and in otherwise fully rehabilitated cases, although maybe not in as obvious a form as in the case just described. Parents or other members of the family may report that the patient can sit for hours staring in front of him, but he will always deny having been daydreaming. In two such cases, the patients were even referred to the hospital, their condition being tentatively diagnosed as psychomotor seizure, which was clearly disproved by description, observation, and EEG. The observation of impulsion is of great importance in the prognosis and therapy. Even in the early remission phases the exercise of all remaining abilities depends largely on sufficient response to outside stimulation. It is of the greatest importance that in the later remission phases all attempts to elicit a response to outside stimulation be constantly made. We have experienced that patients who had made very good progress in an environment geared to rehabilitation lost already-recovered abilities because of a lack of outside stimulation when sent home or transferred to an institution with custodial character. In severe cases, the loss of spontaneous impulsion, in spite of retention of the response to outside stimulation, may result in the patients' succumbing quickly to infections and other intercurrent diseases as soon as the possibilities for stimulation are not used. The question of what is to be done to further impulsion is particularly important in the case of children and adolescents. Cases have been reported in which the patients can be rehabilitated to a very high degree and show an almost unnoticeable defect in intellectual powers. Upon reexamining children who during the first years after the apallic syndrome showed a tendency towards excessive impulsion in accordance with the Kramer-Pollnow syndrome, it was found that a decrease in spontaneous impulsion became noticeable only at the onset of puberty. In these cases, too, the social prognosis is mainly determined by what is done to further impulsion.

Disturbances of Affectivity

As soon as affects appear after the coma vigile has subsided they initially follow a simple pattern. An euphoric joyful mood is predominant, which is triggered by the slightest occasion and which may be expressed in a rough-sounding, recurring, unusually strong laughter not at all differentiated by facial expressions or gesticulation. This kind of behavior, which was also mentioned by Gerstenbrand (1967) and which is distinctly different from the normal organic euphoria, contributes largely to the picture of a "typical" postapallic state. But there is also an opposite mood, which is expressed by many patients, and that is a sham rage behavior. Unpleasant stimuli such as painful procedures performed upon the patient by the doctor or a nurse may result in a shrill, uninhibited screaming and defense movements. The affect is accompanied by vegetative signs such as flushing in the face and upper part of the body, etc. Both emotional states–euphoria and sham rage–are stimuli for motions. Only one or the other may occur in a patient, or both emotional states may be expressed rapidly alternating; anger, for example, may change abruptly to loud laughter. These affective disturbances are also very important in the later remission phases. The fact that euphoric laughter occurs so easily can have a favorable effect upon the family or nursing staff, since it is communicative. Sham range, however, can continue to exist in a somewhat changed manner in otherwise well rehabilitated patients, especially in children and adolescents. These patients break into "fits of rage" for very insignificant reasons. In the case of an otherwise well recuperated 12-year-old girl, the parents reported that the child would break into an "animalistic, inhuman scream of rage" whenever she had to do her homework immediately after lunch or whenever her sister would not immediately give her an eraser upon demand. During such "fits" the patients are "completely beside themselves" and "irrational"; they cannot be calmed by soothing words or punishment. When this outburst has disappeared, after only a few minutes, the patients are completely exhausted. This behavior can lead to very unpleasant social disturbances, since it is not usually treated as pathologic but as rudeness. The patients are often asked to apologize and promise not to do it again, although such a promise cannot be kept.

The first verbal utterances–also closely connected to the affects–are usually expressed in a very undifferentiated manner. "Ouch," "go away," and "leave me alone" may be uttered in anger; "darling" or "come here" when happy. We can see here the relation of the comments on impulsion, and it brings to mind the fact that affect has always been considered a stimulation leading to increased impulsion. It follows that even pathologic affects can be useful in therapy.

In most patients, emotions of anger or joy do not appear spontaneously but occur only as a reaction to stimuli from the environment, as was shown in the brief examples above (a relationship exists between impulse and outside stimulation). The reactions to such stimuli are without any shading or nuances; the emotional behavior is fully expressed at once. We can therefore speak of an emotional hyperpathia by analogy to the neurologic symptoms of pain hyperpathia.

Other emotional expressions such as exaltation, ecstasy, sorrow, enthusiasm, irritation, and grief cannot be observed. This enumeration already indicates that we are dealing with affects that require noëtic object content. This points generally to the relation–emphasized by Störring (1965)–between more subtle emotional states and intellectual behavior. Modesty also belongs to that type of affect which can express culture and personality. For example, the patients initially do not prevent exposure of parts of their bodies, as might occur during exercises in physiotherapy. On the other hand, they do not expose themselves on purpose, and it would thus be wrong to see exhibitionistic tendencies in this exposure, as is occasionally opinioned by the nursing staff. Enuresis and encopresis do not cause any embrassment either, even to the advancedpatient, so that the nursing staff sometimes attributes this kind of behavior to malicious intent on the part of the patients. A female patient who had progressed very well judging from her verbal abilities urinated into her toothbrush glass, for example, in the presence of a neighbor, even though the toilet was not far away. Yet in other cases early existence of modesty has been observed, so that there is no entirely uniform line in this area.

Other emotional states which exhibit a primitive or rather original character in patients with apallic syndrome should be mentioned at this point. Among them is an indiscriminate need for affection. For example, in one female patient after the coma vigile had subsided, her expressions of unhappiness could be quickly appeased by stroking her gently. A year later, this patient would draw any person toward her and would always want to kiss and stroke them, again without any sexual connotation.

Another emotional state is a sympathy-antipathy behavior. In some patients its existence is noticed very early. They will gladly permit some people to approach them–usually nurses–to feed and care for them, whereas toward others they show continued hostility. This behavior, however, is not at all based on experience, since it has been observed that they do not single out people who make a special effort toward them or who develop an emotional attachment to them. This kind of behavior has already been described by Fischgold and Mathis (1959), as well as by Gerstenbrand (1967). Hubach and Poeck (1964) also report such behavior but come to the conclusion that even under such conditions a relationship with the patient is possible. However, we should not forget–and perhaps that is the most interesting aspect–that such sympathy-antipathy emotions are almost entirely reflexive and do not involve the entire personality in interpersonal relationships, since a personality as such is no longer or not yet existent in these patients.

Disturbed Thinking

Thinking and verbal ability also undergo very complex disturbances, from which conclusions might be drawn as to normal thinking, but they have not been examined more closely. To some extent, the apallic syndrome can be considered an experimental field for the examination of centrally caused but not aphasic disturbances of speech. Although the *understanding of words* is disturbed in many patients, it is present again to a surprisingly high degree in a very early phase. Active speech, however, always remains severely disturbed for a long time. A point mentioned in the section on impulsion is also valid here: it is very easy to be deceived by the amount of a patient's verbal expression which seems to suit the situation. In reality, however, every patient's speech without exception is considerably impoverished in a manner not seen, for example, in the dementive processes of disintegration. This phenomenon is most obvious in patients who do not progress beyond a stage where they can only use a few phrases. Even the most advanced patients will always suffer from verbal unproductivity, loss of flexibility, and richness of the spoken language, which leads to the use of set phrases and short sentence patterns. This explains why Möllmann's patient (1940) used exactly the same expressions as one of our patients. When reading the expressions of patients quoted in the case material in the literature, one is always remineded of utterances of one's own patients.

From a linguistic point of view, the following can be stated: the biologically founded ability to learn and use language, the so-called competence (Chomsky, 1968a, 1970), undergoes in practically all patients severe damage to its biological foundation or is lost altogether. Frequently, patients only recover a part of their former style of language. Many lose the ability to extend their vocabulary and to learn new speech strategies. They lose the ability for creative language usage which every adult possesses. This ability is necessary, even in everyday use, to adapt speech to the changing situation. The author's observations have shown that during the remission phases the patients do not learn the language in the same way a child does, even though they have to start all over again, which would suggest the comparison to a child learning a language. But, as Bierwisch (1966) remarked, the child possesses the ability to set up his own rules of speech and to correct them guided by his language experience. It is this loss of competence that is responsible for the formulalike speech of patients with postapallic syndrome.

Gnostic Disturbances

Disturbances occur in the apallic syndrome which can also be found in the same or similar form in severe traumas with different primary symptoms or in severe amnestic syndromes. They appear in different ways in different patients according to the preferred localization of the disturbance. These disturbances, therefore, do not constitute anything characteristic or specific in the apallic syndrome, but by their structural interrelations they add to the total picture of the remission stages of the apallic syndrome.

Gnostic disturbances should be mentioned first. Even in 1940 Kretschmer called the apallic syndrome the ideal case of panapraxia and panagnosia. We can observe genuine gnostic disturbances of various form and expression in the remission phases. The author has repeated in a number of cases the experiments which for example led Bürger-Prinz and Kaila (1930) to their structural-psychologic concepts of the amnestic syndrome. Severe disturbances show up mainly in the comprehension of configuration, in the recognition of symbols, in the reproduction of configurations, and also when wishing to make one configuration stand out more clearly. It can be observed in the matchstick tests (or also in the subtest for matching pictures in WAIS). The disintegration of configuration is clearly demonstrated in individual examples (see Figs. 1 and 2).

Sexuality

The disturbances of sexuality correspond to a large extent to the familiar clinical picture of brain injuries and other organic dementia. The majority of cases develop a total disinterest in all sexual matters. An increase in sexual activity despite otherwise severe disturbances

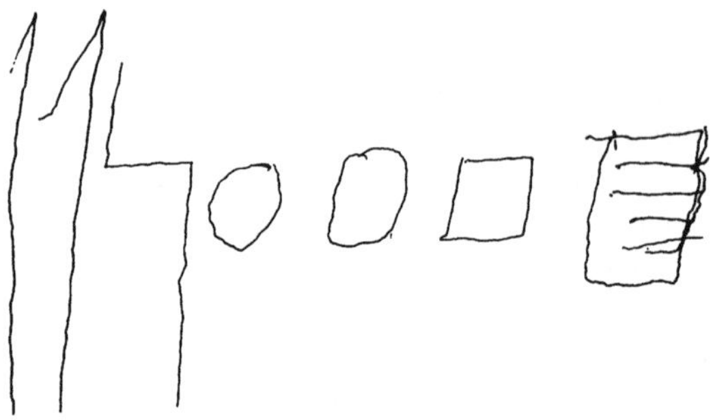

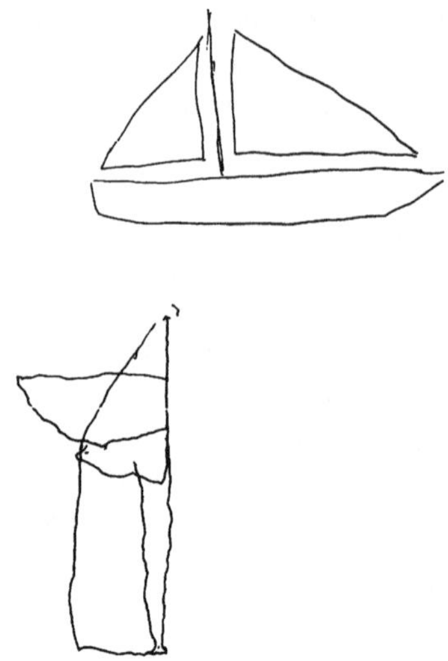

Fig. 1 Fig. 2

Fig. 1. Thirteen months after traumatic apallic syndrome. Patient is given the task of drawing a house. She understands the task and draws half the outlines of a house (*left*) and round and square figures beside it which she identifies as windows and doors, when questioned as to their meaning

Fig. 2. The same female patient. She does not recognize the sailboat in the simple outlines of the copy (although she lives in a port). She cannot name the individual parts, either, since she has not grasped the general content. Recognition does not improve even when hints are given. The task of copying will have to be done, even though she has not understood the content. At first she thinks that her drawing represents a house, then a face

occurs only in a few exceptional cases. One female patient, for example, masturbated every day after lunch at the table, in spite of the presence of other patients. In the establishment of sexuality, however, one can easily be mistaken. One factor is the already mentioned need for affection and the desire for closeness. Another factor is a more or less obvious organic inhibition. The possibility of error here probably accounts for the occasional report in case descriptions in the literature that lively sexuality has been observed, in contrast to the author's own observations.

Tiring and Perseveration

The psychiatrist is accustomed to recognizing an acute, always organic, and diffuse disturbance of the brain in a patient who after only a few questions and answers during an interview shows definite signs of tiring, speaks slower and slower, finds it increasingly difficult to remember, yawns, and repeats himself constantly. This can also be observed in the apallic syndrome. Tiring and persevering tendencies may *initially* and over a longer period of time (several months) dominate the clinical picture to such an extent that a specific examination (apart from simple observation) is practically impossible. The investigation of other psychopathologic phenomena later on may be extensively obstructed by rapid tiring, since achievements that were possible at the beginning of the examination can no longer be produced, even after only a few minutes. This tiring usually remains—but definitely tends to decrease—for a longer period of time, often for several years. The phenomenon of tiring can also be used in the further prognosis. As long as it is still evident, further rehabilitation is possible. In the terminal state the patient does not show any signs of tiring, whereas the tendency to persevere remains as a general somatopsychic symptom in another form.

Memory

Memory is severely affected in all cases. An exact examination, however, is extremely difficult, since other somatopsychic disturbances interfere with those of memory. It is easier to characterize memory disturbances in cases of more advanced rehabilitation. A disturbance of long-term memory is especially noticeable. The patients grasp learning material quickly and are able to reproduce it well after a few minutes. But after a few hours practically all the material is forgotten, and the time needed to relearn it is as long as it was before the first learning. When possibilities for intellectual achievements have reappeared, even those favorably developing cases have to relearn their previous knowledge and abilities, for which a few weeks or months are usually sufficient. More severe cases need a lot more time—often years—to relearn. These patients do not usually succeed in adding new abilities and knowledge to those relearned.

Even in medium severe cases pronounced retrograde lapses of amnesia can be observed. The last events immediately preceding the apallic syndrome are almost completely blotted out, even older object content of memory is thin. In severe cases, only a few memory islands of the former life remain. The patients never refer spontaneously to the past or the future, even when they stay in the hospital for years. They never have any desire to leave the hospital either. These cases, more than any other, have lost the human ability of *Besinnung* (reflection) (Störring, 1965), the possibility of looking at the past and the future, and thus remain tied to the present.

Facial Expressions

The facial expressions of a person do not usually contribute to any great extent to the findings of psychologic examinations because too many mistakes are possible. However, the observation of facial expression can be of valuable assistance in the general context of the clinical picture of a disease. Changes in facial expressions have been observed in all our patients, even in the late rehabilitation phases. These changes are especially shocking to the relatives of the patients. They consist of a loss of individual peculiarities; differentiation disappears and expressions become coarser. These changes are more noticeable in a face that is moving than in one that is still.

Conclusions

The character of the postapallic syndrome, this strange mixture of emotional and intellectual disturbances which differ so greatly from case to case, makes it very difficult to look at and summarize the picture as a whole from a general point of view. Omitting many details, the author has attempted to work out the main features, and still has not been able to establish any kind of regularly proceeding psychopathologic developments. Störring (1965) once attempted a summary from a more anthropologic viewpoint and concentrated on the especially problematic, severe cases, which he entitled *personale Eingleisigkeit* ("one-track personality"). In this study he stressed the fact that man ceases to really exist as a questioning being when all intellectual productivity stops and when all relation to the past and the future disappears. This helplessness might suggest a comparison with a child, but it is a futile one, since a child is especially characterized by his questioning and exuberant spontaneous activity.

12. On the Psychopathology of Postapallic Terminal States

U. BOETERS

Although general interest in the apallic syndrome, especially its posttraumatic forms, has increased during the last few years, relatively little is known even today about the psychopathologic aspects of its late regressive and terminal states. We are still awaiting comprehensive investigations. Hitherto existing publications indicate that one can rarely expect regression of all psychopathologic disturbances when there is further-reaching restitution over a longer survival period. More often defective states will develop.

A synoptic presentation of the terminal states is obviously difficult for several reasons. One feature of the defective states described so far is their remarkable differences. The main point is partly evident, for instance, in a marked intellectual deficiency (Mifka, 1966), this tendency having already been introduced explicitly by Strich (1956) with renewed use of that somewhat controversial concept of "traumatic dementia." What other authors stress, however, is the absence of mental disturbances as opposed to persisting changes in the personality and character of the patient (Stössel, 1966).

Nor do the existing attempts at more precise psychopathologic analyses of the sequelae of an apallic syndrome permit a conclusive interpretation of such contradictory findings, one of the main reasons being that they are founded only on the examination of isolated and interesting cases. Their value for the assessment of the definite final states is limited, since most of these explicitly refer to early regressive stages (Sauter, 1965) or the provisional final stage (Ule et al., 1961). In these cases, a further regression was obviously expected even after long observation periods lasting from several months to several years. Other publications (Vigouroux et al., 1964; Krupka, 1965; Boeters, 1969; Koch, 1969) still indicate the more or less provisional character of the regressive state in spite of an observation which in some cases has lasted for several years. This caution shows that the boundary between functional disturbances and a defect syndrome (Wieck, 1967b) is difficult to locate. An important reason for this problem is the regression which seems to be remarkably delayed compared with other brain lesions. According to the author's observations, the period of restitution may last for 3-4 years, and even then one cannot be sure that in fact all possibilities of restitution are exhausted. This strikingly delayed regression after a single occurrence of brain lesion may by itself make worthwhile a separate study of the postapallic final states in their more practical aspects, although the characteristic initial syndrome, because of its psychopathologic particularities, justifies further pursuit for purely scientific reasons.

The unusually lengthy restitution complicates, of course—also for practical reasons—a careful observation of the cause of the syndrome in comparable conditions. As a rule, it is very difficult in a research-oriented institution to undertake prolonged observation of patients who are in need of constant care. For organizational reasons and many other factors –for instance, particular requests of the patients' relatives–such patients have to be transferred sooner or later to another hospital, thereby depriving the researcher of subjects. As a matter of fact, several of the author's patients whose regression was under observation for several years have, in spite of all possible endeavors, been prematurely removed from our study.

This is why, despite constant endeavors over several years, observations on only 18 patients can be discussed in this paper. These patients, on the one hand, certainly did pass through a phase of posttraumatic apallic syndrome: on the other hand, they reached a degree of restitution which, after long-term control of the cause of the syndrome, can be considered as definitive. It seemed irrelevant to include in this study findings on such patients who, although surviving for several months, never clearly recovered from the apallic syndrome but died of this or another psychoorganic syndrome of the same severity. In addition, all such patients in whom retrospectively the apallic syndrome diagnosed elsewhere could not be definitely confirmed were excluded. Several times it was found that sequelae of brain lesions are apparently being more frequently diagnosed as postapallic transitional and defective states, although initially there is only a prolonged coma or superficial symptoms of a brain stem lesion, but not the characteristic features of the apallic syndrome.

Obviously, the fact that there were only 18 cases does not permit a representative statement on the chances of restitution after a posttraumatic apallic syndrome, especially since a negative selection of patients has to be assumed for other reasons. For, as a rule, patients with brain lesions only come to see the psychiatrist if the initial syndrome is followed by particular psychopathologic complications or if the regression is delayed by remarkable psychic disturbances. Thus, the possibility of a quick and complete restitution after a posttraumatic apallic syndrome cannot be excluded, although individual examinations of such descriptions have indeed led to the conclusion that either the diagnosis was wrong in the first place or that the exact follow-up examination showed longer-lasting and more severe disturbances which had escaped the examiner's attention during the first superficial examinations.

If there is a clear regression with a longer survival period after a posttraumatic apallic syndrome, our experience so far shows that the essential cause may have been an extensive edema of the cerebral medulla. In accordance with this, we usually find later a considerable hydrocephalus with longer-surviving and clearly remitted patients. On the other hand, patients with apallic syndromes due to a primary brain stem lesion have considerably less chance for survival. The third typical pattern of damage in connection with the apallic syndrome–marked cortical lesions–is observed especially with the nontraumatic forms, mainly with anoxemic brain damages (complications induced by anesthesia), with anaphylactic reactions and anabolic disturbances; here, too, the prognosis is unfavorable, often because of the primary disease.

For instance, a patient with a postvaccinal encephalopathy was observed whose apallic syndrome persisted for 21 months without any tendency toward regression under optimal care (Boeters and Reimer, 1970). The clinical diagnosis was later verified by post-mortem findings (Boeters and Korenke, 1972).

Various focal brain disturbances and neurologic complications show, however, that very often we have to take into account focally accentuated contusional lesions, which in the terminal stage, along with brain damage of a more diffuse nature, may also be important from a psychopathologic point of view.

If the later psychopathologic findings on the author's own 18 patients are analyzed, we find, in the first place from the point of view of typology as well as of degrees of severity, more divergent aspects than characteristics in common. Besides complete restitution very severe, otherwise hardly known features of deficiency were found, and in addition to that, several forms of known psycho-organic syndromes, some more marked than others. Our experience shows that this striking variability is recognizable here already in the early stages of regression. It thus permits a limited early prognosis from a psychopathologic point of view. As an example of an especially favorable course of a syndrome, the following case is mentioned:

Case 1: G.U., an 11-year-old boy at the time of the accident. After an initial brain coma of several days, a typical apallic syndrome lasted for 4 weeks. Afterwards a passing apathetic stage was observed, later on considerable excess of drive. There was quick restitution of the disturbances of cerebral function; neurologically there was only a functionally minor hemiparesis of the right side. One year later he returned to school. Certain difficulties with lack of concentration, restlessness and increased irritability arose, but he finally came to a normal conclusion of his primary school education. Then the 16-year-old boy had a severe crisis and the remaining neurologic disturbance made it impossible for him to take up his desired career. After limited psychotherapeutic and psychologic intervention, he was apprenticed as a mason. At 18 years of age he wished to have a driver's licence, and after satisfactory results of an examination of his functional psychology, this was agreed to and the examination was passed with success. At this time there was still a slight alteration in his character in the form of increased irritability and a very slight lack of drive. In addition, he had problems making contact, and had a striking lack of interest in women. Clinically, these symptoms correspond more to a brain-organic defect syndrome than to a pseudo-psychopathy.

Such favorable progress, which if looked at only superficially, corresponds practically to a *restitutio ad integrum*, was only found on three occasions. It is certainly no coincidence that in all of these three cases the apallic syndromes had begun when the patients were still children, since any hitherto comparable observations have only been made on infantile brain damage (Hubach and Poeck, 1965; Ule et al., 1965; Gerstenbrand, 1967). Through close observations, though, a discrete alteration of character was also discovered in these cases. This is an argument against the possibility of a completely defect-free restitution after a posttraumatic apallic syndrome. It is of course difficult to answer the question as to how often such a favorable and perhaps even really optimal progress does occur. We must, indeed, take into account the fact that such patients, with an already primarily recognizable quick regression, will sometimes never be closely examined by a psychiatrist.

Favorable progress after a traumatic brain damage with an apallic syndrome in childhood is not at all the rule, as the following case will show:

Case 2: An 11 1/2-year-old boy, for reasons unknown, jumped in front of a lorry from the railing of a bridge. He had a brain coma lasting many weeks and an apallic syndrome of several weeks' duration. Neurologically paraspasticity of the leg centered on his left side was found, and psychologically a delayed regression of a severe disturbance of drive. The final state was reached after somewhat more than 2 years. The striking features were the persistence of a mixed aphasia, which complicated closer psychopathologic examination. Observable disturbances of expressive behavior showed a considerable decrease in drive and on the other hand an increased irritability and a tendency toward obstinate and aggressive behavior, and regressive tendencies. After a vain attempt at home treatment, the boy had to be transferred to an asylum. The pneumencephalogram showed in this case a strong extension of both lateral ventriculi, especially of the antecornus and the cornu inferius ventriculi lateralis. In addition to this, an extension of the third ventricle was observed.

As in this case, which was complicated by aphasic disturbances, various focal defects with partly psychopathologic, partly more neurologic effects were found with other patients. Aphasic and agnostic disturbances, which have been described for the early stages of regression by Peters (Chapter 11), seem to be dominant. Such focal symptoms as a rule complicate the psychopathologic diagnosis, especially if they are only poorly defined and embedded in relatively rough psychoorganic disturbances. The existence of such "contused focal symptoms" has already been described by Ule et al. (1961) in one of their cases under observation.

In other cases, the features of the defect were rather uncharacteristic and would best be compared to the well-known consequences of diffuse brain lesions–for instance, contused brain traumata.

Case 3: A 20-year-old man at the time of the accident. At the time of the initial syndrome repeated respiratory standstill. Duration of the apallic syndrome was 5 weeks. Later, a paroxysmal disease, neurologic persistence of a tremor as well as complicated remaining pareses partly of the right, partly of the left side of his body developed. In the foreground, however, a severe psychoorganic syndrome with slowing down, loss of initiative, euphoria and retardation was found. Five years after the accident he was at home but in need of care. He finally wanted to get married and asked his mother to put an advertisement in the newspaper.

In this case, the later psychopathologic features are also definitely complicated by late complication of the brain trauma, namely, by a cerebroorganic paroxysmal disease with corresponding progressive alteration in character. Complication by a posttraumatic epilepsy is not at all rare in our series of observations; we were able to locate this five times. Probably depending on the age of the patient, several small, as well as generalized attacks developed. There were also other indirect consequences of apallic syndromes which sometimes led to a secondary influence on the psychopathologic symptoms.

Case 4: A 25-year-old married women. After a traffic accident she had a contused brain trauma with a typical apallic syndrome of a duration of several weeks, in addition to various fractures. In the course of restitution there was extensive transmineralization with the development of considerable "myositis ossificans" and nephrolithiasis. Finally, approximately 1 year after the accident, there developed on both sides nephrolithiasis and relapsing pyelitides and preuremia. At the same time, there was an increasing reduction in drive and return of the apallic syndrome. After a pyelotomy, she quickly recovered from the immediate danger, but there was still a hesitating regression of the psychopathologic symptoms. This ended in the final stage of a very severe Korsakow syndrome which, after an observation period of 5 years, is now stationary.

The exact description of a long-lasting syndrome of an exogenic reaction type and of general and localized brain organic psychosyndromes (Bleuler, 1969) is superfluous here, since these symptoms are known features of various types of brain damage. It may be noted, though, that just such syndromes which are also quite usual after brain traumata of various degrees of severity were relatively seldom found in the final stage.

Case 5: A 41-year-old woman. During regression there had been transitory agnostic focal symptoms. The final stage showed symptoms of orbital damage of the brain with an instinctual disinhibition and disturbances of the central functions of personality. At this point in time no more elementary disturbances of cerebral functions or focal defects could be discovered.

In the final stages of regression, as in the earlier stages, we find in some patients defective features, psychopathologically quite extraordinary and remarkably severe; these seem rather to correspond to the characteristics of the initial syndrome. One had the impression that these very processes had awakened a psychologic interest not only in view of the successive stages of the apallic syndrome but in general for purely scientific reasons.

In a case observed by the author, remarkably defects which penetrated the elementary sphere of concept formation were found. The occurrence of such defects was discussed many years ago but has since been questioned, particularly because of the absence of appropriate observation.

Case 6: G.B., at the time of the accident was a 17-year-old girl who in a traffic accident had been catapulted from a car and buried under it in a ditch. More than 1 h elasped before she was rescued. After that a midbrain syndrome occurred which passed into an apallic syndrome for a duration of 8 weeks. There followed gradual regression over a "silent phase" with only affective and motor reactions, gradual differentiation of the capability of linguistic expression, no remarkable neurologic defects. A regular alpha rhythm in the EEG regressed only after 30 weeks. In the meantime, there appeared a central symptom of a severe disturbance of spontaneous drive. In the second year after the accident her vocabulary, expressive capability, and understanding of the world around her increased only slowly. Advanced fatigability decreased only slightly. The improvement in psychical and intellectual performance was limited to step-by-step restoration of earlier knowledge and capabilities. G.B. kept surprising the examiner with words, expressions, and concepts from her earlier life, whereas more recent impressions were taken up very imperfectly and were then forgotten very soon thereafter. Finally, during continuous observations over 4 years, a steady increase of heterosuggestibility and reactivity of a periodic character developed. This seemed to obscure at times the persisting disturbance of spontaneous drive.

In the final stage the patient showed a remarkable dedifferentiation of her physiognomy (which we later found typical for other cases); her facial expression seemed empty; all reactions were undefined. Psychomotor coordination was severely disturbed, especially on examination of more delicate movements. Further examinations showed that the injured person was unable to conceive the completion of her motor operations. When in a preponderantly euphoric emotional condition, interrupted by occasional and provoked irritation, the patient showed very strange drive behavior. Left to herself, the patient remained completely passive, but she was inciteable, open to stimuli, and showed an unfiltered reactivity (lack of stimulus barrier, according to Goldstein, 1928). Exploratory and psychologic test examinations of her behavior led to remarkable findings. The quick gesticulatory, verbal, and affective reactions, which were not always strikingly disturbed, to the manifold outside stimuli caused the patient's behavior to seem nearly "normal" upon superficial observation. A more in-depth study showed, however, the complete lack of stimulus barrier and the blind and purposeless reaction. The thought processes, still possible, but to a large extent mechanized and reflexlike, were characterized by the reduction of the stimulated imaginatory processes in their illustrative and meaningful features. Very often the conceptual ideas were so rarified that they occurred only as undefined general terms and vague, framelike concepts and were insufficient for developing logical, meaningful thought. The patient appeared to be limited to random and sometimes altogether unconnected partial thoughts or tended to complement her incomplete thoughts with widely different yet reflex-associated concepts, so that anomalies appeared and incorrect expressions and meanings were used, and she could also not follow a thought to its conclusion. Her frequent tendency to fill in the gaps through perseverance, however, was secondary and not caused by the fact that there was a primary inhibition of the conceptual process by fixed associations. It is more the case that the already existing associations were only reproduced when further conceptional parts of the same field failed to appear.

Attempts at solutions by the patient—some of these correct more by coincidence, others incomprehensible—produced the impression of a striking dissociation of psychic performances. The inconstancy did not depend on pleasure- or displeasure-determining influences, nor was it even based on the experience of a successful performance or a failure. Examinations revealed that the disturbance of the thought processes was such that it penetrated the elementary conceptional relationships and their imaginative fundamentals. In the terminology of Gestaltpsychology, there is a disturbance to the degree of dissolution of figure-basic relationships. From the point of view of associative psychology, a disturbance of the basic pattern of concepts can be recognized. Thus, the patient showed disturbances of concept formation, which are still theoretically very controversial, namely, a disjunctive conceptual decay, and an elementary psychopathologic disturbance which was introduced by Heilbronner (1900) and Liepmann (1908) but which was later attacked by Jaspers (1959).

Further observation 9 years after the accident–the patient is now in an asylum–revealed a practically unchanged picture. After being transferred, she became accustomed to her new surroundings within a few days. Still dominant are the strong reactivity towards outside stimuli and a tendency toward angry irritation and aggressive behavior. She still has a very weak memory, and her emotional reaction to impressions is cool and superficial. The patient still consistently shows adjustment behavior patterns–for instance, she has learned to play with dice.

The interpretation of such severe defects creates considerable problems. Secondary damage by environmental influences is hardly probable but cannot be altogether excluded. There is no support, however, for somatic complications, as discussed earlier. That is why we are justified in assuming that the extensive lesion of large pathway systems, which is possibly accentuated by cortical lesions, is responsible for the disturbances even in elementary psychic functions. The extension of the morphologic brain damage is also proven in this case by a considerable hydrocephalus.

If we compare the degree of severity and the typology of the very heterogeneous sequelae in progress after traumatic apallic syndromes, we find that as a rule disturbances of drive regulation appear. It is true that they are themselves strongly pronounced to varying degrees and hardly ever overlooked during careful examination. In the final stage the impression of a frontal lack of drive is dominant, and with it a loss of spontaneity with more or less well preserved, occasionally excessive reactivity to outside stimuli. Some of the patients–for example, the one described in Case 6–even gave an impression of a partial hypervigility. The disturbance of the drive regulation has also been characterized by the axial symptom which can be followed in the course of its regression, as shown in an earlier paper (Boeters, 1969). Of course, in early regression the first impression is that of a more diencephalic lack of drive. Even the psychopathologic picture of the apallic syndromes can be considered, according to Kretschmer (1940), under the aspect of a kind of drive blockage. In support of this hypothesis we will briefly discuss a further observation.

Case 7: A 50-year-old woman with subarachnoidal hemorrhage after rupture of an aneurysm at the right arteria cerebri anterior. As a result of the rupture of an aneurysm there was a closure of the artery. Shortly thereafter, a control angiography of the other side also revealed a closure of the left arteria cerebri anterior. The woman was in a stupor which later intensified. The intense negativistically colored stupor finally passed into an apallic syndrome which lasted for several weeks; coma and finally death followed. This clinical diagnosis of a double-sided closure of the anterior arteriae could be verified pathologicoanatomically. Further substrates for the development of an apallic syndrome such as necroses in the regions supplied by the above-mentioned vessels could not be found.

The dominant disturbances of drive regulation after the onset of the apallic syndrome apparently decisively influence–according to the progress and intensity–the different features of the follow-up and defect disturbances. As the drive functions are of fundamental importance and penetrate far into various psychic regions–even into perceptional functions–it is quite possible that the occasional impression of locally accentuated lesions and even contused focal symptoms could have a relation to these fundamental disturbances. Some behavioral disturbances, and even success or failure in examination situations, must be seen under the aspect of drive disturbances.

Quite often in the final stage the behavior of the patients was altered, that is, it coarsened and there was a tendency toward reflex behavior, one-way affects (Störring, 1965) being dominant, and these corresponded strikingly in their prompt and intensive reactivity with the rest of the patients' openness to stimuli. The term "affectual hyperpathy" chosen by Peters (Chapter 11) seems to be very suitable in this context. Other psychopathologic disturbances are more or less strongly pronounced in the defective stage, and they are—apparently depending on the individual character of the brain lesion—of a more facultative character. Occasionally we find accentuated amnestic disturbances, sometimes also brain-local psychosyndromes and complications from obvious focal disturbances of an aphasic or agnostic character. The psychopathologic late sequelae are sometimes complicated by secondary damage and typically by posttraumatic paroxysmal diseases.

Neurologic disturbances in their final stage show in fact a very high variability and intensity. We may find complicated residual pareses. A special articulatory speech disturbance also frequently occurs which slows down the flow of speech and gives it a monotonous and howling character. This strange speech disturbance, like many other aspects described by Peters (Chapter 11), leads one to at once suspect sequelae after an apallic syndrome. Further neurologic disturbances which can be seen in the defect syndrome involve more the extrapyramidal motor system, dystonias, and tremor, observed on several occasions. The neurologic disturbances after a traumatic apallic syndrome, however, are as a rule less pronounced than the psychic alterations; they are of great importance, especially because of the unfavorable combination of psychic alterations.

The dominant problem in care, therapy, and all attempts at rehabilitation is the disturbance of drive regulation, which even limits intensive and long-lasting endeavors to gain functional compensation. It is true that a comprehensive therapy makes it possible sometimes to exercise the motor and simple psychic functions and leads at least to modest success. The result depends, however, on the duration of the care. If the intensive therapy has to be stopped, the successfully exercised functions are blocked because of the patient's lack of spontaneity.

Based on these conditions, it can be stated that, of the author's patients, five have remained almost completely helpless and in need of care after traumatic apallic syndromes, whereas only three patients have hardly noticeable defects. The remaining patients still showed such severe defects that rehabilitation to the point of taking up a job is not possible. Such unfavorable results would look better if the cases which at first had proceeded favorably could also be included, but we have to take into account the fact that a considerable percentage of these will retain severe permanent effects. Since these cases—at least in the author's own observations—are mainly sequelae of extensive edematous necroses, an early and intensive prophylaxis and treatment of such lesions are more important than controlling the immediate danger in the initial stage.

III. Pathology

13. Neuropathology of the Traumatic Apallic Syndrome

G. PETERS and E. ROTHEMUND

Introduction

Twenty cases of the apallic syndrome have been examined. Nontraumatic cases were not included in this study. The age of the patients ranged 9-53 years, the average age being 31.8 years. Fifteen patients were male and five, female. The duration of the clinical syndrome varied from 3 weeks to 7 years with an average duration of 11 months.

Skull fractures were present in half of the cases; in three of these ten cases both the basis and vault were involved, whereas in two other cases, the mandible was also fractured.

In two cases an intracerebral hemorrhage and in four cases an epidural and/or a subdural hemorrhage were found as space-occupying lesions. In the remaining cases a posttraumatic edema had to be postulated.

In 13 of the 20 cases a severe midbrain syndrome developed following the accident and prior to the onset of the apallic syndrome.

Primary traumatic lesions in the form of foci of cortical contusion were seen in 11 cases; they were mainyl restricted to the base of the brain. With the exception of two cases these foci were rather small.

Death from respiratory paralysis was observed in only one case. The bulbar type of death supervened in the course of a midbrain syndrome caused by recurrent bouts of tentorial herniation with mesencephalic compression. In the remaining cases the cause of death varied as follows: an extracranial infectious process (three cases), development of a pulmonary process with secondary hematogenous encephalomeningitis (one case), pulmonary embolism secondary to thrombosis of the iliac veins (one case), a paralytic intestinal ileus (one case), and suicide (one case). Heart failure superimposed upon a terminal pulmonary illness was listed as the cause of death in the remainder of cases.

As for the traumatic mechanism, in the majority of cases there was evidence of a trauma producing kinetic energy exerted in a sagittal plane, usually in an orocaudal direction, rarely in a caudorostral direction. In seven cases the injured person was a pedestrian. In another case the accident was described as a fall downstairs. The remaining cases were all automobile, motor scooter, or motorcycle accidents.

Neuropathologic Findings

In our material the corpus callosum and the central white matter were the most frequently damaged structures. Callosal lesions were present in all 20 cases; however, they were no more than minor in two cases, lasting 22 and 24 days respectively. The corpus callosum is a favorite seat of traumatic lesions. We think that these lesions are due to a stretching or tearing of the corpus callosum which takes place following distortion and increase in cross diameter of the skull, with corresponding changes of the cranial content when a traumatic force is applied in the sagittal plane. This type of traumatic event appeared to be regularly present in our material. The callosal lesions consisted of circumscribed areas of necrosis, old hemorrhages, patches of diffuse or focal demyelination, often extending also to the septum and fornix (Figs. 1 and 2). Not infrequently a sudanophilic break-

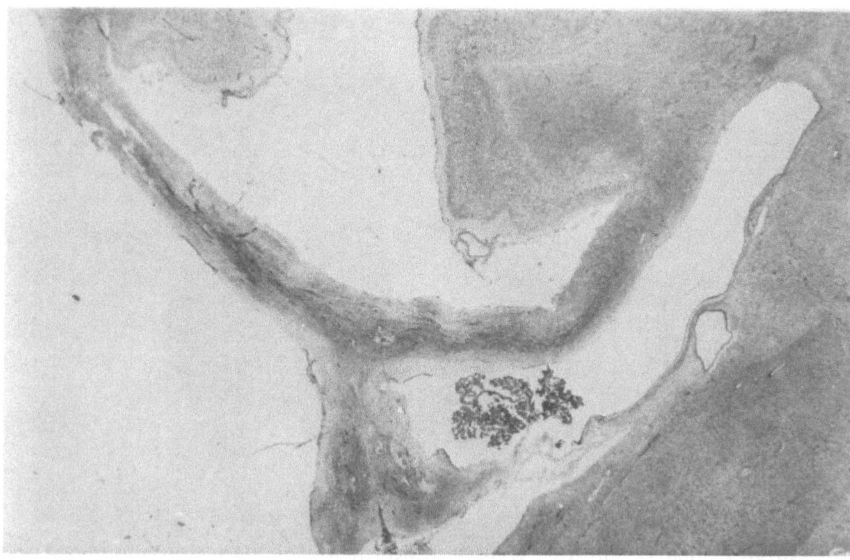

Fig. 1. Survival time 9 months. Severe atrophy, glial proliferation, and collection of macrophages along entire length of corpus callosum. The fornix is also involved

down of the nervous tissue with a peculiar linear configuration running perpendicular to the course of the callosal fibers was seen. The areas of necrosis and old hemorrhages lay most often medially, in the vicinity of the ventricular cavity, along the line of attachment of the septum pellucidum and laterally, at the junction between corpus callosum and central white matter. In only two cases were the lesions bilateral and symmetrical. Small hemorrhages per rhexis were mentioned by Schacht (1965) and Minauf (1966) in exactly the same regions in cases of trauma with short survival time. In a few cases demyelination and lipid disintegration were seen medially in the dorsal layers of the corpus callosum just beneath the falx. In this region Schacht and Minauf have also seen in their own material a circumscribed area of destruction of the upper callosal fibers with small hemorrhagic extravasations in the vicinity. True rupture of the corpus callosum has never been observed in our material.

In the same locations Grcevic and Jacob (1965) have also observed bleeding, edema, focal loss of myelin with lipid breakdown, and secondary organization. Practically in every case a few macrophase were seen lying free in these paraventricular foci. In accordance with what has already been said concerning the pathogenesis, Grcevic thinks that the lesions are due both to the establishment of sharp pressure gradients between the fluid ventricular phase and the solid circumlittoral phase (cavitation effect) as well as to the stretching of the corpus callosum, septum, and fornix following a sudden distortion of the inner liquoral compartments of the central nervous system.

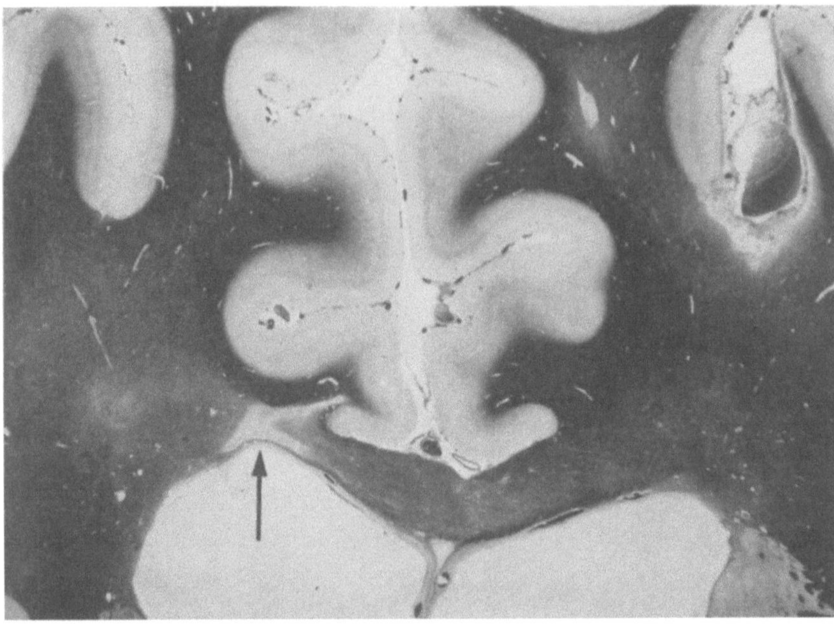

Fig. 2. Survival time 11 months. Well-circumscribed stage III necrosis in junctional area between corpus callosum and the left centrum semiovale (*arrow*). Diffuse demyelination of corpus callosum and cerebral white matter

In cases with a somewhat longer period of survival the corpus callosum was definitely atrophic (Fig. 1), so that an almost complete severance between the two hemispheres, at least at some point in the callosal commissure, could be readily assumed. Regarding the distribution of the lesions, we were able by means of serial sections from the genu to the splenium to demonstrate in our 20 cases that the lesions are most frequent and severe in the middle third of the corpus callosum, i.e., where this structure is the thinnest and least firmly fixed. Only in five cases were there moderate to severe lesions all along the entire length of the corpus callosum; however, also in these cases the most affected regions were never found either at the genual or at the splenial levels. The septum was involved in 13 cases, the fornix in 14; in general, the septal changes were never as marked as the callosal alterations. Of the 51 cases reported by Lindenberg et al. (1955), nine showed a lesion extending throughout the whole length of the corpus callosum; 21 showed widespread lesions stretching over one- to two-thirds of this structure, while the remaining 21 cases exhibited minor changes, mostly in the caudal half of the corpus callosum.

Cerebral White Matter

Demyelination, in the form of a pallor on the myelin stains, was noticeable in every case; however, the degree of pallor varied from case to case (Fig. 2). The astrocytes showed progressive changes in all cases. The latter changes were often focally accentuated, occasionally far more severe than the corresponding myelin loss. Only a few cases failed to show patchy areas of necrosis and old hemorrhage with hemosiderinladen macrophages. In the areas of necrosis the fatty breakdown of the nervous tissue was always marked. In addition, a diffuse lipid breakdown was often noticeable. However, the fatty products seen as crystalline deposits with a polarizing microscope did not stain with an alcoholic Sudan solution. These negative results with Sudan IV, as well as the blackening obtained with osmic acid, prompted Strich (1956, 1961) to conclude that these products are formed at the early stages of the myelin breakdown. However, Holländer (1964) was able to prove histochemically that these products are cholesterol esters, which do not take the Sudan stain at room temperature due to their higher melting point, which ranges from 40° to 42°C. If the slides are heated 38°-40°C, the breakdown products of myelin regularly stain with an alcoholic Sudan solution. Amorim (1934b) saw colorless anisotropic crystals derived from the myelin disintegration products in the degenerative processes of the white matter—for instance, in amyotrophic lateral sclerosis, although the crystals were few in number under these conditions. It is not clear why in the posttraumatic encephalopathy of long duration these crystalloid deposits should be particularly abundant.

Only rarely was the fibrous gliosis of any note; when it was severe it was particularly conspicuous along the ventricular cavities. Far more frequent than the fibrous gliosis was a spotty or streaklike cellular gliosis which could be seen in the paraventricular regions. Paraventricular areas of necrosis and old hemorrhage were apparent in four cases, particularly around the walls of the lateral ventricles (Steiner's angle). The later changes, as well as the paraventricular fibrous and cellular gliosis, should be regarded as a direct result of the primary injury following the sudden building of sharp pressure gradients between the different phases of the intracranial content (cavitation effect). The changes in the inner layers of the corpus callosum should be viewed in a similar manner, i.e., as direct consequences of the traumatic distortion of the ventricular cavities. In contrast, the diffuse white matter lesions, as well as the necroses, should be considered as secondary processes—the former due to local circulatory disturbances likely to occur during a sudden drop in blood pressure, respiratory distress, and profuse sweating. Indeed, the age of the necrotic areas was quite variable in our material. According to our study, the lesions in the cerebral white matter and in the corpus callosum are a constant finding.

Thalamus

The most frequent findings in this region were focal and diffuse demyelination and paraventricular astrocytic proliferation. In six cases there were also small areas of necrosis; in one case the necrosis was much more widespread. These lesions had a variable distribution in the thalamic nuclei. They can definitely be regarded as secondary lesions due to the cutting off of the blood supply to the penetrating arteries of the thalamus and to the posterior choroidal arteries. Even if a more comprehensive study of a greater number of cases had shown a variable measure of focal neuronal loss as well as of swelling and vacuolation of the nerve cells, we would adhere to our present results, and as for the development of the clinical syndrome, we would prefer not to assign any significant value to these merely secondary changes in the thalamus.

One is often tempted to attribute the loss of the normal rhythm of sleep and wakefulness during the apallic syndrome to lesions in the ascending multisynaptic reticular system. Associated with or being part of this system are the nonspecific projection areas of the thalamus, which have no direct connections with the cerebral cortex, the centromedian nucleus, the nuclei of internal medullary lamina, the midline nuclear group or the nucleus reticularis thalami. We feel that if a lesion of the reticular system is to be found, it should be looked for at the pontine and mesencephalic levels rather than anywhere else. Jellinger (1965) also tends to support this view.

The striatum and pallidum were only rarely involved. The pallidum showed areas of necrosis in four cases, the caudatum in two cases. In the latter there was also residual evidence of old, paraventricular bleeding.

Cerebral Cortex

Areas of incomplete and complete necrosis, occasionally penetrating into the subcortical white matter, were found in 11 cases. However, they were of import only in one case in which the patient died 25 days after the trauma. No great emphasis should be laid on the clinical significance of the cortical changes, all of which should be regarded as secondary except for the primary contusive lesions found, as mentioned above, in 11 cases. With the exception of one case, the cortical lesions were definitely not the cause of the "decorticated state." In this single case among our 20 observations there were, anatomically, widespread cortical lesions and clinically, frequent generalized epileptic seizures which occurred during the 25 days of hospitalization. Irreversible gastric bleeding and loss of blood through the tracheostoma caused the hemoglobin values to sink as low as 36%. In addition, a gangrenous hemorrhagic tracheobronchitis developed, and toward the end, an aspiration pneumonia. The anoxia brought about by the many diverse mechanisms was most likely responsible for the extensive areas of total infarction and selective neuronal degeneration found in the cerebral cortex and basal ganglia (thalamus and hypothalamus).

Brain Stem

Alterations in the midbrain and pons were present in all cases. The majority of the alterations encountered in our material were clearly of a secondary nature. Jellinger (1965) also feels that primary traumatic lesions in the brain stem are a rare occurrence. We do not share the opinion of French (1952), Wertheimer and Allegre (1953), and other authors that the primary traumatic lesions of the brain stem represent the essential morphologic substrate of the traumatic apallic syndrome. The hippocampal and uncal lesions (anemic and hemorrhagic infarctions, superficial losses of substance, incomplete necroses), which have been repeatedly demonstrated and which were seen in ten of our 20 cases, indicate that in the great majority of cases–indeed, in all probability in all cases–early in the process the midbrain is compressed either through the medially displaced or through the transtentorially herniated mediobasal portions of the temporal lobes. Less frequently seen were necroses in the occipital lobes, in the drainage district of the vena occipitalis magna, in the supply area of the arteria cerebri posterior (two cases), as well as secondary changes in the thalamic nuclei, in the territory of distribution of the perforating thalamic vessels and posterior choroidal arteries (six cases).

If one can rely on the results obtained by Mayer (1967, 1968) in his systematic examination of the midbrain, then the frequently seen crural lesions and the occasionally encountered necroses of the lateral and medial portions of the substantia nigra should likewise be regarded as a result of the pressure against the free edge of the tentorium and/or as a direct consequence of the clamping off of arteries, but mainly of veins. Also, the often recognized more or less symmetric necroses in the tegmentum, in the brachia conjunctiva, and in the velum medullare anterius are best explained as changes secondary to the impaired venous drainage caused by the tentorial herniation (Fig. 3). The necroses occasionally observed in the regions of the red nucleus and Edinger-Westphal nucleus are also secondary alterations.

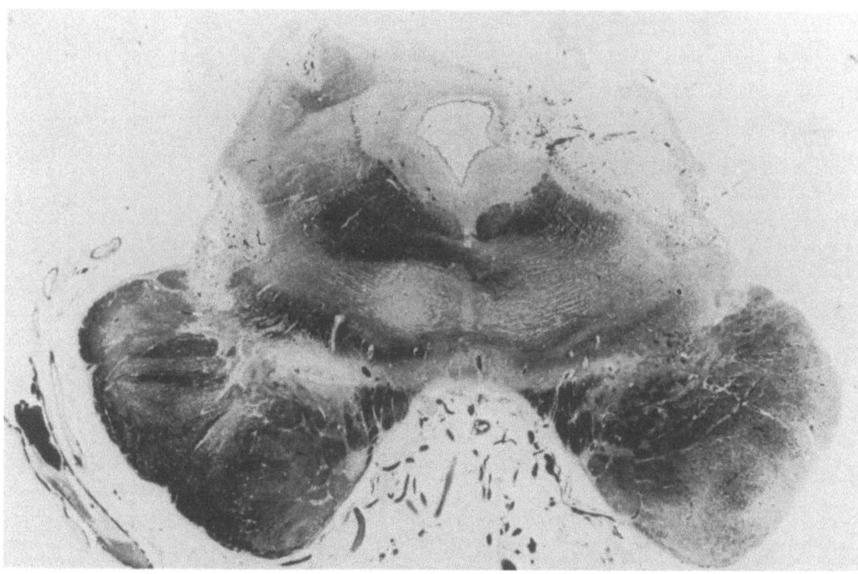

Fig. 3. Survival time 11 months. Stage III necrosis in tectum of midbrain, along fissura lateralis mesencephali and in substantia nigra of one side. Diffuse demyelination of decussation and the cerebral peduncles. Dilatation of aqueduct

As for these circumlittoral lesions, however–including the periaqueductal lesions–in agreement with the results of Mayer (1968), one has to recognize the probability of a primary traumatic change due to the aforementioned cavitation effect. Pathogenetically, these alterations are rather comparable to those found along the shores of the lateral ventricles. In eight of our cases we have observed these periaqueductal lesions, which varied according to the survival time and included old hemorrhages, necroses, and fields of glia proliferation. On the other hand, the bruising not so infrequently seen along the sulcus lateralis mesencephali should also be regarded as a primary lesion. According to Krauland (1950, 1963), and Mayer (1968) this region is a favorite location for hemorrhages per rhexis.

A lightening of the tone of the myelin, almost regularly seen in the central region of the rostral pons and affecting equally the pyramidal tracts and the pontocerebellar fibers (Fig. 4), should be regarded as the direct result of an edematous imbibition of the tissues.

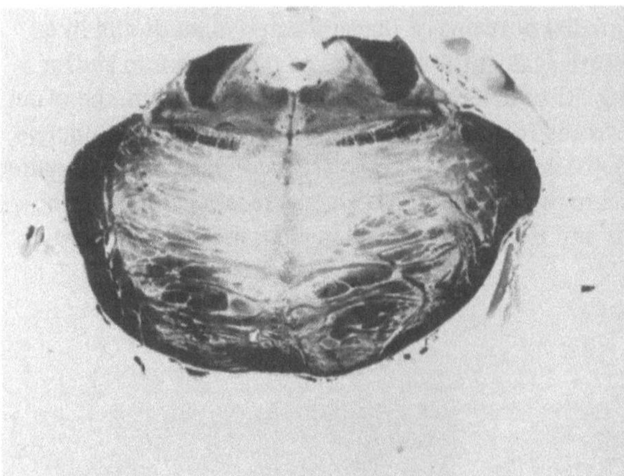

Pons: Section of the rostral portion

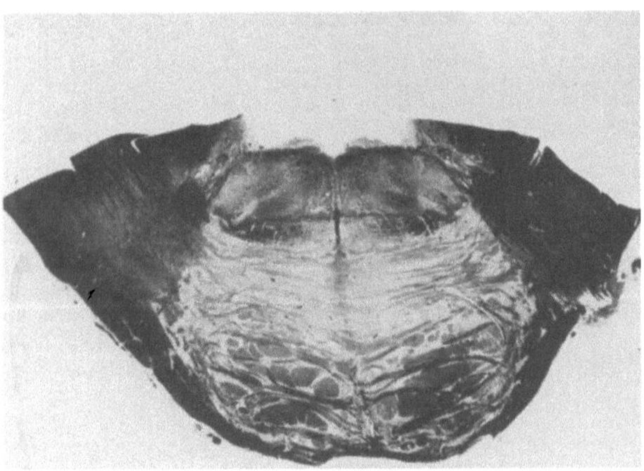

Pons: Section of the middle portion

Fig. 4. Survival time 23 days. Marked diffuse pallor of myelin sheaths in central portions of pons much more evident in rostral third than in middle third

This defect was observed in 14 cases. The glial reaction was frequently related to the degree of demyelination. In many cases the glial changes were, at any rate, minimal. Mayer (1968) was able to observe in his own material centrally located hemorrhages and edema a few hours after the trauma. With increasing survival time he spoke of a "peripheralward spread of the edema." Morphologically, the picture seen in the myelin preparations of our cases recalls the similar picture seen in cases of central pontine myelinolysis, which was first described by Adams et al. (1959).

In five cases the areas of necrosis in the mesencephalic tegmentum spread more or less widely, impinging upon the centrencephalic system. Furthermore, in four cases a focal accentuation of the glial hypertrophy and hyperplasia in the region of the aqueduct and in the deep tegmental gray matter was found. In other cases the intensity of the glial changes in these areas differed in no way from that observed in the remaining outlying regions of the midbrain. It should be mentioned, however, that in three of our cases the area corresponding to the reticular neurons appeared, at least on the slides which had been studied, by and large unchanged.

The glial reaction in the *red nucleus* could possibly be related to the destruction of the dentatorubral tract. However, this finding was equally present in three cases in which the brachia conjunctiva were intact. In one of these cases the glial changes went hand in hand with a rather severe neuronal depopulation of the red nucleus.

The lesions of the *pyramidal tracts* could be followed at different levels from the midbrain through the pons down to the medulla. In nine cases we found a loss of myelin and glial changes of variable degree, with a unilateral or bilateral distribution, in the cerebral peduncles. In 11 cases the pyramidal fibers appeared pale at the level of the pons. This finding was associated in two of these cases with a diffuse, rather severe paleness of the entire pontine basis. In nine cases a partial degeneration of the pyramidal tract of one side or of both sides at the level of the medulla oblongata was observed.

The pyramidal changes can be interpreted as wallerian degeneration of axons damaged at the upper levels by pathologic processes located in the cerebral white matter or in the internal capsule. In other cases the pyramidal changes can be regarded as resulting from purely local injurious events and mechanisms (Kernohan's notch, central edema of the pons, etc.). At the level of the medulla oblongata the pyramidal changes always represent a case of secondary wallerian degeneration.

In the medulla oblongata lesions other than those involving the pyramidal tracts were very modest and always secondary in nature. A unilateral and a bilateral pseudohypertrophy of the inferior olivas occurred in two cases. The nerve cells were extremely swollen, sometimes appearing only as pale discs. In addition, hypertrophy and hyperplasia of the glia with numerous multinucleated cells was observed, by all means far above the degree of neuronal wastage. The olivary hilus, as well as the neighboring tissues, was severely demyelinated, so that an involvement of the olivocerebellar tracts could be readily recognized. A disorder of the subcortical motoricity could also be suspected as a result of the lesions affecting the spino-olivary and olivospinal tracts.

Cerebellum

The cerebellar lesions, which have been discussed elsewhere by Gerstenbrand and Lücking (1970), were always secondary. Anatomically, we like to distinguish the lesions found in the brachia conjunctiva from those found in the vermis and in the cerebellar hemispheres. The superior cerebellar peduncles were damaged in six cases. In three cases the lesions were quite modest. A circumscribed area of incomplete edemanecrosis was seen in one case; in another, a grade II complete necrosis surrounded by a lacunar zone of edema at the upper edge of the brachium conjunctivum of one side could be observed. In both instances the clinical evolution had been relatively short (24 and 33 days respectively). Secondary changes in the nucleus dentatus were not noticeable. In the other three cases, with a survival time ranging from 4 1/2 months to 3 1/2 years, rather extensive areas of necrosis in the peduncles proper (twice bilaterally) and/or in the decussation were found. In the last three cases, retrograde degeneration of the nucleus dentatus was also apparent in the form of a severe loss of nerve cells and myelated fibers. In the single case with an isolated lesion in one of the peduncles there was a corresponding neuronal loss in the ipsilateral nucleus dentatus. One other case with a survival time of 11 months showed demyelination and massive fibrous gliosis of the hilus and fleece of the dentate nucleus of both sides.

In the cerebellar vermis a frequent and essential finding was a loss of Purkinje cells, a variably severe atrophy of the granular layer with a more or less heavy demyelination of the corresponding folia. In four cases the changes were diffusely and equally distributed over the entire vermian cortex; in six cases they were more conspicuous in the dorsal vermis and in three cases in the ventral vermis. Furthermore, in four cases there was a mild to moderate paleness of the central white matter and a limited glial reaction, similar to that observed almost regularly and to a much greater degree in the central white matter of the cerebellar hemispheres.

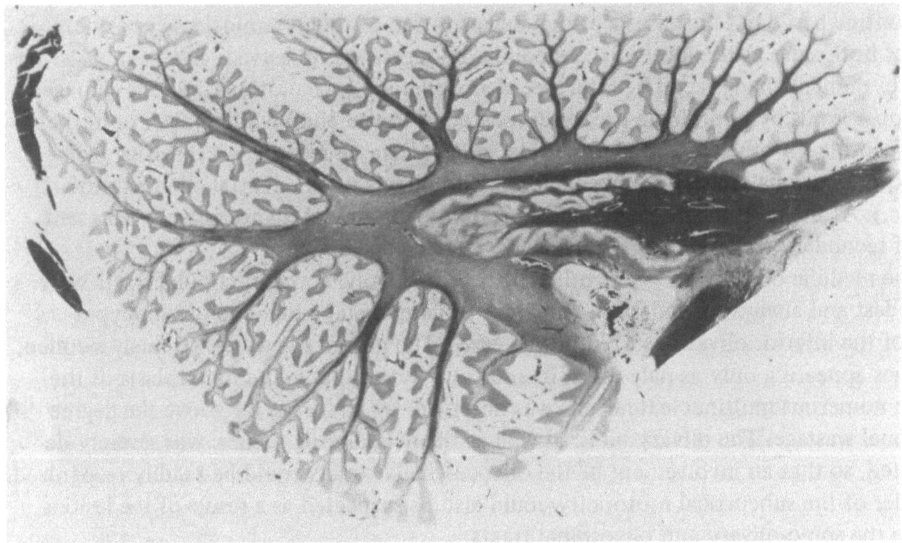

Fig. 5. Survival time 6 months. Diffuse demyelination of central cerebellar white matter. Fibers of the brachium conjuctivum appear well myelinated

Similar to the cerebral lesions, those in the *cerebellar hemispheres* appeared in the central white matter essentially as diffuse and edematous (Fig. 5). These lesions frequently correlated with those observed in the pons. Also, the degree of edematous imbibition was often the same for both regions (with one exception). In this way, in five cases a mild diffuse pallor a slight to moderate glial reaction could be determined, and in seven cases a moderate to profound loss of stainability of the myelin sheaths could be demonstrated. In the latter cases there was a correspondingly more pronounced cellular gliosis, whereas in a few isolated cases the fibrous gliosis was quite conspicuous. With the appropriate staining methods for nerve fibers, the axons in the most severely demyelinated areas often appeared swollen, fragmented, and reduced in number. Fully advanced axonal degeneration spread over larger areas was never observed.

Nothing remarkable was seen in any of the cases at the level of the inferior cerebellar peduncles.

Conclusions

A critical review of our clinical and pathologic data and of that reported in the literature suggests the following pathogenesis of the traumatic apallic syndrome.

The determining factor is the transtentorial herniation which in turn is the result of space-occupying intracranial processes. We are dealing here with epidural and/or subdural hematomas, rarely with intracerebral hematomas. Actually, the most frequent occurrence is posttraumatic edema. The tentorial herniation manifests itself clinically in the form of a more or less fully developed midbrain syndrome. In our experience the latter is not the result of primary traumatic lesions at the mesencephalic and pontine levels. This very finding signifies the reversibility of the clinical syndrome. If the venous and arterial disturbances caused by midbrain compression are promptly removed–hence the life-saving importance of an early and appropriate therapy–irreversible anatomic lesions need not occur, and the midbrain syndrome can resolve itself without ever developing into a full-fledged apallic syndrome. Similarly, in such a case brain edema need not cause permanent damage in the cerebral white matter. But if irreversible lesions in the midbrain and the cerebral white matter do occur, and if a traumatic apallic syndrome does develop, then the clinical syndrome is in essence the result of secondary processes, namely: the consequences of brain edema and of venous and arterial disorders caused by the transtentorial herniation at the level of the pons, the midbrain, the thalamus, the cerebellum, and certain areas of the cerebrum. The lesions in the brain stem can lead to abnormal vegetative reactions, such as a drop in blood pressure, disturbances of body temperature, and irregularities of respiratory function. These disorders can in turn cause bouts of recurrent edema and circulatory disturbances with corresponding tissue changes. Since in the brain stem, as well as in the cerebral white matter, damage to the axis cylinders and myelin sheaths is limited, a clinical recovery is still possible, even though often only partial. Labeling the clinical syndrome as functional decortication is therefore quite justified. The complexity of the clinical picture with its many manifestations of pyramidal, extrapyramidal, and cerebellar deficiency and/or irritation is to be explained by the multiplicity of lesions, including the secondary changes and the retrograde atrophies at the various levels and in the different nuclear masses of the brain. Sufficient proof now exists that the clinical syndrome is caused to a great extent by secondary lesions–which should prompt a measure of therapeutic optimism. The primary traumatic lesions in the cerebral cortex, seen at the most in only 50% of cases, play no determinant role among the cerebral lesions making up the morphologic substrate of the clinical syndrome. As for the development of the clinical picture of the traumatic apallic syndrome, the intensity of the trauma-producing force, which is often probably not particularly great, if one is to judge by the frequent lack of cortical contusions, is far less important than the posttraumatic phenomena leading to a transtentorial herniation.

14. Pathology and Pathogenesis of Apallic Syndromes Following Closed Head Injuries

K. JELLINGER

In patients with severe brain damage resulting from head injury who survived in apallic syndromes and related conditions, neuropathologic examination has demonstrated a large variety of cerebral lesions (Strich, 1956, 1969; Girard et al., 1963; Grcevic and Jacob, 1965; Jellinger, 1965a, 1968; Peters, 1969). However, little is known so far about correlation between the nature and distribution of the anatomic changes in the brain and the course and prognosis of the rather uniform clinical pictures of so-called traumatic apallic states (Gerstenbrand, 1967).

The present report is an attempt to summarize the neuropathologic findings during the apallic syndrome and its recovery states following closed head injury. Special reference will be given to the pathogenesis of the brain lesions and the clinicopathologic correlations, in order to give further insight into the pathophysiologic bases of these severe posttraumatic conditions.

Materials and Methods

Eighty cases of prolonged unconsciousness and apallic syndromes or their defect states were selected from a series of 700 necropsies of closed head injuries with survival times of several minutes to 1 year. The group of apallic patients includes 59 men and 21 women ranging in age from 5 to 86 years (average: 41 years) who either died without regaining consciousness or survived in various states of apallic syndrome for up to 301 days. The trauma was caused by a traffic accident in 82.5% of cases; the remainder were falls and other accidents. A considerable number were riders of motorcycles and scooters. According to the case histories, the skull was often hit in its sagittal axis or, rather frequently, by posterolateral forces which induced deceleration-acceleration trauma or combined translatory rotary acceleration. Pure lateral impact was rare.

All patients were unconscious from the time of the accident or went through initial or remittent states indicating severe brain stem dysfunction with ocular, motor, postural, and respiratory disorders, usually associated with flexor and/or extensor spasms. Five patients died during prolonged coma or midbrain syndrome 12-35 days (average: 23 days) after the accident. Forty-five patients died in fully developed apallic syndromes 12-257 days (average: 72.9 days) after the injury. In 30 cases showing signs of slight clinical improvement, death occurred in various transitional stages: 20 patients surviving 21-301 days (average: 93.5 days) were in the first stage of remission, whereas 10 patients died within 21-293 days (average: 126.7 days) after the accident in a severe defective state (severe stuporous "dementia").

Death was due to extracranial late complications, such as pneumonia, pulmonary embolism, septic states, uremia, or cardiac arrest, and rarely to cerebral complications of infectious or vascular origin (septic metastatic purulent or mycotic encephalitis, thrombosis of the large cerebral sinuses, etc.) which occurred in 20% of the cases but were responsible for the fatal outcome only in eight cases (10%).

Numerous specimens from all brains were examined histologically with special emphasis on elucidating the distribution of the lesions. The cerebral hemispheres, basal ganglia, and brain stems of most of these cases were semiserially sectioned and stained by histologic routine methods. The pathologic findings in 54 cases of this series and their clinical implications have been previously reported (Jellinger and Seitelberger, 1970).

Neuropathologic Findings

The brains usually showed multifocal lesions of both primary and secondary traumatic origin, often associated with late sequelae of these alterations or other late complications.

Primary Traumatic Craniocerebral Lesions

In spite of the severe blow to the skull, which can be assumed from the clinical histories and the type of injury, skull fractures were present only in 47.5% of the apallic patients, expanding intracranial hemorrhages (epidural and subdural hematomas) in 40%, and cortical contusions–often small and superficial–in 67.5% (see Table 1). By contrast, mechanical lesions in the deep cerebral regions were comparatively frequent: *hemorrhages in the cerebral white matter* were seen in 54%, with large expanding hematomas present in 10% of the cases. In addition to small hemorrhages in the subcortical white matter–probably from sheared veins in the frontal and temporal convolutions–multiple bleeding and necroses or their residuals were noted in about 25% of those brains. They may result, at least in part, from a "central caviation effect" (Unterharnscheidt and Sellier, 1965). These and other mechanical lesions, including tearing of nerve fibers, may later result in diffuse degeneration of the white matter (Strich, 1961, 1969). In long-surviving cases, however, the definite etiologic classification of posttraumatic degeneration of the cerebral white matter is almost impossible, as severe edematous and circulatory changes are often superimposed on the lesions of presumed mechanical origin at the moment of injury.

Hemorrhages and necroses in the basal ganglia considered as primarily traumatic in origin were observed in 46.2% of the patients (Table 1) and thus were considerably higher in frequency than in other necropsy series of brain injuries (Minauf and Schacht, 1966; Jellinger, 1967). Large hematomas present in six cases were either localized at the lateral margin of the putamen (Fig. 1A, B), which corresponds to the preferential site of traumatic vessel rupture due to rotation and tearing forces, or in the pallidum resulting from a tear in the branches of the anterior choroidal artery. Multiple small hemorrhages and their residuals chiefly situated in the vicinity of the ventricles were recognized in 35% of the cases. Often they were associated with callosal lesions and tears in the fornices–cortical contusions being absent in eight such brains–indicating "central cerebral trauma."

Table 1. Frequency of primary and secondary traumatic craniocerebral lesions in patients with apallic syndrome

Type of lesion	No. of cases	Percentage
Skull fracture	38	47.5
Intracranial epi- and subdural hematoma	32	40.0
Cortical contusion/laceration +++	7	
++	17	67.5
+	30	
No superficial brain lesion	26	32.5
Only subarachnoid hemorrhage	16	20.0
White matter hemorrhages		
Small	35	54.0
Large	8	
Diffuse white matter damage	50	62.5
Hippocampal lesions (secondary)	57	71.2
Corpus callosum lesion, total	40	50.0
Rupture	6	7.5
Focal damage (primary and secondary)	34	42.5
Basal ganglia lesions, total	58	72.5
Primary traumatic, small	27	46.2
Primary traumatic, large	6	
Secondary traumatic	48	60.0
Brain stem damage (secondary)	69	86.3
Focal lesions	58	
Diffuse damage	17	
Cerebellar involvement (secondary)	30/34[a]	85.0
Diffuse cortical lesion	16	
Focal infarctions	4	
Diffuse and focal lesions	10	

[a] Histologically examined cerebella.

Lesions of the corpus callosum—of primary and secondary traumatic origin—were present in 51.2% of the cases (Table 1), a figure much higher than that found in acute fatal head injuries (Minauf and Schacht, 1965). Strich (1961), on the other hand, noted callosal tears in all cases of severe "posttraumatic dementia." In addition to subtotal rupture of the corpus callosum in six cases, superficial unilateral or bilateral tears and hemorrhages

Fig. 1 A, B. 24-year-old motorcyclist hit by car (no skull fracture). Survival 118 days in ▷ akinetic mute state. Central trauma with cystic hemorrhage in lateral putamen (*x*), bilateral lesion of corpus callosum (*arrows*) with tear of the fornices, and compression necrosis in right hippocampal gyrus (*double arrows*). (A) Heidenhain's stain.
C. 29-year-old motorcyclist surviving traffic accident for 167 days in partial recovery state of apallic syndrome. Diffuse demyelination of left parietal lobe with sparing of the optic radiation. Spielmayer's stain.
D. 23-year-old scooter rider struck by car. Survived 155 days in deep apallic syndrome. Continuous cortical necrosis in medial occipital lobe due to compression of posterior cerebral artery branch. Heidenhain's stain.
E. 32-year-old woman (skiing accident). Survived 257 days after evacuation of epidural hematoma in apallic state. No primary traumatic brain lesions! Cystic compression necroses in supply areas of left anterior choroidal artery and right thalamo-perforate artery. Vascular lesions in corpus callosum and fornix. Compression necrosis in right hippocampal gyrus (*x*). Luxol fast blue

were present. They were often combined with tears of the septum pellucidum and of the columnae fornicis (Fig. 1A, B), with subependymal hemorrhages in the basal ganglia, and in the paraventricular white matter, causing a peculiar "butterfly-like" pattern of lesions (Grcevic and Jacob, 1965). Vascular lesions chiefly confined to the ventral and central parts of the corpus callosum (Fig. 1E) can be superimposed upon the mechanical changes and may obscure them.

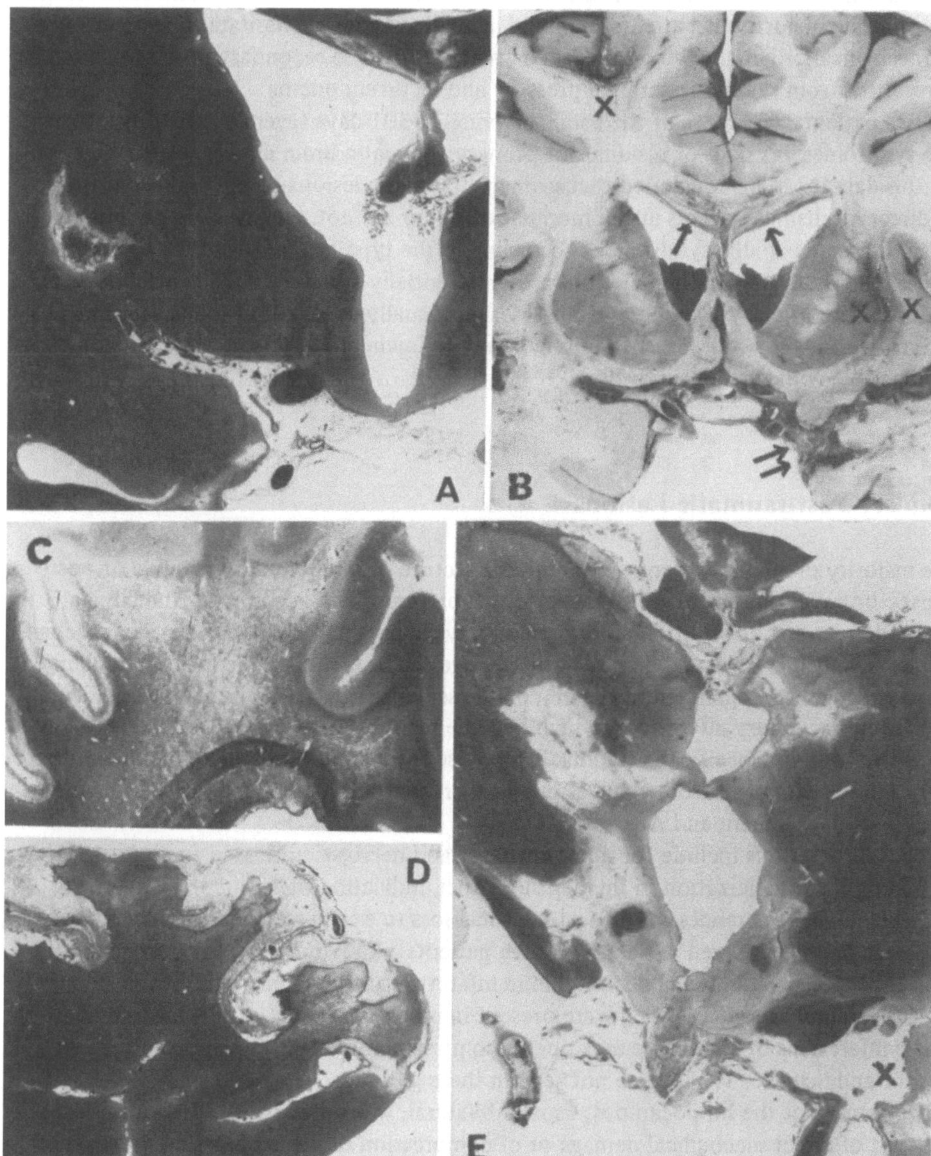

Fig. 1A-E. (Legend see p. 90)

As far as the brain stem lesions are concerned, recent studies suggest that patients with severe mechanical brain stem injuries will usually not survive longer than a few hours (Mayer, 1968; Jellinger, 1967; Peters, 1969), although some exceptional cases of supposed primary traumatic brain stem lesions with survivals of up to many years have been reported (Lindenberg, 1964; Huhn and Jakob, 1970). Although primary and secondary brain stem lesions are claimed to have characteristic patterns of distribution (Mayer, 1968; Crompton, 1971), after long survival a definite anatomic distinction between the residuals of both types of damage will be difficult or even impossible to make. However, for the brain stem lesions observed in the majority of patients surviving in apallic states, we hesitate to assume a primary mechanical origin and would prefer to attribute them to secondary posttraumatic effects resulting from raised intracranial pressure and recurrent edema.

In five patients, i.e., 6.3% of the total surviving 24-301 days (average: 130 days) in apallic syndromes, *no* signs or residuals of primary traumatic brain damage were observed. From this data it can be concluded that primary traumatic lesions of the brain resulting from direct mechanical effects at the moment of injury are not obligatory in patients surviving in traumatic apallic syndromes. According to the type of injury and the direction of impact to the skull, the anatomic lesions are preferentially situated in the central parts of the brain. These primary traumatic cerebral lesions usually account for the acute clinical syndrome with loss of consciousness immediately following the accident, but generally they are compatible with further survival.

Secondary Posttraumatic Lesions

In the majority of apallic patients the anatomic picture is dominated by reactive or posttraumatic brain lesions and their sequelae, which preferentially account for the clinical course and prognosis. In addition to local secondary changes in the surroundings of mechanical defects, multiple focal and diffuse brain damage can be included, the location and extent of which are highly independent of the immediate sequelae of trauma (Schewe and Adebahr, 1970). These secondary alterations, which become manifest after various intervals following the accident, are not specific for trauma. They arise from circulatory and anoxic disturbances, posttraumatic edema and from changes due to increased intracranial pressure (Lindenberg, 1971; Pia, 1957; Graham and Adams, 1971).

Neocortical lesions include focal hemorrhages and necroses unrelated to contusions with predominant localization in the depth of sulci, indicating their vascular origin (Fig. 1B). Ischemic damage ranges from focal neuronal loss to extensive laminar cortical necroses, which were present in seven patients; in three patients a known episode of posttraumatic cardiac arrest occurred. Medial occipital lobe infarcts resulting from compression of the posterior cerebral artery (Fig. 1D) were present in nine such brains (11.3%), while hemorrhagic infarctions of the striate area due to compression of the internal occipital vein (Adebahr and Schewe, 1967) were not seen in these patients.

Involvement of the hippocampus, usually bilateral, was noted in 71.3% of our series. As a result of direct mechanical damage or of compression of vessels crossing the level of the tentorial edge, sickle-shaped hemorrhages, superficial and deep focal necroses in the hippocampal gyri or Ammon's horn and their residuals were observed (Fig. 1A, B), which differ in location from typical hypoxic necrosis in Ammon's horn (Gerhard and Brölsch, 1970; Graham and Adams, 1971).

White matter damage, which has been considered to be one of the basic lesions in traumatic apallic syndromes (Strich, 1956, 1969; Ule et al., 1961; Girard et al., 1963; Osetowska, 1964), was seen to varying degrees in 62% of the author's cases. The following lesions of cerebral white matter could be distinguished: (1) Small focal necroses and glial scars in the subcortical and deep white matter which are assumed to result from tears and microlaceration of the nervous tissue (Strich, 1961; Oppenheimer, 1968). As 15% of our cases had received multiple fractures, the sequelae of cerebral fat embolism should also be taken into consideration. (2) Small perivascular necroses and hemorrhagic scars which may result from vascular tears and secondary circulatory disorders. (3) Flaky demyelination with sparing of the arcuate fibers in the vicinity of traumatic defects due to posttraumatic edema. (4) Diffuse white matter degeneration (Fig. 1C) with little sudanophilic decomposition products and large amounts of birefringent lipids with a large increase in esterified cholesterol (Holländer, 1964), indicating regular degradation of myelin with delayed lipid decomposition. This "posttraumatic leukoencephalopathy" (Osetowska, 1964) shows little astroglial response with minimal fibrillary gliosis. It may result in cyst formation, dilatation of the cerebral ventricles, and secondary degeneration of the large fiber tracts. Although the pathogenesis of diffuse posttraumatic white matter degeneration is still conjecturable, it is thought to result from a complex effect of degenerative changes secondary to mechanical lesions–e.g., shearing and disruption of nerve fibers (Strich, 1961, 1969; Nevin, 1967) and, also to posttraumatic vascular and edematous lesions (Ule et al., 1961; Jellinger, 1965a, b; Peters, 1969).

Posttraumatic hydrocephalus, which was present in more than half the author's cases, may result either from diffuse brain atrophy due to gray and white matter lesions (Fig. 1A and B) or from disorders of CSF circulation and resorption demonstrated by pneumencephalography and isotope cisternography. This high-pressure hydrocephalus promptly improves through ventriculoatrial shunting (Lewin, 1968; Zander, 1969).

Multiple focal damage to the basal ganglia was seen in 60% of the cases (Table 1), often located in the supply areas of branches of the anterior choroidal, posterior communicating and posterior cerebral arteries or in the drainage areas of the internal cerebral or intercrural veins. These lesions range from multiple infarctions in the thalamus, globus pallidus, subthalamus, and anterior hypothalamus (Fig. 1E) to unilateral or bilateral sclerosis of the thalamus or pallidum. Small necroses or hemorrhages in the walls and floor of the third ventricle (Fig. 1E) were noted in 22.5% of the cases. The separation of these lesions–often referred to as Duret-Berner hemorrhages–from residuals of primary traumatic damage may be difficult.

Brain stem damage was observed in 86.3% of the apallic patients (Table 1) and by far exceeded its incidence in acute fatal head injuries ranging from 12.2 to 65% of the cases (Mayer, 1968; Jellinger, 1967; Crompton, 1971). A comparison between the frequency of brain stem lesions, space-occupying intracranial hemorrhages, and other sequelae of increased intracranial pressure indicated clear-cut correlations between both parameters except for acute fatal head injuries (Jellinger and Seitelberger, 1970). These data strongly support the assumption that brain stem damage in posttraumatic apallic syndromes are of *secondary* traumatic nature. Three types of reactive brain stem lesions can be distinguished:

1. Focal damage (hemorrhages and infarctions), (70% of cases).

2. Diffuse damage to the brain stem tegmentum or basis (30% of cases, almost half of which were associated with focal lesions).

3. Central pontine myelinolysis and related lesions (four cases).

(1) *Focal brain stem lesions* are the mechanical and vascular sequelae of transtentorial herniation due to shift and distortion of the brain stem by increased supratentorial pressure and show a characteristic pattern of distribution. Superficial necroses in the dorsolateral mesencephalopontine tegmentum and tectum, including the quadrigeminal plate and brachium conjunctivum (Fig. 2A), result from compression by the free tentorial edge with or without circulatory disorders. Mechanical damage to the cerebral peduncles, particularly

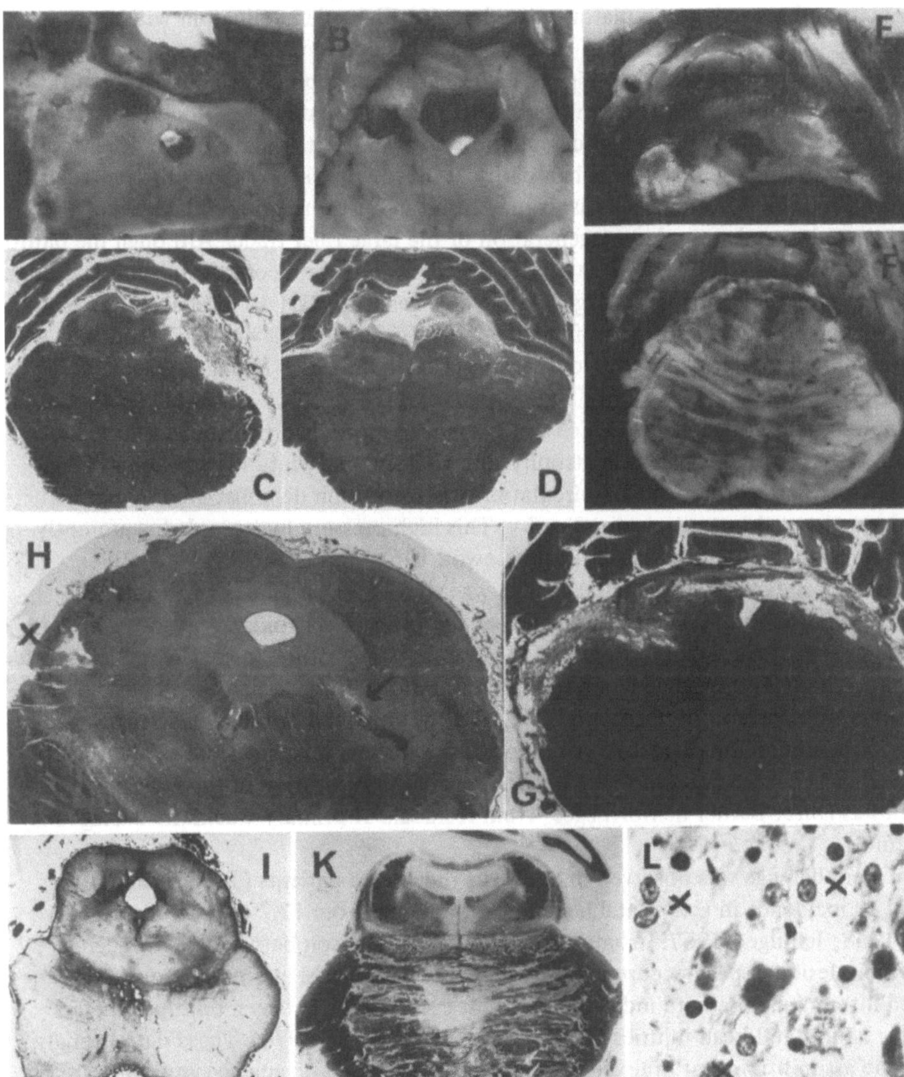

Fig. 2A-L. (Legend see p. 95)

at "Kernohan's notch," was seen in almost half of our apallic patients and was often combined with secondary degeneration of the pyramidal tracts. The majority of the brain stem lesions show a definite and common pattern of distribution indicating their vascular origin.

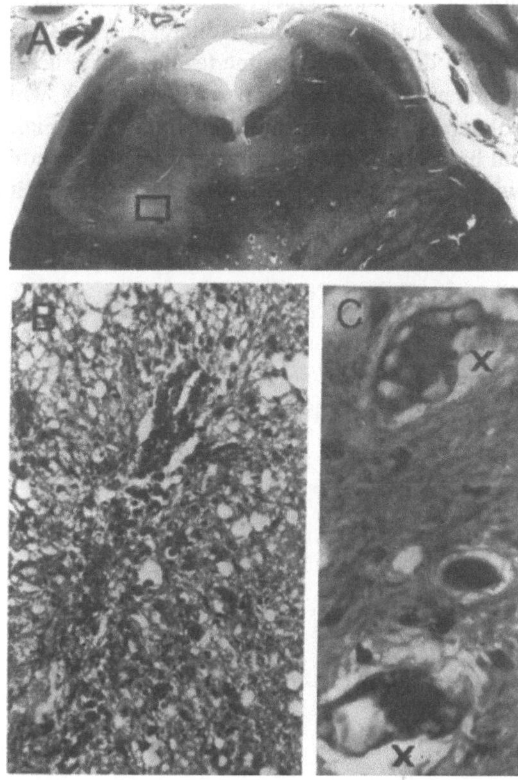

Fig. 3A. Small vascular necrosis in central tegmental tract, (B) histologically showing perivascular hemosiderin pigment.
C. Cytoplasmic vacuolation of degenerating neurons of the inferior oliva (*x*). H & E x 540

◁ Fig. 2A. Woman aged 47, survived fall (evacuated subdural hematoma) 30 days in first recovery state from apallic syndrome. Vascular necroses in posterior pulvinar and inferior colliculus.
B. Woman aged 48, died in deep apallic state 42 days after traffic accident. Necrosis in dorsolateral pontine tegmentum.
C, D. Woman aged 74 surviving car accident for 111 days in apallic syndrome. Compression necrosis of dorsolateral pontine tegmentum, involving rostral pontine reticular nuclei and central tegmental tract. Klüver-Barrera.
E-G. Motorcyclist aged 23, survived traffic accident for 160 days in apallic state. (E) Bilateral necrosis in mesencephalic tegmentum and sulcus mesencephali lateralis. (F) Rimlike necrosis in velum medullare anterius and pontine tegmentum. (G) Superficial necrosis in dorsal and lateral pontine tegmentum; atrophy of adjacent cerebellar gyri. Heidenhain's stain.
H. Man aged 39, survived drunken fall on occiput (without skull fracture or cortical contusions) for 28 days in apallic state, tegmentum and contralateral necrosis (*x*) in lateral tegmentum. Heidenhain's stain.
I. 30-year-old motorcyclist hit by car (no cerebral contusions!). Survived 301 days in partial recovery state of apallic syndrome. Diffuse glial fibrosis in periaqueductal gray matter, rostral pontine tegmentum, and substantia nigra. Kanzler-Arendt stain.
K. 11-year-old boy, survived traffic accident in apallic syndrome 84 days. Small demyelination focus in central pontine basis (pontine myelinolysis). Luxol fast blue.
L. Patient without alcoholic history. Spongy lesion of central basis pontis with incomplete demyelination and many "clear" glial cells (*x*), and preservation of neurons. H & E x 475

This pattern is schematically summarized on six transverse sections and correlated with the vascular supply of the human brain stem (Fig. 4). Many of these lesions follow the course of particular vessels or are situated in their central supply areas. Rimlike necroses in the pontomesencephalic tegmentum (Fig. 2F, G) and paramedian lesions in the midbrain tegmentum, including the periaqueductal gray, in the central gray of the midbrain and pons, and in the dorsolateral pontine tegmentum (Fig. 2B) result from compression of the long circumferential and superior cerebellar arteries, while lesions in the ventrolateral tegmentum, dorsolateral basis pontis, and substantia nigra (Fig. 2H) are due to compression of short lateral branches of the basilar artery. Peculiar median and paramedian brain stem lesions showing the features of incomplete necroses with intense gliovasal reaction are thought to

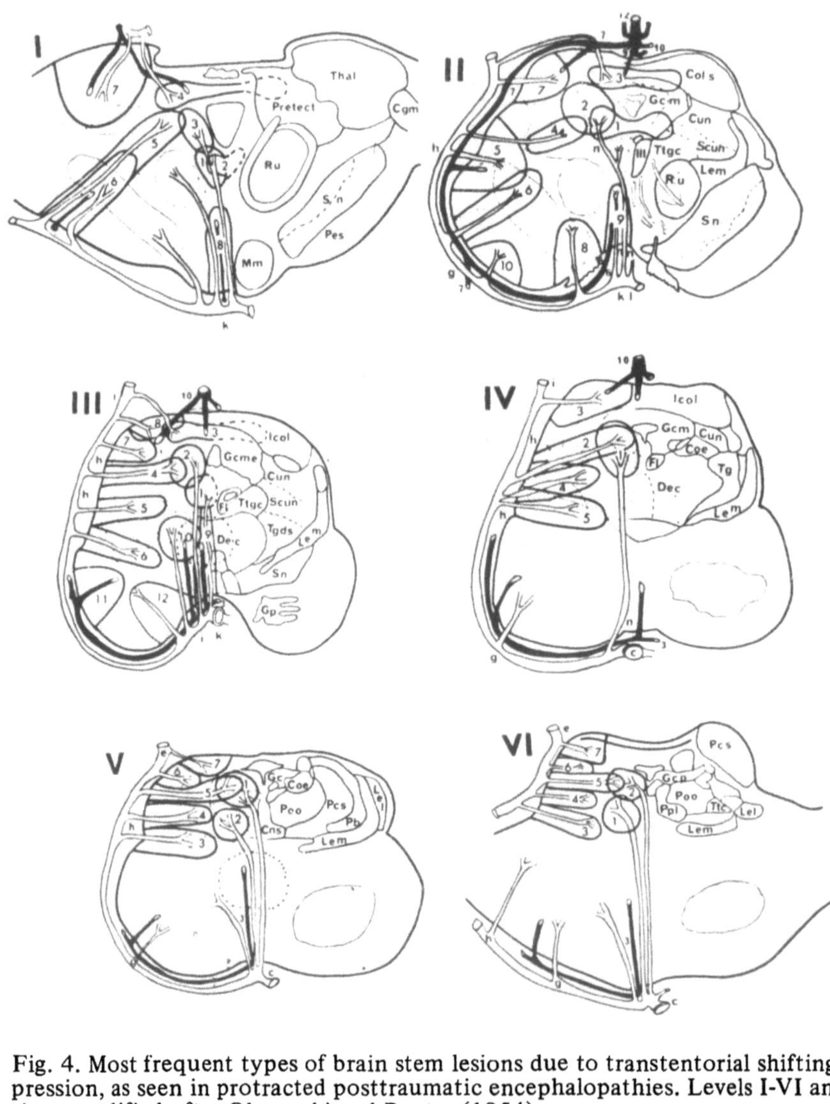

Fig. 4. Most frequent types of brain stem lesions due to transtentorial shifting and compression, as seen in protracted posttraumatic encephalopathies. Levels I-VI and abbreviations modified after Olszewski and Baxter (1954)

result from drainage disorders in the pontomesencephalic veins. Often multiple infarctions in different arterial and venous supply areas are observed.

The posttraumatic brain stem lesions closely resemble those in increased supratentorial pressure of varying origin (Zülch, 1955; Pia, 1957; Klintworth, 1968; Mayer, 1969). They show a local pattern similar to secondary brain stem damage in acute fatal cases of various origin. However, the lesions in long survivors are smaller and have a tendency to be more peripherally located in the lateral and dorsolateral tegmentum, whereas the median and paramedian necroses are usually confined to small central areas supplied by the perforating brain stem arteries or veins. Whereas rhectic hemorrhages and spongy necroses are common findings in acute fatal brain stem damage, ischemic infarctions and paramedian "pseudo-malacias" due to recurrent edema are much more frequent in apallic patients with long survival. From these findings one may assume that secondary brain stem damage, compatible with long survival, results from factors somewhat different than those operative in acute lethal brain stem lesions.

(2) *Diffuse damage and gliosis* of the brain stem without focal necroses were noted in 12 cases (15%). In addition to small spongy lesions, there was a diffuse increase in astrocytes often resembling the Alzheimer-II type of glia (Fig. 2L). After long survival, a dense glial fibrosis was noted in the tegmentum, periaqueductal gray and substantia nigra (Fig. 2I). In another 10 brains these changes were associated with small focal brain stem infarctions or hemorrhages, some of which were only detected on serial histologic sections. These diffuse changes, referred to as glial dystrophy of the brain stem, are considered, therefore, as an *abortive type* of posttraumatic brain stem damage. Chronic edema due to subacute or remittent obstruction of venous drainage and repeated compression of the brain stem in the tentorial hiatus are considered important pathogenic factors.

(3) In the base of the pons, butterfly-like vascular necroses were observed in two cases. They terminated in scars reminiscent of central pontine myelinolysis (Adams et al., 1959), which has been reported in chronic alcoholism, liver disease, malnutrition, after circulatory and endocrine catastrophes, and coma of varying etiology often associated with electrolyte disorders (McCormick and Danneel, 1967; Jellinger and Seitelberger, 1970). This latter type of lesion was seen in two apallic patients–an alcoholic, aged 37, who died 18 days after head injury in a remittent midbrain syndrome (Seitelberger and Jonasch, 1970), and a boy, aged 11, who died 84 days after head injury in an apallic syndrome due to chronic sepsis (Fig. 2K). The topical pattern of this peculiar demyelinating lesion in the drainage area of the anterior pontomesencephalic veins (Holdorff and Cervos-Navarro, 1971) may indicate venous drainage disorders, chronic edema or permeability disorders as important pathogenic factors, but metabolic disturbances of the neuroglia or more complex processes might also be operative. Diffuse myelin pallor and gliosis of the basis pontis, referred to as "diffuse pontine dystrophy" (Seitelberger and Gross, 1969) and which may represent an abortive type of the above lesion, was seen in 15 apallic cases (19%), only five of which had a history of chronic alcoholism.

In the *cerebellum* ischemic damage was identified in 85% of the histologically examined cases (Table 1). In the majority of cases there was diffuse ischemic damage, as shown by varying degrees of Purkinje cell loss or diffuse cortical atrophy; in seven cases circumscribed lobular atrophy was seen. Four cases showed infarctions in the upper cerebellar artery territories, while in about one-third of the cases a combination of diffuse and focal ischemic damage of the cerebellum was recognized.

Late Sequelae

Delayed consequences of primary and secondary traumatic lesions include secondary degeneration of various efferent and afferent fiber tracts (Strich, 1969), particularly of the corticospinal pathways, optic system, medial and lateral lemnisci from the pons upward, the superior cerebellar peduncles, dentatorubral and cerebello-olivary pathways.

Hypertrophy of the inferior olivas, associated with lesions of the dentato-olivary tract, usually of vascular or neoplastic origin (Rondot and Ben Hamida, 1968; Sohn and Levine, 1971) and rarely seen after head injury (Huhn and Jakob, 1970; Vuia and Rothemund, 1971), was recognized in eight apallic patients surviving between 23 and 185 days (average: 89 days). In none of them was palatal myoclonus reported. In two cases unilateral olivary degeneration resulted from focal vascular lesion in the ipsilateral central tegmental tract, in another two from necrosis in the superior cerebellar peduncle. Bilateral olivary hypertrophy due to bilateral damage to the brachium conjunctivum was present in two cases. In another case, it resulted from vascular necroses in both superior cerebellar peduncles and the dentate nucleus and in a further case from combined damage to the brachium conjunctivum and central tegmental tract. The pattern of olivary lesions in relation to the point of interruption of the olivopetal pathway was in full accordance with the topistic relations in the dentato-olivary pathway (Lapresle and Ben Hamida, 1970). The absence of palatal myoclonus rarely reported in traumatic apallic syndromes (Gerstenbrand and Machacek, 1968) could be explained on the basis of concomitant lesions in the reticular formations of the brain stem.

Clinicopathologic Correlations

The great variability and multiplicity of cerebral lesions associated with traumatic apallic syndromes and their defect state allows only limited conclusions regarding their pathophysiologic significance and relationship to the clinical course. In many apallic patients, however, a series of anatomic changes with constant patterns of distribution are obvious, which suggest certain important physiologic and clinical implications. In the present series of traumatic apallic syndromes, an attempt was made to correlate the clinical features with the anatomic brain lesions. In Table 2 the length of survival and the clinical condition at the time of death are compared with the most conspicuous anatomic brain changes regardless of their origin. The total number of lesions is greater than the number of cases which often showed multiple damage. Attempts were made to locate the lesions of the brain stem in precise anatomic structures.

For the classification of the clinical pictures ranging from deep unconsciousness (coma) to severe stuporous defect syndromes, four degrees of severity were recognized, following the clinical criteria established by Gerstenbrand (1967):

4 +: Deep coma or fully developed midbrain syndrome
3 +: Fully developed stage of apallic syndrome.
2 +: Slight improvement to first recovery state of apallic syndrome.
1 +: Severe defect state of partially recovered apallic syndrome.

Among five patients surviving in prolonged coma or midbrain syndrome (stage 4 +), four showed focal necroses in the periaqueductal gray matter or the dorsal wall and floor of the third ventricle. In two of them they were associated with other focal brain stem damage, in three with pallidothalamic infarctions, in one with central pontine myelinolysis, while diffuse white matter damage was present in one patient. Neocortical contusions were seen in four, hippocampal involvement in two cases. One brain showed diffuse gliosis of the brain stem without focal lesions in brain stem and basal ganglia.

From 45 patients who died in a fully developed apallic state (state 3 +), 27 showed unilateral or bilateral lesions at the posterior walls and floor of the third ventricle and/or in the rostral periaqueductal gray. In 19 patients there was associated focal damage to other brain stem areas. In 15 cases focal necroses involved the mesencephalic reticular formation, nine of them associated with other brain stem lesions, while in six cases softening merely affected the dorsolateral mesencephalic tegmentum, which was involved in a total of 17 cases of this group. Damage to the central pontine tegmentum, present in 16 cases, and to the dorsolateral pontine tegmentum (23 cases) almost never occurred without other brain stem lesions. In 12 brains diffuse gliosis of the brain stem was noted, but only in four of them were no focal brain stem lesions conspicuous; two were associated with multiple diencephalic necroses. Among three cases without definite brain stem damage, two displayed thrombosis of the large sinuses with extensive bilateral hemispheral infarctions, while the

Table 2. Clinicopathologic correlations of apallic syndrome and its recovery states

		Clinical condition			
			Apallic syndrome		
		Prolonged coma Midbrain syndrome	Full state	Slight recovery	Defect state
	No. of Cases	5	45	20	10
	Survival (days)	12-35	12-257	21-301	21-244
	Intracranial hemorrhage	2	20	8	4
	Cortical contusion or lesion	4	30	12	9
	Diffuse white matter lesion	1	27	15	7
	Diencephalic lesion	3	24	17	5
Lesions of the rostral brain stem	Floor of 3rd ventricle	1	17	0	0
		4	27		
	Periaqueductal gray matter	4	19	0	0
	Mesencephalon reticular formation	1	15	0	0
	Dorsolat. mesencephalon tegmentum	1	17	4	0
	Pontine reticular formation	2	16	3	0
	Dorsolateral pontine tegmentum	2	23	8	1
	Diffuse glial dystrophy	1	12	10	1
	Central pontine myelinolysis	1	1	0	0
	Hippocampal lesion	2	35	15	5

third showed multiple damage in the diencephalon and callosal rupture. Pallidothalamic necroses, often bilateral, were present in 24 such brains, diffuse damage of the hemispheral white matter in 27, neocortical contusions and ischemic involvement in 30, bilateral hippocampal lesions in 78%, and bilateral damage of the callosum-fornix system in 30%.

Among 20 patients showing slight clinical improvement in apallic syndromes (state 2 +), none displayed lesions within the floor of the third ventricle, the periaqueductal gray or the central mesencephalic reticular nuclei. Four revealed damage, usually combined lesions, in the dorsolateral mesencephalic and central pontine tegmentum, while in eight such brains focal damage was confined to the pons. Five showed involvement of the dorsolateral tegmentum without damage to the central and reticular nuclei. In ten cases diffuse gliosis of the brain stem was present, in only three accompanied by focal lesions. Two patients without definite brain stem damage showed multiple pallidothalamic necroses, which were absent in only three cases of this group. Diffuse white matter damage and bilateral hippocampal lesions were each seen in 75% of the cases, and cortical contusions or lesions and symmetric tears of the fornix were seen in eight such brains.

From among ten patients showing some recovery from apallic syndromes and dying in severe defect states (state 1 +), only one displayed focal brain stem damage, i.e., small necrosis in the brachium conjunctivum and a rimlike scar in the pontine basis. Another brain showed diffuse gliosis of the brain stem withou focal lesions. Multiple diencephalic changes were noted in five, and diffuse white matter degeneration in seven such cases. In three of them the latter was associated with extensive laminar cortical necroses due to cardiac arrest as a late complication. Extensive cortical contusions and lacerations were seen in five such brains, bilateral hippocampal involvement in a further five.

A comparison of the frequency and distribution of the most important anatomic findings in the four clinical groups of the present series of traumatic apallic syndromes and their recovery states provides strong support for the suggestion that brain stem lesions predominantly account for the clinical course and prognosis of these conditions.

Multiple focal, often bilateral lesions in the posterior wall and floor of the third ventricle, in the periaqueductal gray and in the central parts of the midbrain and rostral pontine tegmentum affecting the mesencephalopontine reticular formation were invariably associated with prolonged coma, coma vigile, akinetic mutism, or a complete apallic syndrome without remarkable clinical improvement. None of our patients with such localized lesions regained responsiveness. In addition, severe optomotor and postural disturbances akin to a state of chronic "decerebration" and a disturbed sleeping-waking rhythm were observed.

The first remission phase of the apallic syndrome (Gerstenbrand, 1967) was also seen in cases with partial alteration of the mesencephalic and pontine reticular core associated with lesions in the dorsolateral midbrain and pontine tegmentum or damage to the caudal central pontine tegmentum. Similar clinical conditions were associated with bilateral damage to the pallidothalamo-subthalamic regions. In *none* of these fatal cases, however, could fully developed apallic states be reasonably attributed to diffuse degeneration of the hemispheral white matter alone, because all were associated with focal damage to the diencephalon and/or the rostral brain stem.

The only patient in this group who showed severe white matter damage and laminar neocortical necroses without brain stem lesions slowly improved to incomplete apallic syndrome with some reaction to the environment.

It should be emphasized that only one of those patients who regained consciousness showed peripheral damage to the rostral brain stem tegmentum. On the other hand, severe organic defect syndromes akin to incomplete apallic states (Ingvar and Brun, 1972), or "stuporous severe dementia" (Strich, 1961; Crompton et al., 1966) were associated with diffuse white matter damage and widespread telencephalic cortical lesions with or without pallidothalamic changes, but without any significant damage to the brain stem and its reticular core.

Conclusions

Secondary brain stem lesions, observed in a large number of cases of prolonged coma and apallic syndromes after head injuries (Struck, 1963; Jellinger et al., 1963; Jellinger 1965a, b; Crompton et al., 1966; Mayer, 1968, 1969; Peters, 1969; Jellinger and Seitelberger, 1970), are assumed to play a decisive role in the etiology of these posttraumatic conditions. The damage often affects central parts of the rostral brain stem and basal diencephalon, involving the rostral mesencephalic activating system and/or the nonspecific diencephalic projection system. These lesions account for persistent impairment of responsiveness, "loss of behavior," and conditions comparable to chronic functional decerebration.

The above findings agree with numerous clinical, neuropathologic and experimental data which suggest that the regions upon the integrity of which consciousness depends are situated in the central core of the rostral brain stem, corresponding to the oral parts of the "reticular ascending activating system" (Hassler, 1967; Jouvet, 1969; Ingvar et al., 1970). The same is true for the experimentally induced localization of regulating areas of sleep and wakefulness (Moruzzi, 1972) and of postural mechanisms. Many patients suffering from brain stem damage passed through or died in a condition referred to as "akinetic mutism" or "coma vigile," which is in accordance with other clinical-pathologic and experimental data (Skultety, 1968). In some patients a hypokinetic state with decreased vocal output but intact sleep-waking rhythm could be attributed to bilateral damage to the thalamopallidal system in the absence of brain stem lesions. This agrees with our present knowledge of the role of the "diencephalic nonspecific projection system" (Hassler, 1967). If there is damage to these nonspecific cortical projection systems at the mesencephalopontine or diencephalic level, other lesions in telencephalic regions appear to be of minor importance for the development of apallic states. In the absence of considerable involvement of the central reticular core and other nonspecific projection systems, however, the pattern and severity of lesions in other parts of the brain–particularly in the telencephalic gray matter (neocortex), in the hemispheral white matter, and in the limbic system–will mainly account for the clinical syndrome.

Apallic syndromes due to diffuse destruction of the telencephalic gray matter with relative preservation of the brain stem–referred to as "neocortical death" (Brierley et al., 1971) or "complete" apallic syndrome (Ingvar and Brun, 1972)–have been reported after cardiac arrest with long survival (Amann et al., 1971; Brierley et al., 1971; Ingvar and Brun, 1972). However, these conditions are rarely observed as a result of head injury, except for a few cases with posttraumatic episodes of cardiac arrest. In our material there are three such cases of apallic states associated with extensive destruction of the neocortex. Two of them showing no clinical improvement had additional brain stem damage, while one patient with "incomplete" apallic defect syndrome displayed widespread cortical necrosis and diffuse white matter degeneration without brain stem damage.

The evidence available from the present series and from the findings of other authors strongly suggests that in posttraumatic conditions the clinical course and prognosis depend primarily on the integrity of the rostral brain stem and, in particular, of the nonspecific reticular projection systems. The fact that some improvement of the apallic syndrome was only recognized in the absence of considerable damage to the brain stem and its mesencephalopontine reticular formation favors the major importance of brain stem damage, usually secondarily traumatic in nature, for the clinical course of these conditions. From the available data, we would contend that *lesions in the oral brain stem are the most frequent causes of posttraumatic apallic syndromes and related prolonged disorders of consciousness.* In the majority of cases these conditions can be reasonably attributed to the blocking of cortical functions resulting from damage to the mesodiencephalic activating systems which cause chronic decerebrate states. Only in a fairly small number of cases does diffuse involvement of the truncocortical junctions due to widespread white matter degeneration or extensive destruction of the telencephalic gray matter account for apallic states and related syndromes following head injury. It should be admitted, however, that all the neuropathologic findings mentioned are highly nonspecific and may occur in severe brain damage of different etiology—e.g., as a result of head injury, cerebrovascular accident, cardiac arrest or increased intracranial pressure, associated with lesions either of the ascending activating systems at various levels or in the telencephalic gray matter, all of which may result in rather uniform clinical pictures (Plum and Posner, 1966; Gerstenbrand, 1967). On the other hand, certain differences between coma and akinetic mutism (coma vigile) due to brain stem lesions and the so-called apallic syndrome *sensu strictu* due to neocortical damage (i.e., destruction of the cerebral pallium) have been emphasized (Ingvar and Sourander, 1970; Ingvar and Brun, 1972). Whether or not a definite clinical and pathophysiologic separation of these conditions—usually associated with impaired consciousness—and a satisfactory correlation between the pattern of anatomical brain lesions and the clinical neurophysiologic data, including EEG and cerebral blood flow, is possible remains open for discussion.

Summary

The neuropathologic findings in 80 cases of apallic syndrome and related conditions following closed head injury are reported. The length of survival was from 21 to 301 days. Most injuries resulted from road traffic accidents. The brains showed multifocal damage of primary and secondary traumatic origin, often associated with the late sequelae of these lesions and other late complications. Skull fractures (47%), intracranial expanding hemorrhages (40%), and cortical contusions (67%)—often small and superficial—were less conspicuous than the results of mechanical damage to central parts of the brain, i.e.,basal ganglia (46%), hemispheral white matter (54%), and corpus callosum (51%), while no definite sequelae of primary brain stem damage was recognized. In five cases, no signs of mechanical brain injury were detected. In the majority of cases, the anatomic picture was dominated by secondary or reactive lesions due to posttraumatic circulatory disorders and raised intracranial pressure. In addition to ischemic neocortical lesions and diffuse white matter damage (60%), multiple lesions were seen in the basal ganglia (60%), Ammon's horn (71%), corpus callosum, and cerebellum (80%). The most conspicuous findings were secondary brain stem lesions encountered in 86.3% of this series. These sequelae of transtentorial herniation show characteristic patterns of distribution which differ in some respects from those in acute fatal cases. Brain stem damage includes focal lesions (70%), diffuse changes (30%), and occasional damage to the pontine basis. Comparing the clinical data and anatomic findings, there is evidence that secondary brain stem lesions chiefly account for the clinical features and prognosis of these posttraumatic conditions. Frequent involvement of central parts of the upper brain stem and its reticular core accounts for persistent impairment of responsiveness and conditions akin to chronic decerebrate states. Apallic syndromes due to neocortic and white matter damage without brain stem lesions are rarely seen after head injuries. The possibilities of separating apallic states and related conditions due to lesions at various sites of the CNS (pallium, white matter, brain stem) are critically discussed.

15. Pathomorphologic Aspects of the Nontraumatic Apallic Syndrome and of the Problem of Traumatic Brainstem Lesions with a Survival of Several Decades

G. ULE

We find nontraumatic apallic syndromes after acute incidents with initial coma and sometimes in the final states of progressive organic diseases of the brain. We do not intend to give a complete list of the eligible pathomorphologic equivalents, nor of the "specific" alterations of the brain. In this respect, "specificity" only exists for the topographic pattern of the alterations, not for their qualities. Jellinger (1965a, b) hinted at the fact that the apallic syndrome as a summation of various pathogenic factors is always based on complex organic damage of the brain. This statement is doubtlessly right for most cases. But it does not release us from the duty to investigate the morphologic damage of each case as thoroughly as possible and to identify the *Störstelle* responsible for the apallic syndrome. As we know today, the location of such a fault can vary from the cortex to the white matter, and also to the brain stem. Considering our experiences with the amnestic syndrome, where different locations of release (neocortical, diencephalic=corpora mammillaria, and archicortical=hippocampus) cause different types of clinical symptoms (Störring et al., 1962), we can suppose that also in the apallic syndrome clinical differences result from different topistic patterns.

Upon the suggestion of G.E. Störring, in 1959 Kretschmer's nearly forgotten term "apallic syndrome" was adopted for the traumatic cases (Ule, 1959; Ule et al., 1961). At that time we were totally under the influence of the cases of severe myelin lesions reported by Sabina Strich and ourselves. The term "apallic" seemed to clarify most impressively these damages to the myelin matter, and this fact grew in importance when similar severe lesions of the white matter in our first case of nontraumatic apallic syndrome were found: Grinker's myelinopathy in a woman who died at the age of 68, 5 months after an intervallic CO intoxication. We considered the severe diffuse lesions of the white matter to be the most important pathogenic factor causing the apallic syndrome. Our opinion was confirmed by the next two cases, which also showed identically large destructions. A 7-year-old girl developed an apallic syndrome after a coma of several days following an appendectomy under barbiturate anesthesia. There was no respiratory or cardiac arrest. Thirteen months later she died from an intercurrent disease. The pathoanatomic findings were a pattern of damage of hypoxemic hypoxidosis with myelinopathy (Fig. 1) and bilateral pallidum softening, and an extreme cystic destruction of the white matter extending in both hemispheres from the frontal to the occipital lobes. Except for little foci of softening in the pallidum, no other losses in the brain stem and the cerebellum were found. This type of postnarcotic encephalopathy, which is different from common anesthesia incidents and is reminiscent of intervallic CO intoxication, is pathogenically hardly understandable.

According to Kreuscher (1967), it is possible that during anesthesia, especially with barbiturates, the circulation and intake of oxygen of the brain can be reduced to 50% or

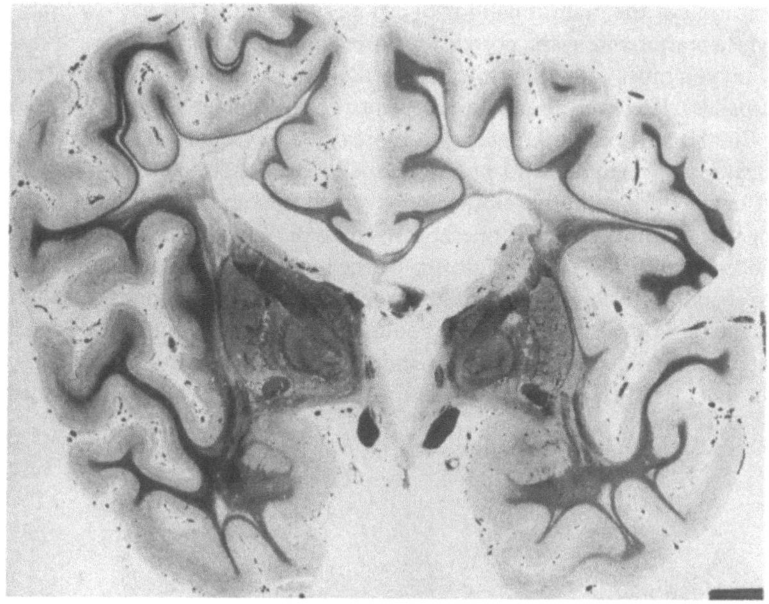

Fig. 1. Postanesthetic encephalopathy of hypoxemic-hypoxidosis pattern; apallic syndrome

even lower. The explanation is perhaps that, in these fatal cases, individual factors are responsible for such an extreme depression of the oxygen intake which causes the pattern of damage of the hypoxemic hypoxidosis.

On the other hand, it must be kept in mind that disturbances of the microcirculation in a postoperative protracted collapse with disseminated microthrombosis and consumption-coagulopathy are capable of producing lesions in the white matter which sometimes resemble the alterations found with the Grinker myelinopathy in the intervallic CO poisoning.

The latter case demonstrates the reverse course of development of the apallic syndrome. It does not originate from an inital coma but develops in the course of a progressive organic brain disease. In this case it was a diffuse form of multiple sclerosis (MS) (Ule et al., 1965) with large merging regions of demyelinization from the frontal to the occipital lobe. The brain stem and cerebellum proved to be completely intact. The 26-year-old patient died after 4 months of illness. His MS had started with neurologic focal symptoms, had led to a complex of anoetic symptoms in the sense of Duensing (1949), then to the apallic syndrome, and finally to a terminal coma with decerebrate rigidity caused by terminal edema. The only morphologic equivalent of the apallic syndrome which had clinically dominated was the large demyelinization of the white matter as the expression of a homogeneous process with the consequence of a blockage of the alternate truncocortical connections. So the situation is much clearer than in the multifactorial constellation of traumatic brain lesions which, moreover, often have a multilocal distribution.

Doubtlessly there are also alterations in the brain stem which lower the levels of function and efficiency of the brain down to those of the apallic syndrome. Nevertheless, such cases have been rare in our Heidelberg subjects. This is surprising, since, according to the organization of the brain, small losses can be sufficient in the narrow brain stem area. In the white matter and in the cortex the corresponding structures have spread out. Therefore, a lesion must be bigger here than in the brain stem in order to cause similar functional disturbances. However, there are exceptions to this rule, which will be explained in the last case. Firstly, two cases of apallic syndrome caused by bilateral foci in the brain stem: *First case:* A woman of 72 lost consciousness 1 week after an appendectomy without complications. After another week the coma turned into an apallic syndrome which lasted until her death 2 months after the operation. Anatomic findings: Increased stenosing sclerosis of the aa. vertebrales, subtotal closing of the hypoplastic aa. communicantes posteriores with pseudocystic cortical infarct in the left occipital region, and encephalomalacias of identical age in the brain stem [left peduncles and tegmentum of the mesencephalon, hypothalamus, and bilaterally in the medial nuclei of thalamus, in the region of the a. thalamoperforata (Fig. 2)]. The brain stem lesions with the involvement of the formatio reticularis

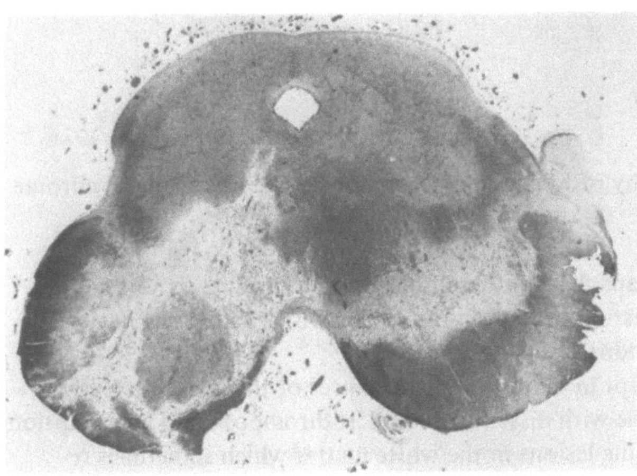

Fig. 2. Arteriosclerotic softening in brain stem; apallic syndrome

are comparable to the case of Lehrmitte et al. (1963). *Second case:* Bilateral necrosis of nucleus lentiformis can also result in an apallic syndrome–for example, in a 16-year-old boy who for 18 days survived a suicidal intoxication with potassium cyanide (Fig. 3). The secondary circulatory brain stem lesions after upper transherniation in respect to apallic syndrome have been thoroughly discussed by Peters (Chapter 13) as well as by Jellinger (Chapter 14).

The importance of large cortical damages in respect to apallic syndrome (Grünthal, 1941) has often been emphasized in the last few years. To support this I will cite two slightly difficult cases.

Eleven days after a proctologic operation a man of 38 went into a coma with respiratory and cardiac arrest, necessitating instant reanimation. In the days that followed, the coma turned into an apallic syndrome. Bronchopneumonia caused death 1 1/2 weeks after cardiac arrest. The autopsy showed a coronary sclerosis of the juvenile type with severe stenosis, but no myocardial infarction. In the brain, ubiquitous pseudolaminary cortical necrosis, especially in the third and fourth layer, and a bilateral "pseudomalacia" in the corpora

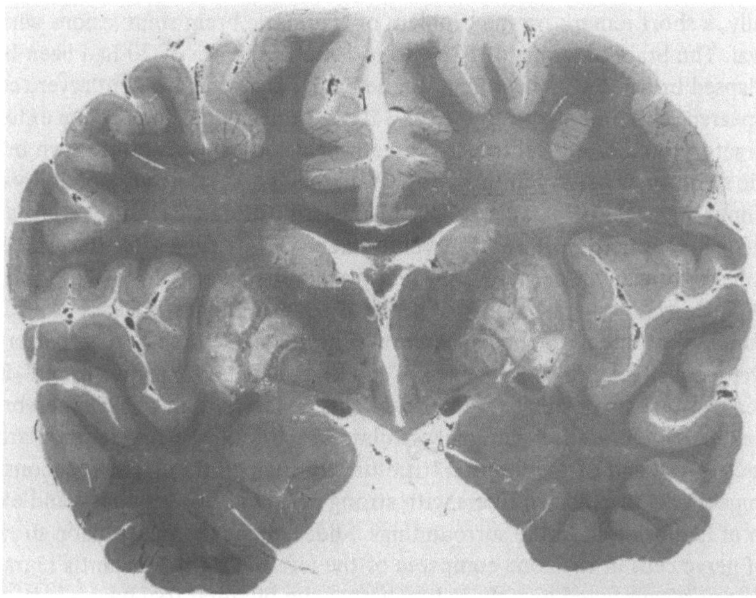

Fig. 3. Bilateral necrosis of nucleus lentiformis after potassium cyanide intoxication; apallic syndrome

mammillaria was found. Also, the putamen and thalamus were disparenchymized. Thus, in this observation cortical and truncal lesions were combined, and in my opinion, pure cortical forms of apallic syndrome will be rare. The alterations of the corpora mammillaria memtioned above could lead to another interpretation. In view of the chronic alcoholism of the patient and his intolerance to alcohol during the last weeks, the possibility of a Wernicke encephalopathy must be discussed. The other locations of predilection in the Wernicke syndrome, however, were intact. Consequently, the alteration of the mammillary bodies should be due to anoxic-vascular damage.

The next case appears to represent a very rare pattern causing apallic syndrome. Four years before her death, a woman of 41 underwent a portocaval shunt operation because of bleeding esophageal varices after cirrhosis of the liver. She developed a so-called ammonia encephalopathy with 430 gamma% ammonia in her blood serum, concomitant neurologic symptoms, and in the last 2 years repeated precomatose states which could always be therapeutically compensated until 6 weeks ante mortem, when she developed a coma which lasted a few days and subsequently an apallic syndrome. The neuropathologic findings revealed two different alterations of the brain. Firstly, a hepatogenic encephalopathy with Alzheimer II glia and spongy degeneration in the striatum, but rarely in the cortex, was found. Secondly, there were vasocirculatory anoxic cortical lesions dating to the last coma, but limited to the valleys of the sulci. The size of these additional cortical lesions alone cannot explain the apallic syndrome. Obviously the additional, relatively small ischemic cortical losses unbalanced the already altered brain (hepatogenic encephalopathy) in such a way that, in spite of amelioration of the serum ammonia level, the coma could be improved only to the degree of an apallic syndrome. The patient died 4 weeks later of pneumonia.

Finally, a short remark on the problem of traumatic brain stem lesions with many years of survival. The brain of a man of 52, who in 1936 at the age of 20 had been buried alive by a collapsed bridge,[1] was examined. Immediately after the accident severe cerebral symptoms appeared, with unconsciousness for 3 days, tonic convulsions of the extensors, wide light-refractory pupils, and centrogenic breathing disorders. It is not known if he developed an apallic syndrome. After 4 months he was discharged in relatively good physical condition without any signs of paralysis. Only inconstant differences in the reflexes of the legs remained. There is no report on his psychic state. A short time after the accident he gave up his job as a bricklayer because of headaches. He then worked in a store and as a packer until 1965. He was not drafted in World War II. During the last 9 years of his life he suffered from hypertonia with clinical cerebral symptoms. He died 37 years after the accident from pyelonephritis. As a consequence of the original head injury we found–in the absence of cortical contusions or other traumatic defects–bilaterally in the crus cerebri old foci, partly callously indurated, including rostrolateral parts of the substantia nigra, parts of the corpus Luysi, and of the internal structures of the pallidum. The foci consisted centrally of a compact part of collagen fibers with strong perifocal fibrous gliosis and exuberant deposition of hemosiderin in the surroundings. Slides of the mesencephalon showed focal losses of nerve cells in the zone compacta of the left and right substantia nigra.

It cannot be answered exactly as to whether the bilateral foci have a primary traumatic genesis or whether they are secondary consequences. But it is remarkable that the mechanical influence on the skull came from above (the patient had been standing under the bridge before it collapsed) and that the clinical mesencephalic symptomatology obviously occurred immediately after the accident. Sub- or epidural hematomas did not exist, and there were no other contusions which could have led to a posttraumatic brain edema with transtentorial herniation. The compact scars with collagen fibers and many deposits of hemosiderin show more evidence of an old rhexis bleeding than of a secondary softening.

Therefore, these foci seem to have a primary traumatic genesis, although a subsequent secondary transtentorial herniation cum sequelibus cannot be excluded. Another remarkable aspect of this brain stem contusion, which allowed survival for 32 years, is the discrepancy between the clinical findings and the anatomical results; in spite of grave losses in the substantia nigra the patient never showed clinical Parkinson symptoms when being neurologically examined. Thus, as Eicke found as early as 1943, negative clinical findings do not necessarily exclude grave morphologic losses in the substantia nigra.

---

[1] Case report by Huhn and Jakob: Nervenarzt **41**, 326-334 (1970).

16. Neuropathologic Correlates of Supratentorial Lesions in Traumatic and Nontraumatic Apallic Syndrome

N. GRČEVIĆ

Since it is impossible to produce experimentally a clinical condition which would correspond to the apallic syndrome in man, the only reliable source of information remains the human model, i.e., the clinicopathologic correlation of human cases. However, there has not yet been a general agreement on the various aspects and criteria of definition for the syndrome. Because of this, the clinical data received by the neuropathologist may vary from place to place giving the correlation a rather subjective flavor. The other problem on the clinical side of the correlation is the technical value and grade of precision of clinical data. The apallic patients with long survival are sometimes too routinely followed and recorded in the latter stages of the disease. In such cases it is sometimes difficult to reconstruct precisely the course of the disease and the chronology of events, which may be of great importance for the later anatomic analysis. On the other hand, the acute cases—especially traumatic and ischemic ones—are often, during the whole first phase of the disease, treated in general hospitals or emergency units of general surgery, where some of the special neurologic examinations may not be carried out, with the result that important information may later be missing. Taking into account the fact that the apallic syndrome is essentially a transient clinical phenomenon, a syndrome of unpredictable onset, of variable course, and of varying duration, it is understandable that we have to be able to operate with very accurate records on the course of the clinical disease in which the apallic syndrome occurred. Otherwise, we are correlating a certain morphologic picture with an uncertain or not clearly defined clinical phenomenon which was only temporarily a part of the clinical symptomatology. In other words, the anatomic substrate of the apallic syndrome in a given case may be only a small part of an otherwise very widespread pathologic process. The division of the apallic syndrome into various phases—as Gerstenbrand (1967) did—may be of help in the anatomicoclinical correlation if the criteria for such division are generally accepted and if the "phases" of chronologic development are promptly and precisely identified and recorded.

The clinical difficulties, however, also arise from the fact that the apallic syndrome may occur in various diseases and at very different times or stages of the clinical course of such diseases. Thus, in some cases the apallic syndrome occurs in earlier phases and disappears gradually in the further process of recovery or remains arrested for long periods of time. In other cases, however, the apallic syndrome displays an opposite chronologic pattern, occurring in the late stages, or even as a terminal sign in fatally progressing cerebral disease. The "phases" valid for the traumatic apallic syndrome may be quite reversed in some nontraumatic examples. In such a complicated and variegated problem the results of clinical observations and study are not only subject to the precision of recording but also to the number of observations. Thus, the statistical significance can only be achieved if a large amount of material is studied by the same methods and according to the same criteria.

The main problem on the neuropathologic side of a correlative study of the apallic syndrome is in the methodologic approach to the examination of the brain. Complete information on the pathologic process in the brain can only be obtained if the whole brain is histologically examined. Several types of lesions and various changes have been described in the brains of patients who had the apallic syndrome. The localization and spreading of the lesions vary substantially, but some typical patterns of distribution have been established.

The conditions in which the apallic syndrome most frequently occurs have the bulk of the pathologic process localized in the supratentorial areas of the brain. Following is a brief discussion of some of the most frequent models of supratentorial correlates of the apallic syndrome, such as subacute sclerosing panencephalitis, diffuse sclerosis, cerebral hypoxia, closed brain injury, and glioblastoma of the corpus callosum.

In the case of *subacute panencephalitis* we are searching for the anatomic correlate of a late or terminal clinical phenomenon within an extremely widespread pathologic process in the brain (van Bogaert, 1965; Nagel et al., 1959; Weingarten and Seitelberger, 1953). This means that the reconstruction of the pattern of distribution will be of little use without a good evaluation of the chronology of the lesions. The pattern of distribution of the process in subacute panencephalitis is well known. Although the gray matter (cortex) is also attacked, the bulk of the process is in the hemispheral white matter, which undergoes severe morphologic changes. The observations from our study of a series of cases with various survival times showed that the progress of the disease is not followed by expansion of the pattern of distribution of the lesions, but rather by qualitative deterioration of histologic changes within the basic and original pattern. The qualitative deterioration of the histologic picture in cases with long survival times extends to almost complete destruction, demyelination and even spongy and lacunar disintegration. The glial proliferation is sometimes so pronounced that in one of our cases who survived for 7 years the picture in low magnification looked like diffuse sclerosis. In none of our cases could we find evidence of the spread of the process toward the new regions in the late stages of the disease. This fact makes the model of panencephalitis especially interesting for correlation with other models and indicates that the "apallic phase" of the disease has its basis within the standard pattern and not in some other "new lesions."

The model of *diffuse sclerosis* (Fig. 1) is much less known, and only a few cases have been described with a clinical picture of an apallic syndrome (van Bogaert and Scholz, 1932; Born and Binder, 1962). Diffuse sclerosis makes up the bulk of the pathologic process in the paraventricular white matter, centrum semiovale, and corpus callosum. Here, too, the substrate of the apallic syndrome is located within this pattern of lesions similar to that of later stages of panencephalitis.

Quite the opposite is the well-known model of the apallic syndrome in *hypoxic encephalopathy* due to cardiac arrest or other causes of sudden reduction or stoppage of the blood supply to the brain (Brierley and Cooper, 1962; Gross et al., 1955; Haberland, 1961; Hornet and Petrescu, 1961; Lindenberg, 1963; Sayk, 1961; Scholz et al., 1959; Steegmann, 1961). Here the main pathologic process develops in the cerebral cortex and in the gray matter although the white matter may be involved secondarily. The chronology of the process is also different in these cases. The apallic syndrome occurs if the patient survives the initial

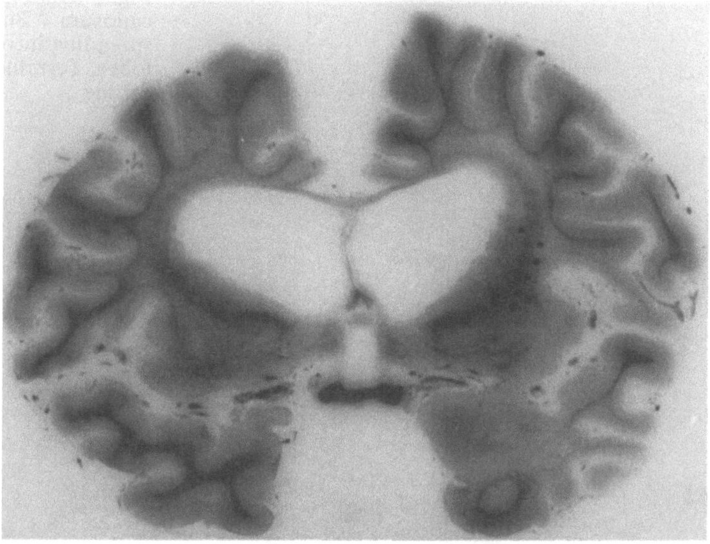

Fig. 1. Diffuse sclerosis. Apallic in last stage of disease. Severe demyelination with typical sparing of U-fibers. Destruction of corpus callosum. Weil staining

stage of deep coma and is often a transient syndrome to further recovery. It could be said that the hypoxic damage is most intensive in the initial stage. A good part of this damage, however, is reversible in nature, and such tissue may return to its normal function. The process of recovery takes place within the large pool of reversibly damaged parenchyma, and its development depends on various secondary factors which may act upon such reversibly damaged tissue. The basic shape of the distribution pattern of the lesions is quite specific, and it indicates the site of the primary action of ischemia. The anatomic substrate of the apallic syndrome obviously lies within this basic pattern. Correlative neuropathologic studies of our cases of cardiac arrest with survival times of from 2 days to 2 years showed that, the longer the survival, the more distinct becomes the pattern of distribution of the lesions. This pattern shows a clear correlation to the angioarchitecture of the gray matter and with the hemodynamic conditions in the areas of the border zones and terminal fields. This pattern, naturally, is also dependent upon the length of actual ischemia, but again, only in its size and extent and not in its basic shape. This "cortical model" of the apallic syndrome, in the author's opinion, offers a lot more information than has already been collected.

We have had the opportunity to observe an apallic syndrome-like picture in a few cases of *glioblastoma of the corpus callosum* (Fig. 2) with butterfly-like spreading into the white matter of the cerebral hemispheres. This picture developed in the last stages of the clinical disease, as a transient sign toward the terminal coma. There was no doubt that the development of the apallic syndrome coincided in these cases with the growth of the tumor into the white matter of the cerebral hemispheres, similar to the above-mentioned leukoencephalopathic model of the apallic syndrome. It also coincided, however, with the increase in intracranial pressure, which means that the secondary mechanisms within the brain stem could also have been responsible for it. The active growth of the tumor makes this model

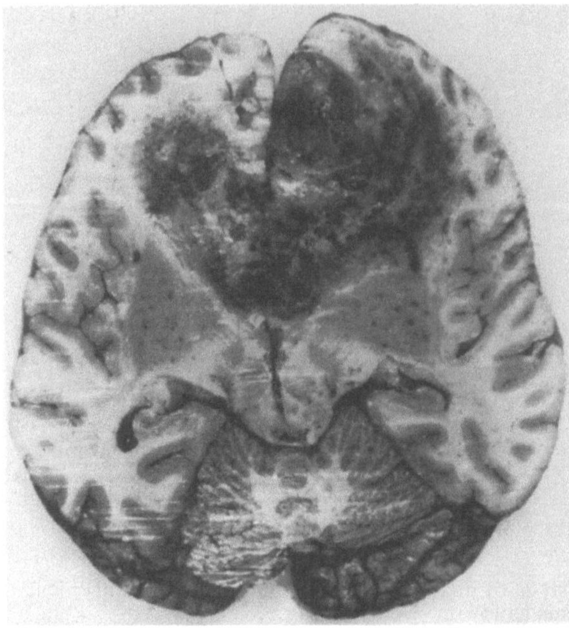

Fig. 2. Glioblastoma of corpus callosum. "Butterfly-like" spreading into both frontal lobes. Terminal apallic syndrome

different and less acceptable as a model for study of the anatomic substrate of the apallic syndrome.

Of all the models of the apallic syndrome the *traumatic model* (Adebahr, 1959, 1963a, b; French, 1952; Gemsenjager, 1960; Gerstenbrand, 1967, Girard et al., 1963; Gosztonyi et al., 1965; Grčević and Jakob, 1965; Grüner, 1965; Holländer, 1964; Jellinger, 1965a, b; Jellinger et al., 1963; Lindenberg and Freytag, 1960; Nyström, 1960; Osetowska, 1964; Peters, 1951, 1955; Rosenblath, 1899, Strich, 1956, 1961; Trillet, 1949, 1961; Ule, 1959; Ule et al., 1961) seems to offer the best possibilities for correlation.

The first series of cases of posttraumatic apallic syndrome which we studied (Grčević and Jakob, 1965) had survival times ranging from 15 to 847 days after the accident. The main constituents of the pattern of lesions were "paraventricular lesions" with predilection in the midline-corpus callosum-septum pellucidum-fornix zone as well as in the axial lateral paraventricular white matter (the "butterfly" pattern). From this area the damage fanned out into the white matter in a rather diffuse manner. There was strikingly little cortical damage in all of these cases and very little pathologic changes in the brain stem. The process in the brain varied from case to case in its size, quantity, and stage of the lesions, but the essential pattern could always be recognized. The chronologic development of the tissue changes clearly indicated that a similar pathogenetic mechanism took place in all cases and that the sequence of events was always the same. In order to further substantiate our hypothesis that practically all of the lesions within the pattern of "internal cerebral trauma" (Grčević and Jakob, 1965) are of primary traumatic origin, we examined brains from patients who had survived for very short times or who had died instantly after closed acceleration injury in the fronto-occipital direction. The results showed that the "acute pattern" of lesions strikingly corresponded to the "subacute pattern" of the "internal cerebral trauma" as far as topography of the supratentorial lesions was concerned. The differences were in the character of the process and the stage of the tissue lesions; only the hemorrhagic ones could be detected in the earliest posttraumatic phase. A significant topographic difference between the cases with short and long survival times was in the lesions of the brain stem.

The cases with short survival had, as a rule, extensive changes in the upper brain stem. Those of our cases who developed a typical apallic syndrome and survived longer had the best pronounced supratentorial pattern of the internal cerebral trauma with very little change in the brain stem. Our study indicated that, the longer a patient survives a severe fronto-occipital acceleration head injury, the fewer changes he is likely to have in the brain stem, but the more likely he is to develop the full picture of the apallic syndrome. The lesions in the brain stem can, therefore, be correlated with coma and death.

The brain process in the traumatic apallic syndrome begins as a result of the action of physical forces upon the brain as a whole. The clinical correlate of the early posttraumatic phase is, therefore, a correlate of a maximal effect, with coma and an extremely severe clinical picture, from which the size of the actual irreparable brain damage cannot be predicted. The apallic syndrome occurs after a certain period which can already be considered as some sort of "recovery." It is therefore chronologically similar to the postischemic apallic syndrome and opposite the apallic syndrome caused by panencephalitis, diffuse sclerosis, tumors, etc.

If the acceleration brain injury is in a physical sense a total attack on the brain, it is difficult to further retain a rather doctrinary view on "primary" and "secondary" lesions. The author feels more justified in building the pathophysiologic correlate of such injury on the basis of "reversible" and "irreversible" damage and their interrelation during the posttraumatic development. In addition to the lesions which are visible immediately after the accident (classical primary lesions), there are many changes taking place at that time which are not yet visible. Some are irreversible, but the majority are reversible. This large pool of reversible changes represents the points of least resistance to various noxious agents. This is actually the pool in which the development of the disease will be decided, but its origin is basically traumatic. The greatest role in the secondary mechanisms is played by hypoxia, but its action is mainly on the tissue already affected by the mechanical forces of injury, where it causes the normally reversible changes to become irreversible. A similar explanation can be given in the case of edema, which is certainly a secondary phenomenon, but its primary cause is not yet clear and requires further study. How much damage in the white matter is due to edema as the so-called edema necrosis, and to what extent edema is due to the primary damage to the parenchyma, remains to be explained.

In conclusion, it can be said that the constancy with which the above-described pattern of supratentorial lesions occur offers good evidence of the importance of these patterns in the development of the apallic syndrome. It seems reasonable to assume that the physiologic correlate of the apallic syndrome lies in the interference of lesions within these patterns with certain projecting systems of the brain. The existence of a cortical model and even more distinct subcortical models suggests that this interference may take place at various levels. This allows for the possibility of the existence of other models of the apallic syndrome, like the brain stem model (French, 1952; Gerstenbrand, 1967). Thus, the supratentorial anatomic patterns, i.e., the supratentorial models, do not exclude the possiblity of an eventual role played by the brain stem in the physiologic organization of the apallic syndrome.

IV. Pathophysiology

17. An Attempt at Interpretation of the Apallic Syndrome on the Basis of Experimental Findings

G.F. ROSSI

Introduction

If the experimental basis for the apallic syndrome is to be an exact experimental reproduction of the complex symptomatology characterizing the syndrome itself, then such an experimental basis is lacking. Based on the author's personal experience and reports in the literature, the apallic syndrome is typical of man and cannot be artificially reproduced in animals.

This difficulty in establishing analogies between clinical and experimental findings is implicit in the definition of the syndrome itself, that is, in the adjective "apallic." According to what has been repeatedly stated by several authors, the origin of the clinical manifestations of the syndrome is the functional exclusion or limitation of telencephalic structures (or "pallium"). The great difference in the development and therefore in the functional importance of these structures in man and animals is in itself sufficient to explain the difficulties mentioned above. It should be remembered that, in the original description of the syndrome given by Kretschmer (1940), the abnormalities of higher nervous activity characterizing the apallic syndrome were described as panagnosia and panapraxia, which are abnormalities that can hardly be studied in the laboratory animal.

This report, therefore, will be limited to a discussion of a possible experimental basis, not so much of the whole picture of the apallic syndrome, but rather of *some* of its aspects which can be compared with some findings of experimental research.

In the author's opinion, there are two main aspects of the apallic syndrome which can be considered for such a comparison: (1) some of the peculiar symptoms of the so-called full stage (*Vollstadium* according to Gerstenbrand, 1967) and (2) the characteristic mode of evolution of the syndrome, from its beginning to the so-called remission stage (Gerstenbrand, 1967).

Experimental Analogies with the Full Stage of the Apallic Syndrome

The complex of clinical signs characterizing the full stage of the apallic syndrome has been described in detail by Gerstenbrand (1967). If focal neurologic deficits are not taken into consideration, the most important of these symptoms can be summarized as follows.

1. Disturbances of consciousness, leading to coma vigile; wakefulness and sleep manifestations can be present, but the sleep-wakefulness cycle is usually altered.

2. Reaction to physiologic stimuli is characterized by movements of a primitive motor pattern; emotional reactions are usually lacking.

3. Abnormalities of posture.
4. Vegetative disturbances.

While the study of the second, third, and fourth of these groups of symptoms can be approached even in animals, the recognition of the first group and its analysis appear to be difficult. The disturbance of consciousness in the apallic syndrome is characterized by the loss of activities and contents of consciousness and at the same time by the preservation of vigilance. Obviously, activities and contents of consciousness cannot be studied in animals. The experimental analysis of this aspect of the problem, therefore, has to be limited to the study of vigilance.

On this basis, the attempt to find experimental analogies with the full stage of the apallic syndrome should be aimed toward finding an experimental situation having the following main characteristics:

1. Presence of signs of vigilance. Periods during which the animal appears to be vigilant alternate with periods during which it appears to be asleep. A sleep-wakefulness cycle is therefore present, despite abnormal temporal characteristics such as a longer duration of sleeping time or a lack of relationship between the sleep cycle and time of day, or a fragmentation in brief repeated cycles.
2. Reactions to peripheral stimuli limited to simple movements, often scarcely coordinated; lack of signs indicating an emotional content in the reactions of the animal, such as signs of fear or rage.
3. Postural disturbances.
4. Vegetative disturbances involving respiration, circulation, temperature, bladder, and rectal functions.

Do experimental situations reproducing the above-described picture exist? To remain as close as possible to the human apallic syndrome, the answer should be sought in experiments based on "chronic" cerebral lesions, i.e., in experiments in which the animal has been kept alive after the occurrence of the cerebral lesions for a period of time long enough to allow the disappearance of transitory phenomena (such as cerebral edema) and the appearance of compensatory events.

A. Total Sections of the Neuraxis

With the aim of reaching a primary orientation, it seems useful to start by taking into consideration those experiments in which the cerebral lesion is a total transverse section of the neuraxis. We shall consider later the experiments based on more discrete lesions limited to one or the other cerebral structure or region.

Figure 1 reproduces schematically on a sagittal section of the cat's brain cerebral transections largely used in experimental neurophysiology. These sections start at the highest level (the decortication) and succeed each other at progressively lower levels to reach the spinal cord. We shall summarize the effects of each section and look for possible analogies with the group of signs of the apallic syndrome already described. We shall take into consideration only behavioral signs, leaving aside the electroencephalographic ones, which—because of their complexity—require separate discussion. Only the effects produced by the cerebral section "caudally" to the section itself will be considered.

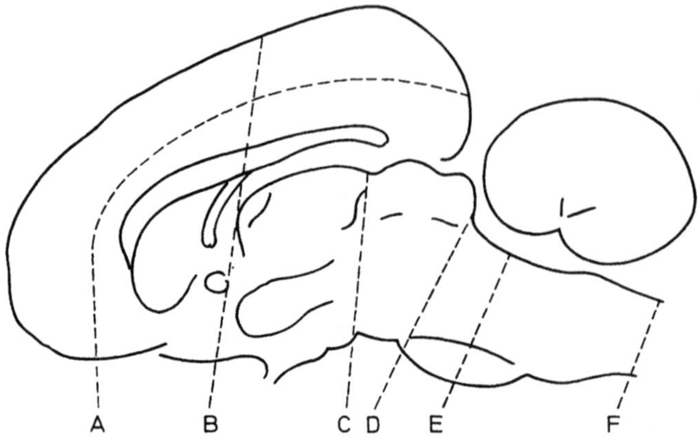

Fig. 1. Schematic representation of the level of the most utilized complete transections of brain in experimental neurophysiology

A - Decorticate B - Thalamic
C - Mesencephalic D - Rostropontine
E - Midpontine F - "Encêphale isolê"

1. *Decortication* (*A*), i.e., the complete surgical isolation of the cerebral cortex from subcortical structures (Bard and Rioch, 1937; Patton, 1960; Jouvet, 1962): Vigilance, as well as sleep-wakefulness cycles, are present. The animal reacts to peripheral stimuli with the appropriate movements; its reactions are often characterized by emotional content. When the animal is suspended the limbs show extensor rigidity. Rigidity disappears and deambulation is possible when the animal stands on the floor. Vegetative disturbances are lacking.

I do not believe there are sufficient elements in the decorticated preparation to permit analogies with the apallic syndrome.

2. *Thalamic preparation* (*B*), i.e., brain transection just in front of the thalamus: The preparation does not differ much from the preceding one (Bard and Macht, 1958), except for the fact that the emotional content of its reactions to even weak stimuli is always quite evident (typical "sham rage").

Even in this preparation, therefore, there are not sufficient similarities to the full stage of the apallic syndrome.

3. *Mesencephalic preparation* (*C*) or *cerveau isolé* (Bremer, 1935): After an initial period of continuous somnolence, behavioral signs of vigilance reappear (Bazzet and Penfield, 1922; Keller, 1932; Rioch, 1954; Bard and Macht, 1958; Batsel, 1960, 1964; Jouvet, 1962; Hobson, 1965; Villablanca, 1964; Sprague, 1967), and sleep-wakefulness cycles can be recorded. The animal reacts to external stimulation with more or less coordinated movements; it is capable of grasping an object placed close to its mouth; deglutition is possible. Extensor rigidity is noticeable; however, with the passage of time, it does not prevent the animal from crouching down and even walking. Neck and labyrinthine reflexes are clearly evident. Emotional reactions can be provoked, but only at a high threshold. Vegetative conditions are altered, mainly because of a loss of thermic regulation. Urinary retention often occurs.

On the whole, therefore, the mesencephalic preparation presents certain analogies with the complex of symptoms of the full stage of the apallic syndrome.

4. *Rostropontine preparation* (*D*): The brain stem is transected at the level of the rostral part of the pons. This preparation, together with the midpontine one—to be described below—have been the subject of detailed analysis (Rossi, 1957; Rossi and Zanchetti, 1957; Batini et al., 1958, 1959). The rostropontine preparation is similar to the mesencephalic one in many aspects. The differences are that (1) the resumption of movements with the passage of time are more limited and (2) emotional reactions are lacking.

Therefore, the similarity between chronic effects of experimental rostropontine transection and symptoms of the full stage of the apallic syndrome appears even more evident than for the mesencephalic preparation.

5. *Midpontine preparation* (*E*): The brain stem transection is carried out at the level of the middle pons, just in front of the trigeminal roots (Rossi, 1957; Rossi and Zanchetti, 1957; Batini et al., 1959). In contrast to the rostropontine preparation the midpontine one is almost continuously awake. Moreover, complete suppression of the REM sleep phase occurs if the brain stem transection encroaches upon the caudal part of the pons (Jouvet, 1962).

Analogies with the full stage of the apallic syndrome are difficult. A decrease in time spent sleeping does not appear to be common in the apallic patient. However, it may occur in some subjects.

6. *Encéphale isolé preparation (F):* The neuraxis is transected between the medulla oblongata and the spinal cord. Apnea and fall of vasomotor tone obviously follow. Comparison with the apallic full stage is not possible.

In summary, this brief review of the effects of experimental chronic complete transection at different levels of the neuraxis seems to indicate that behavioral signs following transections performed at brain stem level are in some way reminiscent of the human apallic syndrome. In particular, pontine transections appear to be the most interesting. The effects of transections rostral to the brain stem—at diencephalic and telencephalic levels—are not comparable to the characteristic symptoms of the apallic syndrome. As stated above, the limits of such a comparison should be kept in mind.

B. Partial Cerebral Lesions

If one accepts the conclusions reached above, the second step of the analysis would be to examine the brain stem partial lesions responsible for behavioral signs correlating to the full stage of the apallic syndrome. For what was reported in section A above, such an analysis should take into consideration the lesions located at rostropontine level.

Schematically, brain stem structures can be subdivided into "specific" and "nonspecific" or reticular ones [see critical reviews in Brodal (1957) and Rossi and Zanchetti (1957)]. The classic experiments carried out 20 years ago by French (1952), Lindsley et al. (1950) and Moruzzi and Magoun (1949) in the cat and monkey revealed the importance of nonspecific reticular structures for the maintenance of vigilance. The extensive destruction of these structures, in fact, is followed by a comatose state. Figure 2 depicts the location and extent of such destruction in one of the author's experimental preparations. However, subsequent studies (Genovesi et al., 1956) showed that, at least in the cat, the depth of the

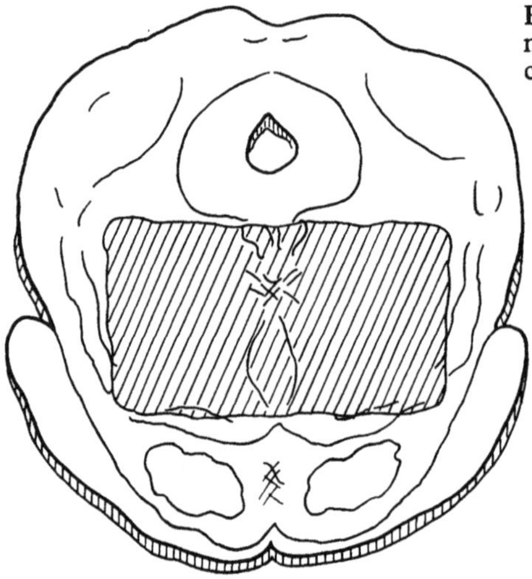

Fig. 2. Extensive reticular destruction at ponto-mesencephalic junction in the cat followed by comatose state

coma gradually decreases with the passage of time until vigilance is resumed. The return of vigilance is paralleled by the return of some spontaneous and reactive motor activities.

On the other hand, the selective destruction of specific structures in the brain stem does not alter vigilance (see review in Rossi and Zanchetti, 1957). This does not mean that specific structures do not contribute to the mechanisms responsible for the maintenance of vigilance (Roger et al., 1956). However, they are certainly less important than the nonspecific ones.

At the present time it does not appear possible to recognize a functional hierarchy among nonspecific structures of the pons as far as maintenance of vigilance is concerned. All of the reticular structures or nuclei appear equally important. The experimental work of Magliani et al.(1963), based on the effects of reticular lesions on the experimentally induced pseudo-affective manifestations, appears to support such a view. A certain differentiation among reticular nuclei with respect to their role in the mechanisms of REM sleep has been found (see Jouvet, 1962; Moruzzi, 1963; Rossi, 1963).

In view of the well-known importance of the reticular formation–not only for the mechanisms of vigilance but also for the mechanisms regulating postural tone and movements as well as visceral functions–the following conclusion has been reached: Most of the previously described effects produced by the complete transection of the brain stem and for certain aspects similar to the full stage of the apallic syndrome appear to be due mainly to the lesion of nonspecific or reticular structures.

C. Remarks

The first part of our analysis, designed to find relationships between the results of chronic experimental cerebral lesions and the complex of symptoms of the full stage of the apallic syndrome, leads us to the following conclusions:

1. The complex of symptoms of the full stage of the apallic syndrome for which a relationship with the data of chronic animal experimentation is possible seems to be the consequence of the suppression of telencephalic, diencephalic, and mesencephalic functions, i.e., of most cerebral functions. It follows that, strictly speaking, the adjective *apallic* does not appear to be sufficient or adequate to define the above-mentioned complex of symptoms. The functional exclusion of the pallium certainly occurs, but in addition functional exclusion of the diencephalon and mesencephalon should be considered.

2. Nonspecific or reticular formations of the pontine part of the brain stem appear to be the most important cerebral structures the chronic destruction of which lead to the experimental situation more closely reminiscent of the full stage of the apallic syndrome.

3. Cases of apallic syndrome following anatomic damage to the brain stem are reported in the anatomicoclinical literature. These cases fit in well with the conclusions of our analysis of experimental findings. However, in many other cases of human apallic syndrome no anatomic damage to the brain stem has been found (Gerstenbrand, 1967). This appears to contradict the interpretive hypothesis made above on the basis of experimental findings. It is possible, therefore, that the hypothesis of the importance of the brain stem in the mechanisms responsible for the apallic syndrome is not correct or is incomplete. It must be noted, however, that anatomic integrity does not necessarily mean functional integrity. We shall reconsider this point later.

Experimental Contribution to the Interpretation of the Evolution of the Apallic Syndrome

One of the characteristics of the apallic syndrome is its particular mode of evolution through different successive stages or phases. The consequences of experimental brain stem lesions also show particular changes with the passage of time.

a) Analogies Between Evolution of the Apallic Syndrome and Evolution of Signs Produced by Experimental Brain Stem Lesions

The initial phase of the apallic syndrome is described as the "mesencephalic syndrome." In animals, the rostropontine transection is also immediately followed by a complex of signs quite similar to those seen after mesencephalic transection (acute rostropontine preparation).

Later, both in man and in animals, the development of the syndrome may take one of two directions: (1) toward the bulbar syndrome or (2) toward the so-called full stage syndrome. The full stage is followed by what may be called the regression stage. At its beginning it is characterized by a better organization of behavior and motor reactivity, and by the appearance of emotional signs. This occurs in a surprisingly similar manner in both man and animals.

Subsequently the human apallic syndrome shows a stage characterized by behavioral manifestations reminiscent of the Klüver-Bucy syndrome. Some of these manifestations have also been observed in animals with chronic lesions in the nonspecific brain stem structures (Sprague et al., 1963): hyperphagia, tendency to seize and grasp any object with the teeth, hypersexuality (hetero- and homosexuality), and lack of fear or rage signs. These behavioral disorders do not occur in animals with total brain stem transections.

In man the further evolution may go through a Korsakoff stage and then a psycho-organic syndrome. For these stages, a comparison with that which occurs in the evolution of the chronic experimental syndrome is no longer possible.

Finally, it is possible to have an apparently complete remission of all pathologic signs—i.e., a complete recovery—both in man and in animals with circumscribed brain stem lesions. Complete recovery is not possible in animals with complete brain stem transections.

It is remarkable that both in man and animals the evolution of the syndrome appears to develop through progressively higher levels, in a jacksonian sense (Gerstenbrand, 1967: Bricolo and Dolce, 1969). As schematically illustrated in Figure 3, it seems that each re-

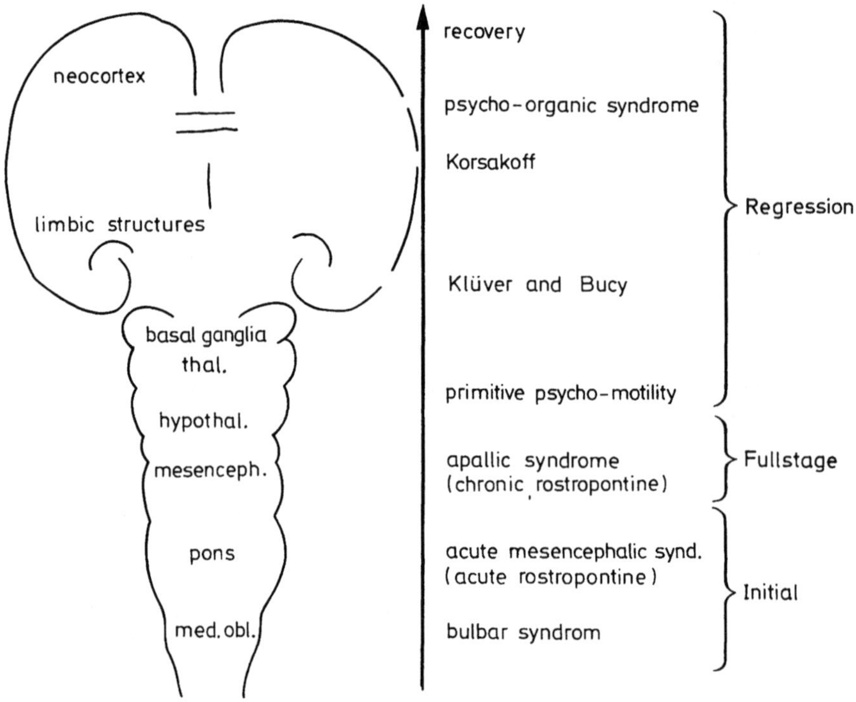

Fig. 3. Different stages (or evolution) of apallic syndrome in relation to different levels of encephalic functional organization

mission stage or phase corresponds to the functional recovery of a progressively higher cerebral level. This is true both in man and in animals. However, the time necessary for this evolution is different; several weeks or even months are necessary in man in comparison to a few days or weeks in animals. In general, the lower the level of the animal species, the shorter the recovery time (Woods, 1964).

b) Mechanisms of Recovery of the Apallic Syndrome

One of the most interesting findings of animal experimentation concerning the evolution of the effects of cerebral lesions is the great capacity for functional recovery following damage to the nonspecific structures of the brain stem. However, recovery is much more limited when specialized or specific cerebral functions are involved.

The explanation of this difference is difficult. Schematically, two hypotheses can be advanced:

1. The neurons of the nonspecific structures, probably because of their nonspecific nature, are capable of good autochthonous functional activity even if deprived of their synaptic connections with other nonspecific or specific neurons (Sprague, 1967). Following extensive mutilation of the nonspecific structures of the brain stem, the spared nonspecific neurons appear to be capable of carrying on the entire functional work and compensating for the damage. It must be remembered that nonspecific neurons are located at all levels of the brain stem–in the medulla oblongata, pons, and midbrain–and even rostrally to the brain stem itself, in the diencephalon. Therefore, it is unlikely that a lesion–even a large one–would destroy the whole nonspecific neuronal population.

2. It is likely that the effects of brain stem lesions are due not only to the suppression or alteration of neuronal mechanisms–as conceived in the classic neurophysiologic sense–but also to the alteration of neurochemical mechanisms. We know, for instance, that important neuronal aggregates having serotoninergic and cathecholaminergic functions are located in the brain stem, mainly in the pons (Falck et al., 1962; Dahlström and Fuxe, 1964). We also know the relevant role of amines in the mechanisms underlying the change in vigilance (Jouvet, 1967). The previously described effects of brain stem lesions, therefore, might be partially due to the alteration of amine metabolism. With the passage of time such a metabolism might recover; spared brain stem neurons or neurons located elsewhere in the brain might supply the neurochemical functions of those destroyed. This hypothesis is obviously highly speculative. However, it appears to fit in with two types of phenomena: (a) The treatment of chronic syndromes of altered vigilance with products correcting a supposed deficiency of the amine metabolism may yield good results (Gerstenbrand, 1967; Bricolo, personal communication; personal data). (b) Some apallic patients can reach a complete recovery (Gerstenbrand, 1967; Rosadini and Gentilomo, 1967; Bricolo et al., 1968b); such a complete recovery would hardly be compatible with an organic cerebral damage of such an extent as to justify by itself the appearance of a pathologic state as severe as the apallic syndrome. It is better explained on the basis of recovery of a metabolic alteration.

Conclusions

A true experimental basis of the apallic syndrome cannot be found. The attempt made to find in the pertinent experimental data an interpretation of some of the manifestations of the apallic synrome has shown evidence of the importance of brain stem damage, and in particular of the nonspecific structures of the pons. The statements made regarding the temporal evolution of the syndrome, from the moment of the occurrence of cerebral damage to recovery, and on the relationship between this evolution and that of the symptoms following an experimental lesion of the brain stem's nonspecific structures, appear to support the above-mentioned hypothesis.

The nature of the phenomena responsible for the variations during the course of the apallic syndrome and of the experimental syndrome due to brain stem lesions is not known. The possible importance of a neurochemical factor has been stressed. It is likely that the development of research in this direction—both in the clinical and in the experimental fields—might contribute to a more accurate interpretation of the complex phenomena under discussion. The hypothesis that the altered function of the nonspecific brain stem structures is the most probable causal factor of the apallic syndrome appears in contrast to several anatomicoclinical observations showing lesions elsewhere—for instance, in the diencephalon and the telencephalon—while the brain stem is apparently left intact. One could maintain that anatomic integrity does not necessarily imply functional and metabolic integrity. However, the author prefers to stress again the insufficiency of experimental data for a statisfactory interpretation of the apallic syndrome of human pathology.

18. Experimental Studies with Cats to Produce a State Similar to the Apallic Syndrome

G. DOLCE and H. FROMM

The incidence of all typical symptoms of the apallic syndrome with the possibility of a gradual or fair restitution has hitherto only been described in man. In Rossi's (1970) opinion, the apallic state is an event exclusively reserved for human pathophysiology.

In man, after an acute midbrain or bulbar brain injury an initial coma may turn into an apallic syndrome. As described by Gerstenbrand (1967), these patients are completely unspontaneous. There is no activity or reactivity of mind, yet these patients are not unconscious in a normal sense, since periods of obvious wakefulness and sleep are observed clinically and in EEG patterns (Dolce and Fromm, 1967). Additionally, the apallic syndrome is characterized by severe vegetative disorders, a great variety of abnormal postural reflexes and the reappearance of primitive mechanisms. These typical clinical symptoms imply a serious breakdown of normal telencephalic functions, while uncontrolled mesencephalic and diencephalic functions prevail.

On the other hand, we know from numerous post-mortem examinations that, in spite of this uniform clinical syndrome, highly varied combinations of primary and secondary traumatic lesions were found. Thus, a wide variety of cortical lacerations, lesions of the corpus callosum, and of the fornix are reported, as well as hemorrhage and necrosis in the white matter, in the basal ganglia, in the midbrain, and in the brain stem (reviewed by Gerstenbrand, 1967).

In other words, these findings imply that the apallic syndrome can scarcely be restricted to certain lesions within strictly localized anatomic structures. Furthermore, it is assumed that the apallic syndrome is related to serious disorders within structures of the ascending activating systems. These disorders may be caused by anatomic lesions, or functionally, by edema, or vascular or metabolic disorders. It is of interest to recall that Jellinger (1968) observed rostropontine lesions in 84% of his cases.

In our investigations (Dolce and Fromm, 1967, 1972), in order to obtain an animal of reduced spontaneous motility and behavioral activity, but of preserved vigilance, for a long-term study, six groups of cats with different standardized lesions were prepared:

1. Bilateral stereotactic coagulation of the pallidum
2. Large biparietal resections
3. Bilateral lesions at a quadrigeminal level
4. Split-brain
5. Split-brain combined with a unilateral extensive midbrain lesion
6. Split-brain combined with an hemicerveau isolé

Most remarkable seems to be the behavior of animals in the fifth experimental group, which the authors observed for up to more than 16 months. A split-brain was performed in these cats by means of a specially designed spatula which was introduced stereotactically by an infratentorial, occipital approach. Additionally, a half-sided midbrain lesion at a quadrigeminal level was carried out by means of a stereotactically guided hook. Figure 1

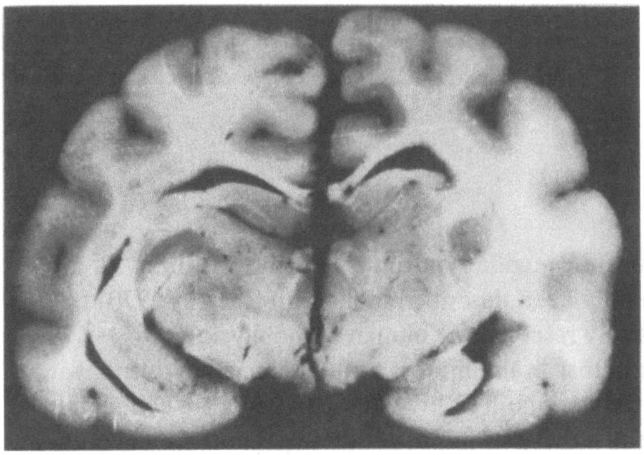

Fig. 1. Split brain of cat. Split through midline structures almost reaches mammillary bodies and extends caudally to rostropontine area

demonstrates the extent of these lesions. The split through the midline structures almost reaches the mammillary bodies and extends caudally to the rostropontine area. At the quadrigeminal level multiple lesions and hemorrhages are seen on the left side. During a deep initial coma lasting up to 3 days a strong extensor rigidity, as in Sherrington's (1947) description of decerebration, was observed in these animals. Apart from stretch reflexes there was no reactivity to stimuli. Severe dysregulation of body temperature made it necessary to keep the animals in incubators for weeks. After a slight lessening of the depth of the coma the animals remained completely adynamic. The only response to different stimuli was a stereotyped, explosive rage response observed for about 10 days. At the same time, catalepsy occurred. The animals remained for hours in bizarre postures molded by the observer.

During progressive recovery from catalepsy the animals remained in a quiet, hypokinetic state over a period of weeks. A flexor position of the limbs was then preferred. Alternating periods of sleep and wakefulness were observed in accordance with slow and rapid EEG patterns. The animals did not react to normal mild tactile and auditory stimuli or to moving objects, nor to mice or rats (Fig. 2). There was no vocalization. At this time the rage response had largely disappeared. The animals did not eat spontaneously; they were fed by tube 3 times a day. When their lips were touched, chewing movements were sometimes observed. Later, a progressive recovery could be noticed. The animals responded to petting and recognized the animal keeper. They raised their heads and trunks spontaneously and showed an increasing interest in events outside the cage. They also started eating spontaneously after 40-70 days. Upon stimulation they exhibited purposeful movements in spite of severe palsy and ataxia. They pushed their food bowls into a convenient position. Finally, a normal hunting response to the presence of a mouse reappeared (Fig. 3).

The authors agree that the term apallic syndrome should not be used without reservation when describing a behavioral state in animals. However, it is believed that there is such a wide range of similarities between the postoperative course in these animals and

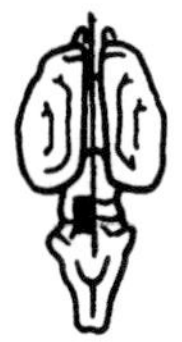

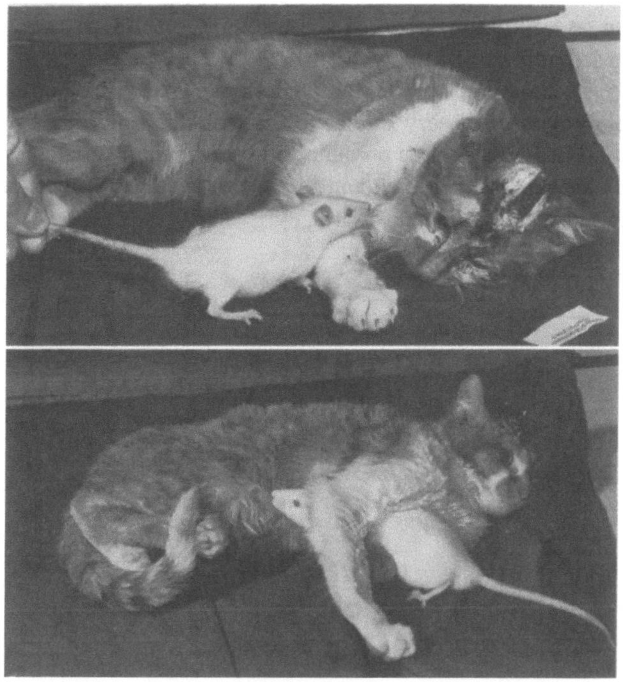

Fig. 2

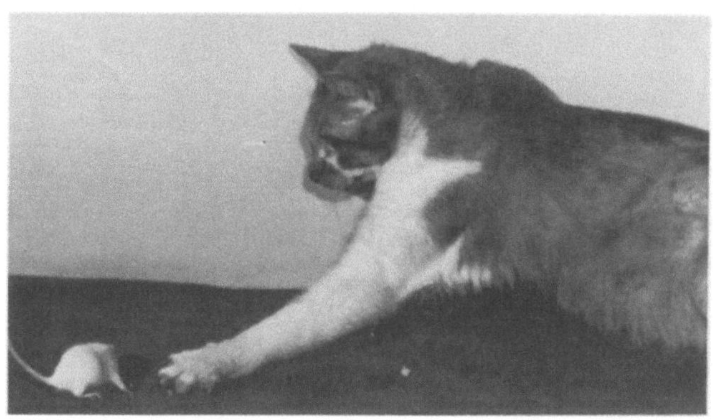

Fig. 3

Fig. 2. Cat in coma vigile (20 days after operation). Loss of motor activity, no response to moving objects or to free-moving mice or rats.

Fig. 3. Same cat in good recovery (152 days after operation). Normal hunting response

the pattern of recovery in the human traumatic apallic syndrome that the term apallic syndrome is justified.

All neurologic signs, deficits, and behavioral alterations which could be observed during this long-term study are well-known from the literature (reviewed by Sprague, 1967) and may be related to lesions within certain structures of the brain stem, midbrain, and diencephalon, as well as to functional alterations of specific pathways and severe dysregulations of the ascending activating systems.

Thus a combination of extensive lesions in subcortical midline structures may produce complete syndromes very similar to those apallic syndromes seen after severe head injuries in man. Furthermore, it is possible to observe certain analogies between the recovery from the apallic syndrome in man and the different stages of recovery after such extensive lesions in experimental animals.

19. Clinical Pathophysiology of the Apallic Syndrome

C.H. LÜCKING

In order to carry out pathophysiologic analyses of the apallic syndrome and to correlate single functions with specific cerebral structures or levels, findings from animal experiments (Sherrington, 1949; Bremer, 1935; Moruzzi and Magoun, 1949; and others), from cases of anencephalus (Gamper, 1926; Monnier and Willi, 1947, 1953), from the analysis of human developmental stages (Monnier and Willi, 1947; Peiper, 1949; Prechtl, 1956), and from chronic disintegration processes (Pilleri, 1961b; Pilleri and Poeck, 1964) will be taken into account in this chapter. The pathoanatomic investigations of the apallic syndromes (Jellinger, 1967; Peters, 1969) did not provide evidence of homogeneous lesion patterns. But obviously the degree of functional lesions can largely surpass that of the perceivable morphologic alterations. Gerstenbrand (1967) was the first author to discuss in detail the pathophysiology of the traumatic apallic syndrome.

The separated susceptibility of wakefulness and consciousness as found in the apallic syndrome is explained by the fact that these functions are linked to different structures. By wakefulness we understand a state in which the eyes are open, the vegetative functions are in an ergotropic condition, and the muscles are in tonic innervation. This pattern alternates with periods of sleep associated with closed eyes and a trophotropic vegetative functional state. This wakefulness-sleep function is linked to the intactness of midbrain structures (activating system of the formatio reticularis mesencephali et pontis), the intactness of the cerebral hemispheres not being a decisive condition. From the anencephali the mesodiencephalic anencephalus of Gamper showed a periodic sleep-wakefulness rhythm (Gamper, 1926); the mesorhombencephalic anencephalus had no sleep-wakefulness periodicity, but could be awakened (Monnier and Willi, 1953), and the pontobulbospinal anencephalus (Monnier and Willi, 1947) presented a continuous state of sleep. The importance for the state of wakefulness of the mesencephalopontine activating formatio reticularis is confirmed by the results of animal experiments (Bremer, 1935; Moruzzi and Magoun, 1949; Batini et al., 1958). A midbrain section leads to the loss of wakefulness (cerveau isolé, Bremer, 1935); a section through the caudal pons or the medulla oblongata does not affect the activating ascendent formatio reticularis, and a state of wakefulness is maintained.

While a state of wakefulness is possible without consciousness, consciousness without wakefulness is inconceivable. Consciousness, as the highest nervous performance which registers, evaluates, processes, accumulates, and responds to sensory afferent flowing in from the periphery, is bound to the cerebral cortex and possibly also to the thalamus, the activity of which is crucially dependent on the ascendent activation (wakefulness) of the formatio reticularis. The isolated extinction of consciousness associated with maintained wakefulness thus can only be the result of a functional loss in the region of the cortex, the thalamus, the thalamocortical connections, or the ascending activating system above the midbrain level. Therefore, the origin of such damage may be non-specific; decisive is the damaging pattern. Hence, coma vigile can be observed in all inflammatory, toxic, anoxic, metabolic, traumatic, and possibly also degenerative processes which lead to a diffuse functional impairment of the cerebral hemispheres. An involvement or isolated damage of the mesodiencephalic structures, however, would have to lead, by suppresion of the awakening systems, to pathologic sleep or coma. Coma vigile as a symptom, e.g., of the traumatic apallic syndrome, evolving as a consequence of an increase in intracranial pressure with tentorial herniation, might not only be a result of a midbrain damage by strangulation but may rather be induced by a diffuse pressure or edema of the cerebral hemispheres. The inflammatory damage to the mesodiencephalic region in lethargic encephalitis does not lead to coma vigile but to pathologic sleep.

Besides coma vigile, the lack of any perceivable emotional reaction is a further symptom of the apallic syndrome. An emotional reaction requires the capability both to recognize and to evaluate a stimulus and to give an adequate motor or vegetative response. The stimulus perception is—as consciousness itself—supposed to be a function mainly of the cortex. It is therefore to be expected that, in coma vigile, emotional reactions do not become prominent. Possibly there exists a primitive evaluation system in the sensible relais nuclei of the ventroposterior thalamus which, after suppression of the cortex, is responsible for the distinct defense responses to pain and temperature stimuli. Gamper (1926) sometimes observed in the mesodiencephalic anencephalus (with parts of the thalamus) a spontaneously appearing whining, but also smiling expression, perhaps as a reaction to endogenous, visceral or vegetative stimuli. Furthermore, a contraction of the face after salty and bitter flavors was observed. Similar manifestations did not appear in the pontobulbospinal anencephalus (Monnier and Willi, 1947).

The inability to recognize, evaluate, and respond to a stimulus—i.e., the loss of the thalamocortical function—also makes it impossible to "perform a meaningful action formula of a learned nature" (Kretschmer, 1940). Certain motor patterns, however, are more or less maintained as reflex responses to external stimuli. Prevailing are motor sequences related to food intake such as chewing automatisms, snout, sucking and grasp reflexes, pollicomental reflexes, and often an intact act of swallowing. They can be elicited by exteroceptive stimuli in the hand-mouth area, also by interoceptive stimuli, and they occur in a patternlike way (motor pattern, Kretschmer, 1953). Here elementary food intake functions remain integrated which are already developed in the first fetal months (Minkowski, 1928; Hooker, 1952) and which with their completion in the 7th fetal month are the prerequisite for the viability of the premature infant (Monnier and Willi, 1947). These early ontogenetic functional elements probably remain intact during the development of the cerebrum and under its permanent control or inhibition (Pilleri, 1961). A disintegration or suppresion of the cerebral functions—particularly those of the forebrain and of the temporal lobe—reactivate these "automatisms" without their acquiring a vital function again.

The nervous substrate for the above-mentioned motor patterns is probably located in reticular formations of the brain stem. Monnier and Willi (1947) observed in the pontobulbar anencephali sucking, snout and lip stroke reflexes, and sometimes also a turning of the head toward the stimulus.

Grasp reflexes and also more complex escape and flexor reflexes to an external stimulus would have to be based on a similar functional level. The position and posture reactions of

Magnus and De Kleyn (1930), however, seem rather to be integrated in the upper brain stem. They were not observed in the pontobulbospinal anencephalus but were quite prominent in the mesodiencephalic anencephalus of Gamper (1926).

The completely developed apallic syndrome is dominated by two forms of body posture: a flexed posture of arms and hands and a stretched position of the legs, or a flexed posture of all extremities. These postures are reinforced by a spastic-rigid hypertension of the muscles. The flexion-stretching posture, as well as the general flexion posture of the apallic syndrome, are preceded by a general stretching posture of the extremities in the acute midbrain syndrome. Since Sherrington (1898), it is known from animal experiments that a functional and anatomic section of the brain stem below the nucleus ruber leads to a stretched posture as a consequence of the predominating vestibospinal influences–which almost exclusively affect the motoneurons of the extensor muscles (Sprague and Chambers, 1953). The nucleus ruber, on the other hand, mainly affects the motoneurons of the flexor muscles (Pompeiano and Brodal, 1957), so that a disinhibition of the rubrospinal influences (e.g., in case of a thalamic preparation with a section below the thalamus) leads to a flexed posture of the extremities. The general flexion posture thus requires intact midbrain structures. It was present in the mesodiencephalic anencephalus of Gamper (1926). The flexion-stretching-posture as a decortication posture (Fulton, 1952), on the other hand, can be induced in animal experiments by removal of the motor cortex. According to Denny-Brown (1966), "decorticate rigidity" is a frequent phenomenon in man after severe anoxia as well as metabolic and inflammatory processes of the cerebrum. These observations point to the fact that the general flexion posture as well as the flexion-stretching posture of the apallic patient must be a consequence of a suppression of the cortex and the basal ganglia, but at the same time they require intact midbrain structures, especially of the rubroreticulospinal system.

Composing another important symptomatic category are the vegetative disturbances. Whereas in the state of sleep the apallic patient presents an equilibrated vegetative functional situation, extreme disinhibition reflected in an increase in pulse rate and blood pressure, tachypnea, and often profuse sweating is observed in the state of wakefulness or with increased external stimulation (e.g., nursing measures, tracheotomy tube). At the same time, a considerable increase occurs in the basal metabolic rate, which can only be compensated for by hypercaloric food intake. This explains the often observed formerly in rapidly beginning cachexic states and trophic disturbances apallic patients. A dysregulation in diencephalic-hypothalamic structures must be assumed to be the origin of these unstable vegetative functions showing a massive disinhibition to external stimuli. Certainly of the same importance is the misprocessing of external stimuli which, due to a lack of inhibition, extremely irradiate and feign an emergency situation. Vegetative disinhibition always runs parallel to an increase in muscle tone with increased flexion and stretching innervation; the pupils are dilated and often motor sequences occur, mainly in the form of oral automatisms.

The main symptoms of the apallic syndrome are (1) coma vigile with maintained sleep-wakefulness rhythm; (2) lack of emotional reactions; (3) reappearance of primitive motor patterns; (4) fixed body posutre; (5) and extreme irradiation of vegetative reactions. This leads to the conclusion that in apallic syndrome mainly the reticular structures of the midbrain and of the pontobulbar brain stem must be intact. This is supported by animal experiments and by observations on human anencephalics. The basis for the apallic syndrome must be seen in an anatomic or functional suppression or disintegration of the cerebrum. This also explains the quite uniform clinical picture observed in completely different underlying diseases of the cerebrum. The traumatic apallic syndrome is not exclusively a result of isolated damage of the midbrain, but rather is a result of cerebral damage due to traumatic hemorrhage or to diffuse brain edema. Additional signs of the optomotor or the extrapyramidal system (e.g., parkinsonism) can be explained by simultaneous lesions of the respective structures and are not to be considered obligatory components of the apallic syndrome. Accompanying symptoms of the upper brain stem are obviously more frequent after a midbrain strangulation than with primary brain processes. The pathoanatomic investigations by many authors (e.g., Jellinger, 1967; Peters, 1969) have shown a corresponding variety of damage patterns which always included the cerebral hemispheres as well.

A strong analogy with animal experiments and attempts to develop experimental models are problematic. The pontobulbospinal anencephali (Monnier and Willi, 1947). for instance, present a hypertension of the flexor muscles, whereas decerebrated monkeys, after section above the pons, show an extensor hypertension called "decerebration rigidity." Apart from the specific organization of the species, the additional traumatic and secondary degenerative processes in the operated animal must be taken into account. A systematic analysis of acute as well as of chronic cerebral disintegration thus provides more information on the organization of the human brain than do animal experiments.

V. Additional Diagnostic Methods and Investigations

20. Temperature Regulation in Acute and Chronic Mesencephalic Syndrome and in Apallic Syndrome

G. LAUSBERG

Acute transverse lesions of the brain stem resulting in functional disturbances are accompanied by typical spontaneous variations of temperature, depending on the caudal or oral localization of the lesion. Clinically and experimentally observed patterns of temperature curves were correlated with special thermoregulatory patterns.

Wilson (1920) pointed out hyperthermia as a constant symptom in acute decerebration states due to midbrain herniation. This observation was confirmed in the following years in different ways; however, the particular character of the temperature curve was not mentioned (Erickson, 1939; Pia, 1957; Frowein, 1958, 1961; Loew and Wüstner, 1960; Müller, 1965; Gerstenbrand, 1967, and others). The rise in temperature in these forms of hyperthermia is characterized by a steady increase, with a changing slope of the temperature curve. Harmonic variation of the temperature curve, seen in the humoral form of hyperthermia, is absent. Regulatory mechanisms become recognizable through the appearance of a plateau in the temperature curve only when pyrexia reaches 40°C. This is considered evidence of the existence of a second regulatory emergency circuit, already suggested by Dubois (1949) on the basis of the clinical analysis of pyrexia. General circulatory and respiratory dysregulation occurs primarily independently of hyperthermia; however, secondarily untreated hyperthermia combined with tachypnea, causes circulatory collapse with tachycardia and hypotension which is sometimes fatal within a few hours after the appearance of the syndrome. Hyperthermia was so prominent in the clinical picture that Pia (1957) considered its occurrence in decerebration states a lethal sign. The advances in intensive care of decerebrate patients brought about the possibility of interrupting the vicious circle of hyperthermia and accompanying dysregulation of other vegetative functions; cases of early death due to hyperthermia are no longer encountered. The therapy aims towards diminishing the vegetative storm, convulsions, metabolic rate, and restoring the fluid balance. The diminution of the metabolic rate and ganglionic blockage not only stabilizes the vegetative functions and improves the prognosis in the first few days but also leads to a decisive decrease in heat production influencing the decerebrate rigidity. Appropriate fluid balance supports the therapy during the first few days, but its effect on the prognosis becomes evident when the fluid reserves of the organism become exhausted. Previously, this state usually occurred within the first week.

According to van't Hoff's rule regarding the speed of chemical reactions, a rise in body temperature of 1°C increases the energy metabolism by 20-30%, which means that at a temperature of 41°C it is almost doubled. An additional rise is caused by increased muscle action due to the increased tonus and spontaneous extension automatisms. Both of these factors can increase the energy metabolism to 6000-8000 cal/day and the fluid loss by evaporation from 900 ml/day to approximately 2500 ml/day, assuming that 42 ml of fluid is lost with the production of 100 cal (Grosse-Brockhoff, 1969). Additional fluid loss through profuse sweating and urination can lead to a critical loss of 15% of the body fluid within the first week.

Twenty years ago it was thought that the restoration of fluid balance might reduce the coexisting brain edema and it was therefore advised to limit the fluid intake to 1000-1500 ml per day. The treatment of brain edema with adequate fluid balance and electrolyte substitution, first recognized empirically and recently confirmed by experimental studies (Reulen et al., 1969; Wesemann et al., 1970), resulted in a definite improvement of the early prognosis.

Studies on the temperature course in decerebrate states revealed a parallel increase in core temperature to surface temperature. As early as 1950 Kautzky and Buchard questioned the original thesis of von Kroll (1935) and Griesel (1939) that the dissociation between core and surface temperature was apparently characteristic for central hyperthermia.

The duration of hyperthermia is directly related to the duration of the decerebrate state. Rapid elimination of the cause of decerebration, i.e., removal of traumatic hematoma or decompressive procedure of the tumor, quickly leads to normalization of the temperature course. In cases where an acute decerebration state becomes a chronic one, the temperature course usually returns to normal at the end of the second week (Fig. 1). The tendency towards hyperthermia, however, remains and can be proven experimentally.

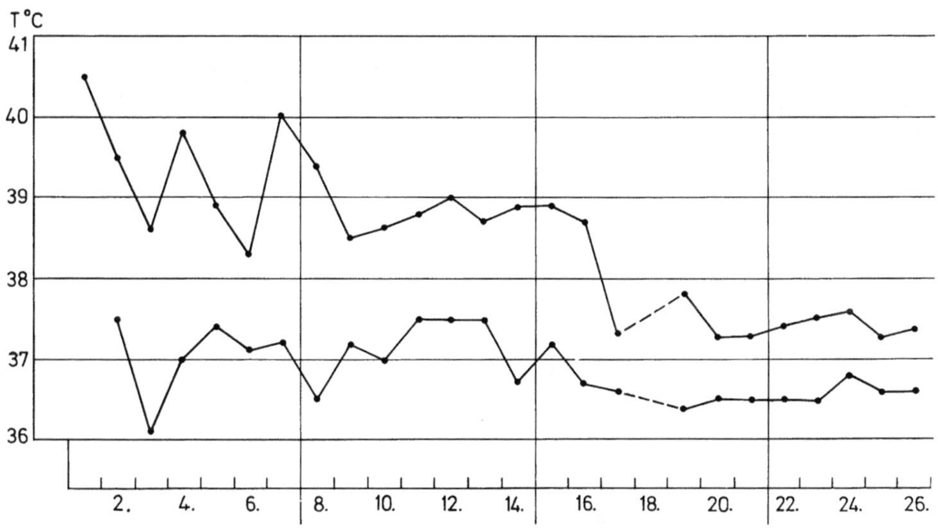

Fig. 1. Maximum and minimum values of body temperature in posttraumatic decerebration states without intracranial bleeding. Days after injury

A rise in room temperature to 40°C over a period of 7 h produces a similar temperature course to that seen in acute decerebration states (Fig. 2). The rise in temperature is preceded by increasing pulse frequency and pulse pressure, whereas the impairment of respiration is concurrent with the rise in temperature. This hyperthermic reaction to the increase in room temperature is highly significant in cases with a mesencephalic syndrome. The temperature curve corresponds in its steepness to that observed in hyperthermia in an acute mesencephalic syndrome.

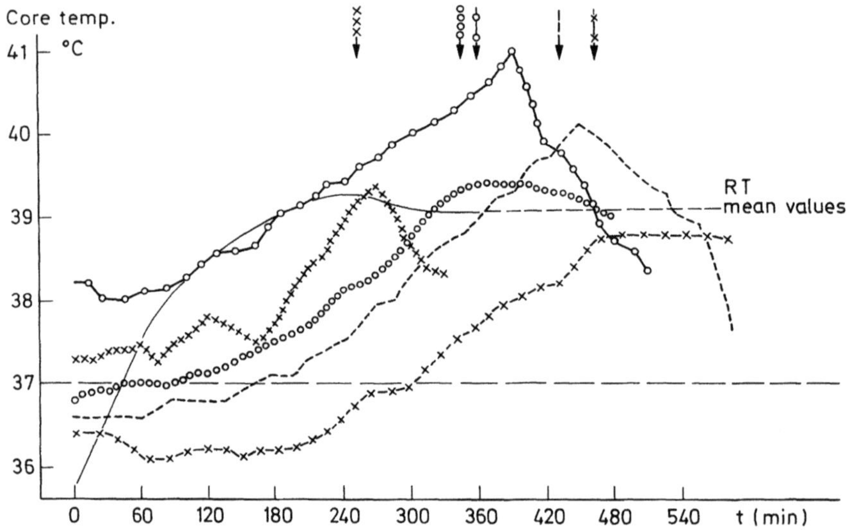

Fig. 2. Heat stress (max. 40°C) in decerebration state. *RT* = room temperature; ↓ = end of stress; n = 5

In the apallic syndrome and under heat stress the behavior of the temperature course is similar to that seen in the mesencephalic syndrome, although less uniform (Fig. 3). Compensatory mechanisms, however, are stronger, and the steepness of the curve and its peak can be clearly distinguished. It is worthwhile to note that hyperthermic reaction to external heat stress has been observed during the remission period in a case with a Klüver-Bucy syndrome.

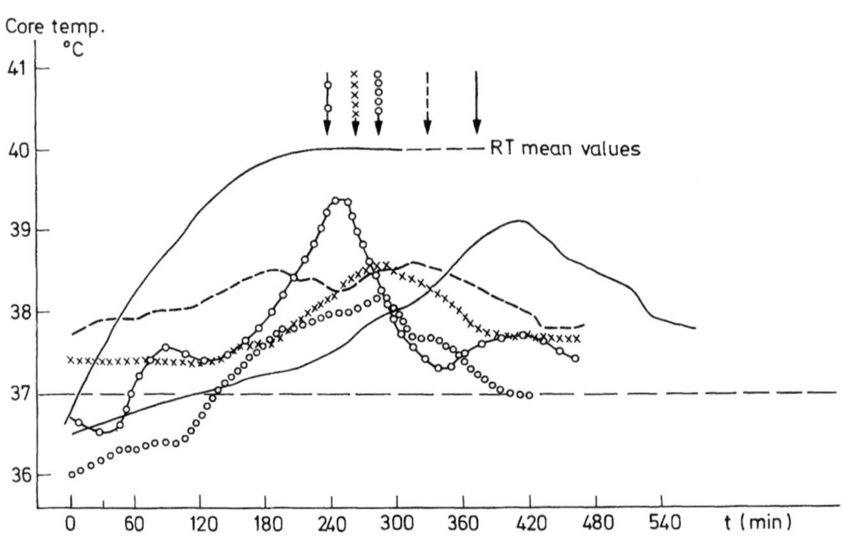

Fig. 3. Heat stress (max. 43°C), apallic syndrome. *RT* = room temperature; ↓ = end of stress; n = 5

Our studies provide evidence of a disturbed regulation of temperature during heat stress in cases of decerebration and postdecerebration states. The temperature course is characteristic of the decerebration syndrome.

However, there is no clear answer to the question as to which part of the temperature regulation circuit is disturbed. The possibility of a displacement of the central thermostat could be excluded on the basis of the temperature curve. The processes of the regulation of heat output in cases of spontaneous and induced hyperthermia are manifested by the rise in surface temperature and by profuse sweating. On the other hand, there is a manifold increase in energy metabolism due to typical extension automatism and muscle rigidity. Thus the increased production of heat cannot be compensated for by an increase in activity of heat-loss mechanisms, resulting in a relative disturbance of the heat output.

The pattern of hyperthermia described above is closely related to other functional disturbances in the mesencephalon. Examples of temperature courses identical to those observed in cases of decerebration were found in cases of suprasellar tumors involving the mesencephalon. Although the mesencephalic lesion as a cause of disturbance in temperature regulation is most probable, the exact morphologic substrate or site of the above disturbances has not yet been clearly identified. Nakayama and Hardy (1969) found that thermal stimulation of regulation centers in the preoptic and anterior hypothalamic area produces increased activity in the reticular formations of the upper mesencephalon. It could be speculated that in cases of mesencephalic and apallic syndromes,the pathways of leading impulses for heat output become blocked in the mesencephalon, resulting in hyperthermia. Our clinical and experimental findings confirm the results of animal experiments in dogs conducted by Keller and McClaskey (1964). These authors sectioned the mesencephalon at the junction between the anterior third and posterior two-thirds. The increase in room temperature from 30°C to 38°C over 6 h on the 10th day after the section resulted in the development of marked hyperthermia. The same result was obtained when the section was performed immediately below the hypothalamus. These findings correspond to our observations in cases of suprasellar tumors invading the mesencephalon. The authors point to the disturbance in heat-output mechanisms as the cause of externally induced hyperthermia and discuss the raising of the threshold for heat-output mechanisms.

The opposite phenomenon, hypothermia–encountered in certain decerebrate conditions–is connected without exception to the fatal brain stem syndrome. Hypothermia was observed and analyzed clinically in 61 of our cases. The analysis of the temperature curves in cases of transverse lesions in the brain stem at the midbrain level enabled us to distinguish three different types of temperature curves, which show a definite relation to the clinical syndromes (Fig. 4).

1. Undulating curve–typical for mainly orally localized lesions in the brain stem
2. Steplike declining curve–seen mainly in caudal lesions of the brain stem
3. Steeply declining curve reflecting brain death

In 1952 Kaplan et al. described slight hypothermia in mesencephalic lesions; these findings, however, did not evoke much interest in subsequent years. On the contrary, spontaneous deep hypothermia has aroused much more attention in recent years, undoubtedly because of the interest taken in the problem of brain death (Schneider, 1970; Butenuth, cited after Schneider, 1970).

The slightest form of disturbance of temperature regulation is reflected in the undulating curve of the temperature course. This form is characterized by good compensatory mech-

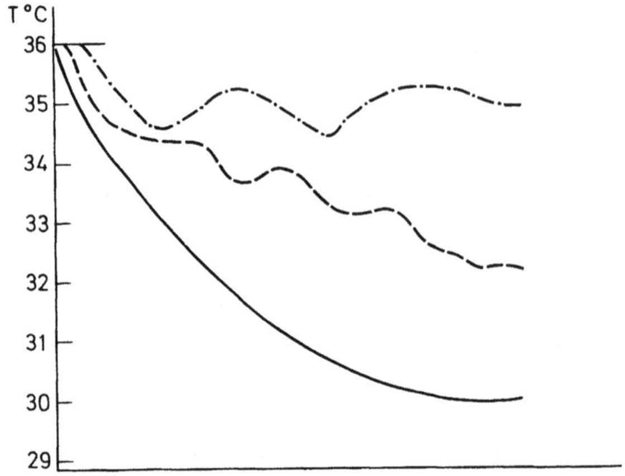

Fig. 4. Temperature curves in central hypothermia. —.—.— Undulating curve, – – – steplike curve, ——— steep declining curve

anisms and to a certain extent by a slight decrease in temperature. The concept of a lower sensitivity threshold of central heat receptors—analogous to the increase in sensitivity of these receptors as seen, for example, in unspecific postoperative hyperthermia—could not be confirmed. The lowest temperature observed in these patients was in the range of 35.9-33.0°C, with a mean temperature of 35.0-35.9°C. The neurologic picture corresponding to this form of hypothermia is comprised in two-thirds of the cases of patients with a mesencephalic syndrome and incomplete bulbar syndrome. Until their deaths none of these patients showed any significant changes in their neurologic symptoms.

A further encroachment upon the temperature regulation is reflected in the steplike decrease in the core temperature. The final temperature falls in one-third of the patients with this temperature course to a level below 33.0°C. At the beginning of such a temperature course the ratio of patients with an incomplete or complete bulbar syndrome to patients with a mesencephalic syndrome is 2:1. However, in this group—contrary to the situation in patients showing undulating temperature curves—all patients displayed a bulbar syndrome in the final stages.

A "uniformly falling" temperature curve reflects a total loss of temperature regulation. Such curves can be seen in 75% of cases with a bulbar syndrome at the beginning of hypothermia. In the final stages approximately 90% of patients with this type of temperature course also reveal a bulbar syndrome. This temperature course, combined with the clinical picture of the bulbar syndrome, could be considered an expression of central death. The course of the core temperature in such cases is poikilothermic, and the temperature adjusts itself to the temperature of the environment (Lausberg, 1970a, b).

If the course of body temperature is correlated with the progression of the brain stem syndrome, one finds that in patients with a mesencephalic syndrome the developing hypothermia is usually slight but that approximately 50% of these patients develop a bulbar syndrome at a later stage with a corresponding change in the temperature course. Uniformly falling temperature curves in patients with incomplete bulbar syndromes indicate further deterioration and a development of complete bulbar symptomatology. A primary bulbar syndrome is characterized from the beginning by a low hypothermic course. The abovementioned observations indicate the importance of the extent of the temperature regulation disturbance for the clinical course. The typical temperature curves corresponding to further deterioration in brain stem function precede the development of neurologic signs.

21. A Neuroradiologic Study of Traumatic Apallic Syndrome*

A. BENATI and A. BRICOLO

Our research was carried out with 11 patients of both sexes (eight males and three females) with ages ranging from 8 to 64 years, who had been admitted to our Neurosurgical Department following severe head injuries. All patients had a midbrain syndrome with coma and stretch cramps which developed either at the time of the trauma or shortly thereafter.

Angiographic cerebral examinations showed signs of extensive traumatic focal lesions in six cases that underwent surgery immediately. Five patients had cerebral lacerocontusions with acute subdural hematomas, and one had an extradural hematoma. Carotid angiography of the remaining five cases did not reveal lesions requiring neurosurgical treatment.

All cases included in this research showed the clinical picture of the transition stage up to the full picture of the apallic syndrome, which set in within 25 days to 6 months after the head injury.

Results

The results obtained from the neuroradiologic studies, together with the data obtained by following the clinical evolution of each patient, led to several findings.

In six cases (Fig. 1) the pneumoencephalographic examination performed during the full stage of the apallic syndrome revealed a more or less severe dilatation of the lateral ventricles due to a central cerebral atrophy (Lindgren, 1951). Four of these patients with the most severe degree of enlargement of the lateral ventricles (Evan's index: beyond 0.40 and up to 0.70) showed a clear dilatation of the fourth ventricle as well as the cerebral aqueduct. In one case, we found not only ventricular dilatation, but also a parietal poroencephalic cavity. The dilatation was always bilateral, although with modest asymmetries. It involved the entire ventricular cavity, often predominating in the frontal horn.

Unfortunately, we are unable to draw any conclusions regarding the period of onset and the evolution of the atrophy, since we lack a seriated longitudinal pneumoencephalographic study. It should be pointed out, however, that in one case the atrophy appeared after only 4 months from date of injury. In a second case, the pneumoencephalogram was repeated 47 months after the trauma, compared with the preceding examination (which had been performed after 20 months) and it was found that there was a further increase in the already severe cerebral atrophy.

---

* Supported by the Marastoni Foundation

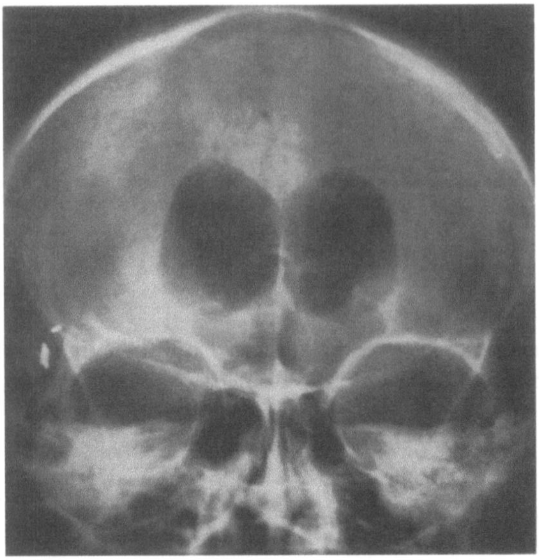

Fig. 1. Umberto F., age 32. After 25 days of posttraumatic coma, he went into an apallic syndrome which has been present for 11 months, showing signs of partial remission. Pneumoencephalography performed 1 year after injury reveals rather severe dilatation of the ventricular system (Evan's index: 0.36)

From a clinical point of view, these six patients all had different evolutions: the apallic syndrome remained unvaried in four patients and may now be considered irreversible (time elapsed: 21, 41, 42, and 78 months, respectively). In two cases there were early signs of partial remission, thus allowing a favorable prognosis. It must be emphasized that these latter two patients had a degree of atrophy which was definitely less severe than the four patients with an unfavorable prognosis.

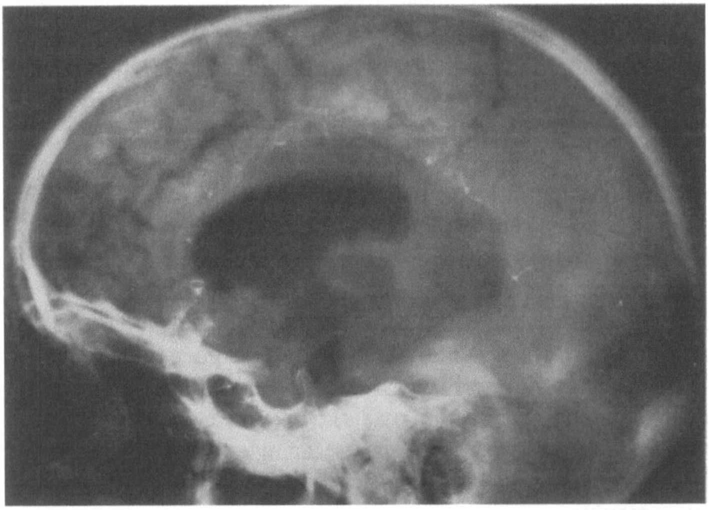

Fig. 2. Chiara C., age 32. After 45 days of coma, she remained in an apallic syndrome for 7 months, showing a slow remission which reached almost complete recovery. Pneumoencephalographic examinations performed 8 months after the trauma reveal a normal ventricular system (Evan's index: 0,26), with dilatation of the subarachnoid spaces of the vault

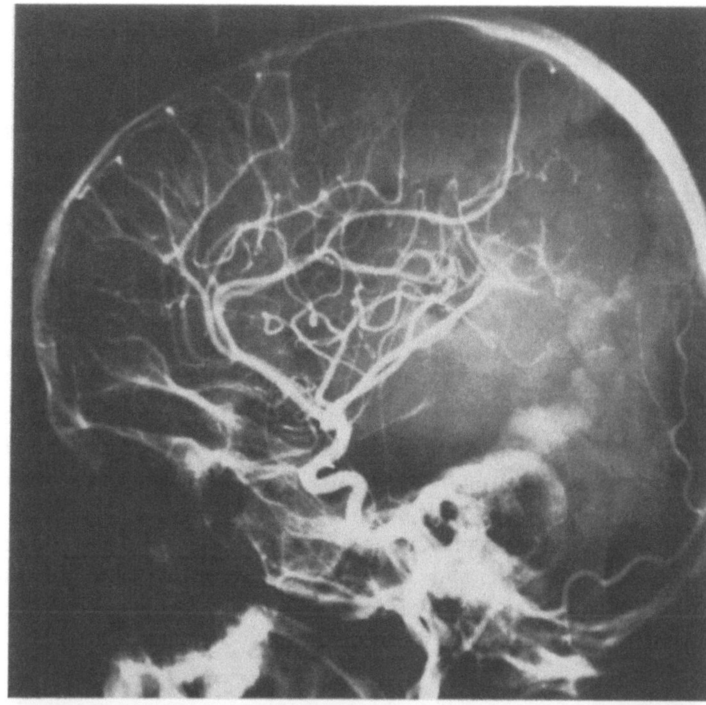

Fig. 3a

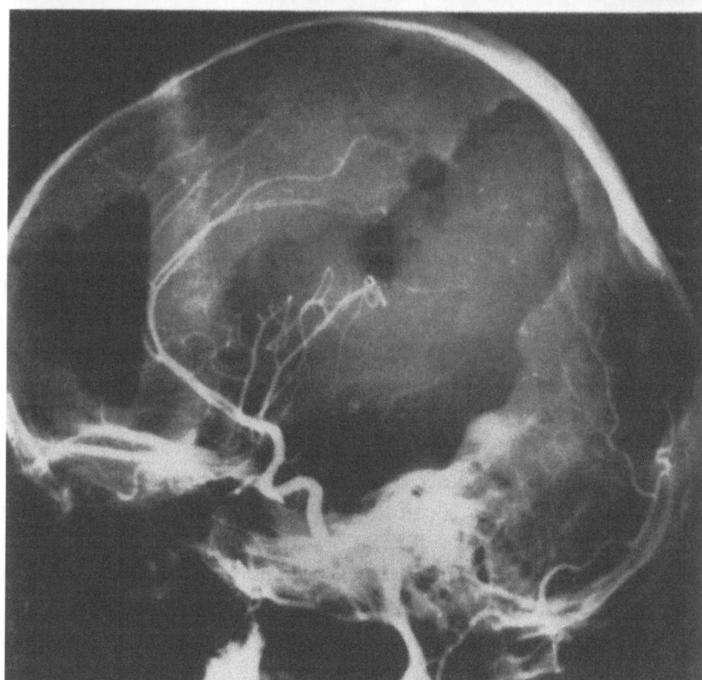

Fig. 3b

Fig. 3. Marina M., age 14. Comparison between carotidangiography performed at time of trauma (a) and one performed 4 years later (b) reveals very conspicuous thinning and impoverishment of arterial tree, the branches of which are stretched by hydrocephalus (i.e., picture of "bare" or "dead tree"). Caliber of inner carotid also appears reduced

The remaining five patients (out of the 11 cases comprising this group) revealed a surprisingly normal ventricular system (Evan's index: below 0.30). Only two patients had cortical atrophy (Fig. 2). The clinical evolution of this group was favorable, with complete recovery in two cases, but without any signs of remission in the other three. The manometric data on liquoral lumbar pressure was normal in all 11 patients. Only seven out of these patients underwent carotidographic examinations during the apallic stage. Five cases showed hydrocephalus, while two cases were normal, thus agreeing with the data revealed by the pneumoencephalographies performed on them.

The comparison of the follow-up angiographies with those performed immediately after the head injury allows for some further very interesting comments. In six cases an impoverishment of the cerebral arterial branches (i.e., the picture of "bare" or "dead tree") was found with a more or less severe narrowing of the diameter of the large arterial trunks. At times this was also evident in the inner carotid. The most important vascular impoverishment was noted in patients with cerebral atrophy (Fig. 3), while a narrowing of the caliber of the inner carotid and its trunks was also observed in one case showing no ventricular dilatation and having a favorable evolution. Carotidographic and pneumoencephalographic findings were perfectly normal in one of the seven cases that also had a favorable evolution.

In two cases carotidographic examinations performed during the early evolutionary stages of coma revealed the onset of hydrocephalus, which was later confirmed by the pneumoencephalographic examination performed during the apallic state.

Conclusions

1. The apallic syndrome does not reveal coherent neuroradiologic pictures, since the pneumoencephalographic and angiographic findings can be either of cerebral atrophy with ventricular dilatation or entirely normal.

2. When a central cerebral atrophy reaches a severe degree (Evan's index: beyond 0.40), it almost always has a negative prognostic significance. On the other hand, when the atrophy has reached a lesser degree, there are possibilities of partial remission and even complete recovery.

3. There can be pneumoencephalographic findings of normal ventricular systems in apallic syndromes with favorable evolution and complete remission as well as in apallic syndromes which turn out to be irreversible. We can thus deduce that nonpathologic encephalographic findings cannot reveal useful data with which to formulate a prognosis.

4. Even though angiography is less valuable than pneumoencephalography in the evaluation of cerebral atrophy it can furnish other useful data in the study of the apallic syndrome. The most significant information revealed by our group of patients is that an irreversible apallic syndrome causes a constant impoverishment of the cerebral arterial tree and a narrowing of the internal carotid and its large trunks. Patients with a protracted but favorable evolution were also found to have a decreased arterial caliber. Normal findings were obtained only in patients who experienced a complete remission within a few months.

5. In the early stages of the syndrome it seems most advisable to perform carotidographic rather than pneumoencephalographic examinations. The former is indeed less traumatic and not at all dangerous, and it furnishes extremely important information regarding the period of onset of the hydrocephalus. An early finding of ventricular dilatation allows the surgeon to perform an early liquoral derivation, thus limiting the spread of the atrophy.

22. Electroencephalographic Findings in the Apallic Syndrome

C.H. LÜCKING, E. MÜLLNER, K. PATEISKY, and F. GERSTENBRAND

Introduction

The electroencephalogram (EEG) records the activity of cortical neurons which are in close contact with thalamic structures and under the permanent synchronizing or desynchronizing influence of the formatio reticularis of the brain stem. Alterations in the cortical region, and also in the basal ganglia, the brain stem and the connecting pathways may modify normal EEG activity. The EEG, however, always reflects only the *functional state* of the cortex without providing information on the degree and localization of morphologic alterations in the individual cases. At the same time, the general viewpoint prevails that EEG activity is strongly correlated with wakefulness, as evidenced by the fact that (1) normal basic alpha activity of 8-13/s is observed only in the relaxed waking state, (2) increased attention leads to desynchronized EEG activity by activation in the ascendent formatio reticularis mesencephali, and (3) a decrease in wakefulness, in sleep or coma is accompanied by synchronized slow EEG waves. A reservation must be made with regard to this view concerning certain phases of sleep (REM phases) as well as comatose states due to lesions in the region of the pons of the brain stem (Loeb et al., 1959).

The apallic syndrome confronts us with a clinical picture pointing mainly to a functional disturbance in the region of the cerebral hemispheres. Initially it may be caused by modifications in the cortex itself or in subcortical structures and in the connecting pathways. Coma vigile as the cardinal symptom is characterized by maintained wakefulness and sleep-wakefulness rhythm and by the suppression of consciousness. This requires intact awakening systems in the upper brain stem (ascendent activating system of the formatio reticularis). The dissociation of wakefulness and consciousness and the other signs of the apallic syndrome, as well as the assumption of an underlying functional disturbance mainly in the area of the cerebral hemispheres, point toward the importance of undertaking a systematic study of the EEGs recorded during the completely developed apallic syndrome, during the individual remission phases, and during the defect stage.

Only those patients with a traumatic apallic syndrome which in all cases had developed after a midbrain syndrome caused by tentorial herniation were chosen for the present investigation. EEGs from apallic syndromes of other etiology (e.g., metabolic, anoxic) are only rarely discussed in other papers (Vigouroux et al., 1964).

Materials and Methods

Twenty-three patients who had been treated for a traumatic apallic syndrome in the rehabilitation ward of the Psychiatric and Neurological University Hospital in Vienna were followed up clinically and electroencephalographically. At the time, 18 patients were between the ages of 20 and 29 years, 3 patients between the ages of 32 and 38 years, 1 patient was 43 years old and another was 54 years old, making a total of 21 men and 2 women. At the time of follow-up examination, the craniocerebral trauma had existed for 1-2 years in 7 patients, for 3-4 years in 11 patients and for 5-6 years in 5 patients. After hospital treatment the patients had repeatedly been examined clinically and electroencephalographically, so that exact notes on the clinical course were available. On the basis of this documentation and according to the criteria formulated by Gerstenbrand (1967), the clinical development was divided into different stages: (1) acute midbrain syndrome, (2) transition stage evolving into the apallic syndrome, (3) completely developed apallic syndrome, (4) remission stage of the apallic syndrome, and (5) defect stage following the apallic syndrome. Of the 23 patients, 14 were largely resocialized, 4 patients were completely disabled, and 5 patients showed disablements of varying degrees.

Due to repeated follow-up examinations, 119 EEGs were available from the 23 patients. An EEG was recorded from 1 patient during the acute midbrain syndrome, during the transition stage from 3 patients, and during the completely developed apallic syndrome from 4 patients. Twenty-two patients were examined electroencephalographically during the remission stage, some of them repeatedly, and altogether 45 recordings were performed. Several recordings were made during the defect stage, so that in this stage 65 EEGs from the 23 patients were available. All of the 119 curves were evaluated by three of the authors independently from one another according to the following criteria: *basic activity* (generalized background activity); degree of *generalized changes* (s = severe generalized changes with predominant theta and delta waves; mo = moderate generalized changes with predominant theta waves and interposition of delta waves; m = mild generalized changes with increased theta activity; 0 = no generalized changes); *foci* and their localization in relation to the site of trauma; *irritative phenomena* in the form of paroxysmal delta waves and/or sharp waves; and *epileptic phenomena* in the form of spikes or spikes and waves.

Results

The analysis of the clinical course reveals developments of varying rates for the 23 patients, from the acute midbrain syndrome to the transition stage and to the completely developed traumatic apallic syndrome. Also, the duration of the completely developed traumatic apallic syndrome, and especially that of the remission stage, vary considerably. Table 1 demonstrates the shortest, average, and longest duration of the individual stages. The beginning of the defect stage, in which no more appreciable clinical remission took place, was observed on an average after 350 days, at the latest after nearly 800 days, and in one case as soon as 60 days after the accident. The onset of the defect stage and thus the end of remission could for some patients be stated only approximately because sometimes even after discharge from the hospital a further remission took place, the termination of which could not be exactly ascertained in time. For this reason, the beginning of the defect state has perhaps been assumed too late in some cases.

Table 1. Duration of the clinical stages in 23 patients with traumatic apallic syndromes

	Shortest duration (days)	Average duration (days)	Longest duration (days)
Acute midbrain syndrome	0.5	2.7	6
Transition stage	2	11	19
Completely developed TAS	2	20	50
Remission stage	54	316	775

The correlation of the individual EEGs with the clinical stages for each of the 23 patients revealed considerable differences between individuals, but generally the same developmental trend was seen for the whole group. The different severity of EEG changes in relation to the individual clinical stages is shown in two examples. Figure 1 shows the

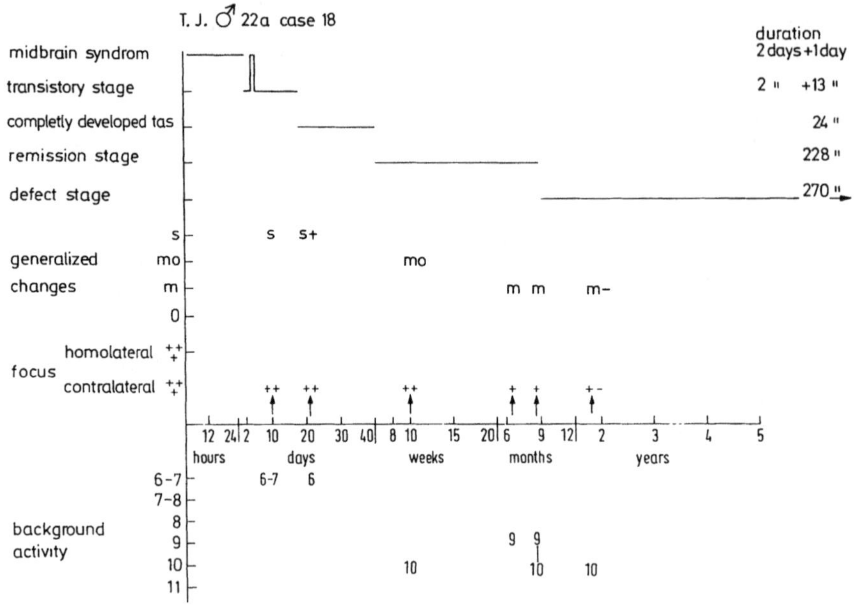

Fig. 1. Clinical and electroencephalographic course of 22-year-old patient (T.J.) with traumatic apallic syndrome (*tas*). Trauma left-frontally. *s* = severe (*s+* = more severe), *mo* = moderate, *m* = mild (*m–* = slighter). ++ = severe focus, + = mild focus, +– = barely perceivable focus

clinical and electroencephalographic course of a 22-year-old patient. The duration of the individual clinical stages corresponds approximately to the patient collective (see Table 1). During the transition stage there is a short-term relapse to the acute midbrain syndrome. The first EEG was recorded during the transition stage and indicates severe general disturbances, a distinct focus contralateral to the site of trauma, and a basic activity of 6-7/s. At the onset of the completely developed traumatic apallic syndrome the generalized changes have even increased. Ten weeks after the accident—already in the remission stage—generalized changes of a moderate degree with still-distinct signs of a contralateral focus and an acceleration of the basic activity to 10/s are observed. After 6 1/2-8 1/2 months following the accident the patient is still in the remission stage: the EEG patterns are largely the same, except for a somewhat slower basic activity. After 9 months the patient reaches the defect stage. More than 1 year later the EEG is nearly normal and presents only discrete generalized changes and focal symptoms.

Figure 2 shows the clinical and electroencephalographic development of another 22-year-old patient who, after a relatively long-lasting midbrain syndrome, went through the

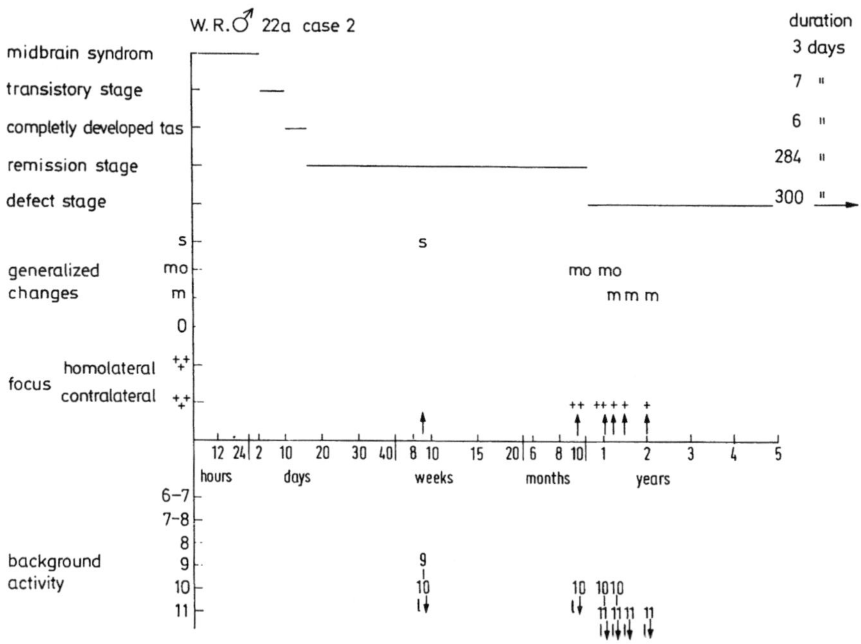

Fig. 2. Clinical and electroencephalographic course of 22-year-old patient (W.R.) with traumatic apallic syndrome (*tas*). Trauma right-fronto-temporal. For abbreviations see Figure 1. l = at left less marked

transition stage and the completely developed traumatic apallic syndrome very rapidly. During the remission stage (9 weeks after the accident), the EEG shows severe generalized changes with a less marked background activity of 9-10/s at the left and without other focal symptoms. Seven months later, toward the end of the remission stage, the generalized changes have slightly regressed, whereas a significant theta-delta focus is observed contralateral to the site of trauma. Three months later, already in the defect stage, this picture was found to be unaltered except for a slight acceleration in basic activity. In three further examinations, performed in the following years in which no further clinical improvement took place, the generalized changes had further regressed, the focus was only insignificantly marked, and the basic activity was stabilized at a frequency of 11/s with a further slight decrease over the left hemisphere.

Figure 3 shows representative EEG tracings for one patient with a traumatic apallic syndrome, taken from recordings performed during (1) the transition stage from the acute midbrain syndrome to the traumatic apallic syndrome, (2) during the completely developed traumatic apallic syndrome, and (3) during the defect stage, which was reached 9 months later. In the transition stage (*A*)—associated with the clinical picture of a marked brain stem lesion—sections of flat activity with a well-maintained basic activity of 7-8/s alternating with sections of diffuse delta interposition of a higher amplitude can be seen. The EEG in the completely developed traumatic apallic syndrome (*B*) is dominated by the theta waves and by delta waves which are more pronounced on the left. Almost 11 months after the accident, in the defect stage, the EEG has normalized to a great extent (*C*).

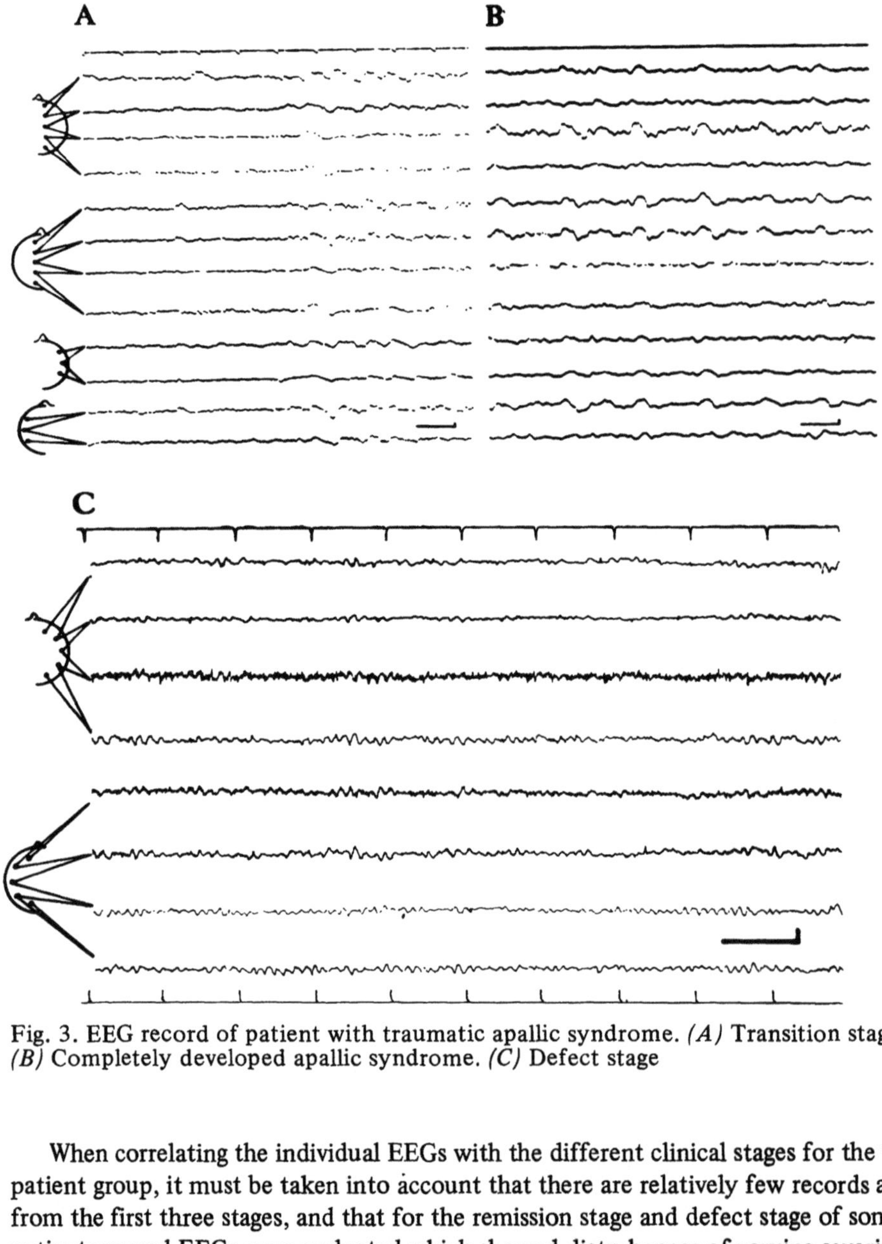

Fig. 3. EEG record of patient with traumatic apallic syndrome. *(A)* Transition stage. *(B)* Completely developed apallic syndrome. *(C)* Defect stage

When correlating the individual EEGs with the different clinical stages for the whole patient group, it must be taken into account that there are relatively few records available from the first three stages, and that for the remission stage and defect stage of some of the patients several EEGs were evaluated which showed disturbances of varying severity. An alteration in the EEG patterns is to be expected, especially in the course of remission, because in this often very long-lasting stage a considerable improvement in the neurologic picture often may take place. In Figure 4, the degree of the generalized changes (for definition, see *Materials and Methods* above) in the 119 EEGs from the 23 patients is correlated with the clinical stages. The only recording made in this group of patients during the acute midbrain syndrome shows only mild generalized changes. This finding has been reported elsewhere (Lücking, 1970b). In the transition stage and in the completely developed

Fig. 4. Degree of severity of generalized changes in EEG in the individual clinical stages of 23 patients with traumatic apallic syndromes. For abbrevations see Figure 1

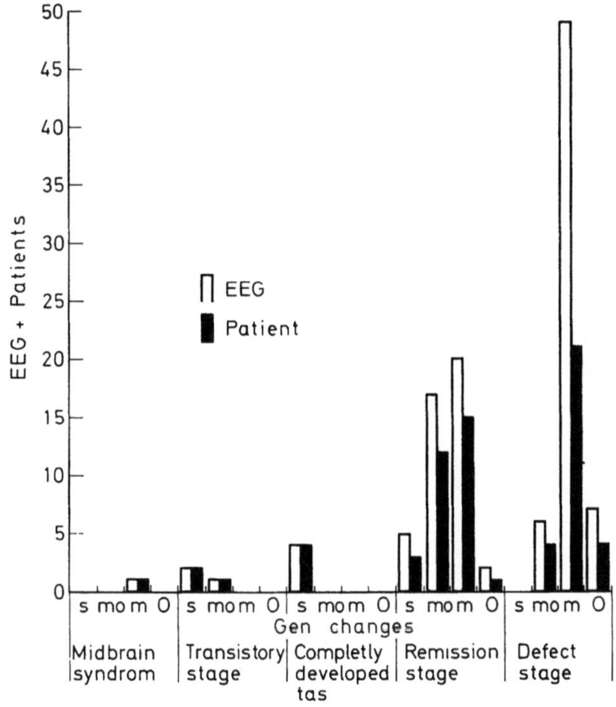

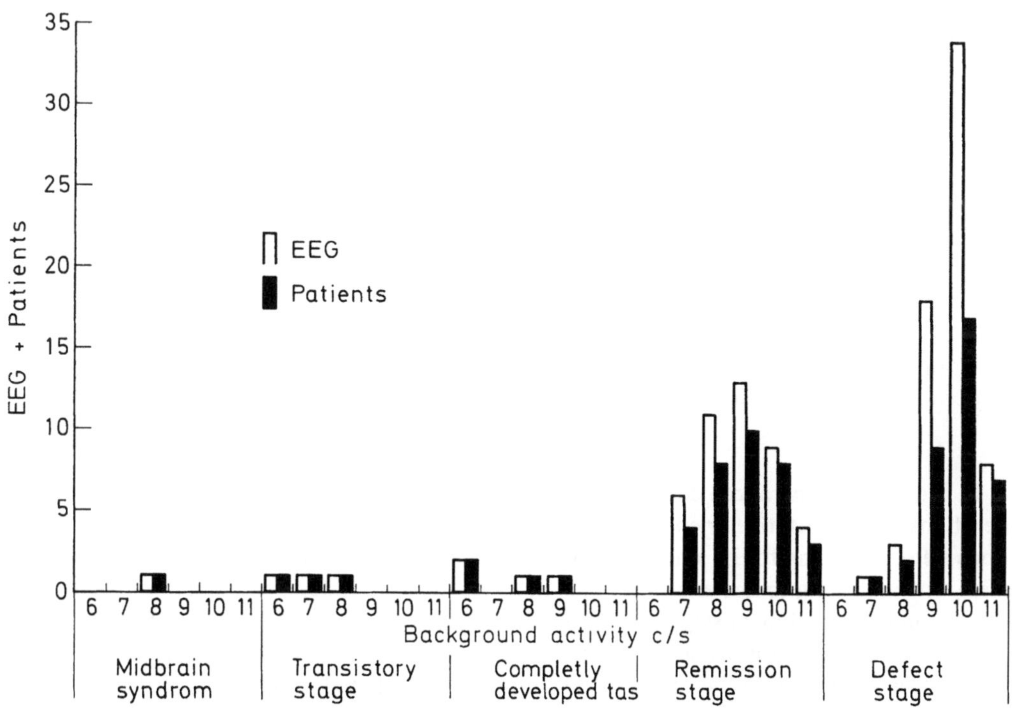

Fig. 5. Background activity in individual clinical stages of 23 patients with traumatic apallic syndrome (*tas*)

traumatic apallic syndrome moderate and severe generalized changes predominate. In the remission stage moderate and mild generalized changes predominate; only in rare cases one may see severe generalized changes. In the defect stage, on the other hand, we have not observed any severe generalized changes; a high percentage of patients show mild to just perceivable generalized changes, some patients show moderate abnormalities or even a normal EEG.

A quite similar development is found by correlating background activity with the clinical stages (Fig. 5). In the acute midbrain syndrome, in the transition stage, and in the completely developed traumatic apallic syndrome, the basic activity has a frequency of 6-9/s, in the remission stage mainly 8-10/s, and in the defect stage 10/s. Sometimes a normal curve with well-pronounced basic alpha activity with a normal distribution and without perceivable generalized changes is observed even before the onset of the remission stage (Fig. 6).

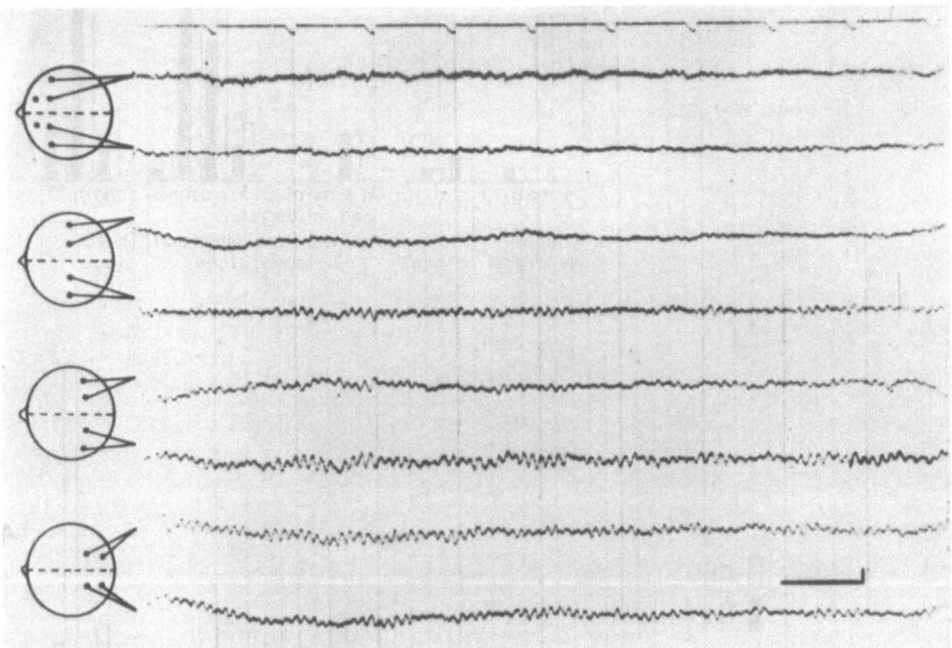

Fig. 6. EEG record of patient in remission stage of traumatic apallic syndrome 4 weeks after craniocerebral trauma; well-pronounced basic alpha activity

In addition to generalized changes and background activity the appearance of focal alterations and of irritative or epileptic phenomena have been analyzed. The focal alterations were, according to the amount of focal theta and delta activity, classified as mild and severe, and according to the site of trauma, in homo- or contralateral foci and correlated with the individual clinical stages. Bitemporal foci were taken into account separately. Table 2 demonstrates this classification in detail. It shows a significant predominance of the contralateral foci with the onset of the completely developed traumatic apallic syndrome. Compared to the remission stage, fewer patients in the defect stage suffered from severe contralateral foci (eight compared with the three patients), but during this time severe and mild homolateral foci are observed more frequently. Figure 7 shows a slight focus over the left posterior quadrant in one patient at the beginning of the defect stage *(A)*, 7 months after the accident with a right frontal trauma. Two years and 3 months later *(B)*, still in an unaltered defect stage, the focus can be seen more clearly and has expanded more precentrotemporally. Bitemporal foci are found relatively seldom; they can manifest themselves only in the late course.

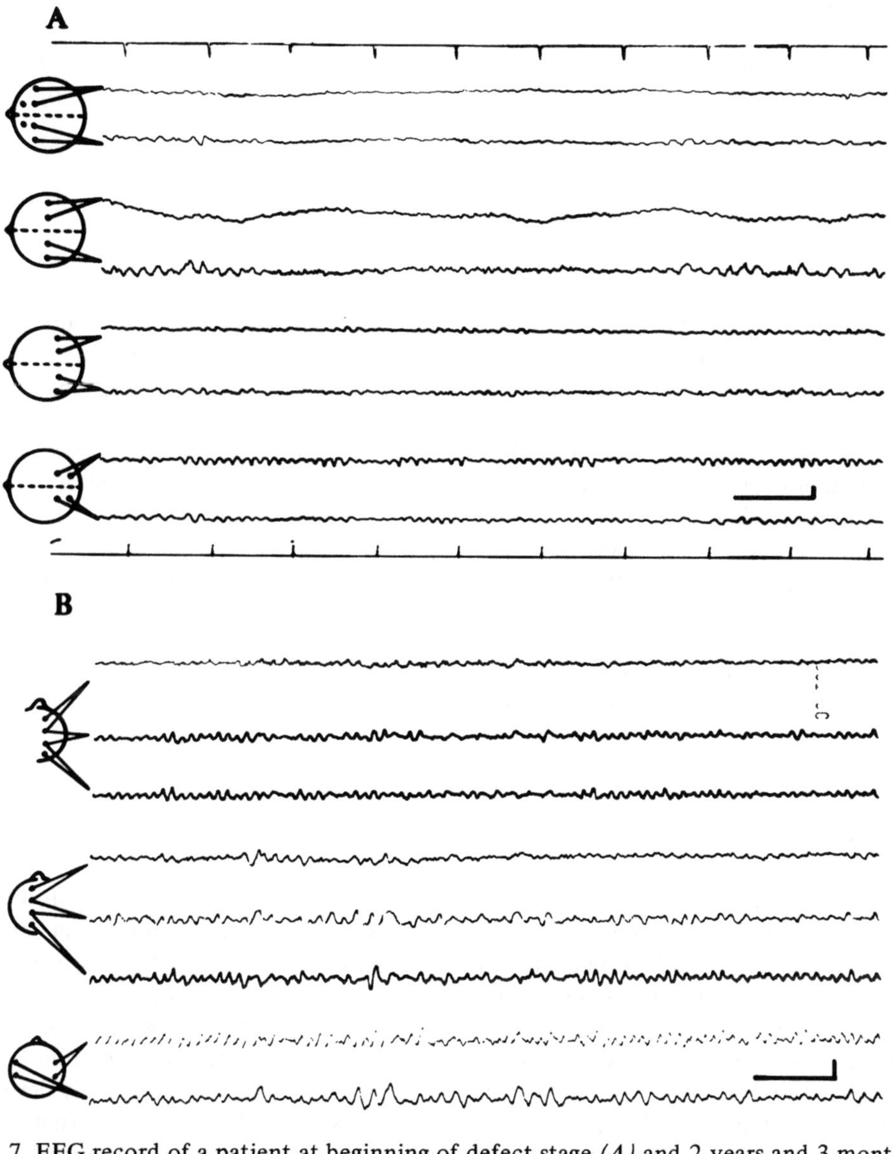

Fig. 7. EEG record of a patient at beginning of defect stage *(A)* and 2 years and 3 months later *(B)* after traumatic apallic syndrome following craniocerebral trauma. Focus above left posterior quadrant *(A)* has become more marked and expanded *(B)*

Table 2. Degree of severity and localization (in relation to the site of the trauma) of foci and appearance of irritative or epileptic phenomena in EEG during individual stages in 23 patients with traumatic apallic syndrome.

Clinical stage		Midbrain syndrome	Transition stage	Completely developed TAS	Remission stage	Defect stage
Number of EEG/ patients		1/1	3/3	4/4	45/22	65/23
Homolateral focus	severe	1/1	–	–	4/4	8/5
	mild	–	1/1	–	1/1	10/4
Contralateral focus	severe	–	1/1	2/2	8/8	3/3
	mild	–	–	–	17/12	31/12
Bitemporal focus		–	–	–	4/3	10/6
Irritative phenomena		–	–	1/1	4/3	8/6
Epileptic phenomena		–	–	–	3/2	10/5

Number of EEGs in relation to the number of patients is indicated EEG/patient)

A number of patients (Table 2) showed irritative or epileptic phenomena. In the completely developed traumatic apallic syndrome irritative phenomena were observed in one out of four patients. In three patients these patterns were observed in the remission stage, in three others only in the defect stage. Epileptic activity was observed in two patients in the remission stage, in five patients in the defect stage. During the remission stage one patient showed isolated spikes above the left centroparietal region immediately after photostimulation, which were found to exist unaltered in the defect stage more than 2 1/2 years later. Clinically this patient had never had an epileptic seizure. The second patient who showed epileptic activity in the remission stage had suffered from one jacksonian attack a few days after the accident. Another patient had a jacksonian attack during the defect stage 3 years after the accident and then showed isolated epileptic activity for the first time. Focal seizures were reported in three other patients without irritative or epileptic phenomena having been observed in former or later EEGs.

Discussion

This is a retrospective study. In order to be able to investigate an etiologically uniform patient group, only the traumatic apallic syndrome was taken into account, which developed in all cases as a result of tentorial herniation. With respect to possible prognostic criteria, patients were mainly chosen who presented a favorable clinical course and had been followed up with exact clinical and electroencephalographic examinations for several years (in most cases, 2-5 years). However, only a few EEGs were available from the early phases of the disease (midbrain syndrome, transition stages, and completely developed apallic syndrome). Chatrian et al. (1963) and Lücking (1970b, 1972) reported on the prognostic value of EEGs recorded in an early stage after a severe craniocerebral trauma with tentorial herniation. In these reports it was shown that the EEG sometimes allows relevant prognostic statements even at that early stage. It must be taken into account, however, that in spite of an initially favorable electroencephalographic and cerebral development death can occur due to extracerebral complications.

The EEG findings from several months of observing apallic patients with mainly lethal courses are reported by Jellinger et al. (1963). During the first few weeks most severe generalized changes–including a flattening of the curve without any reactivity to external stimuli–were observed, and in the following months (during the completely developed apallic syndrome) a predominating theta activity with interpositon of delta waves without alpha activity was observed. In the late phase (5-6 months after trauma) further marked generalized changes with a low index of alpha waves and an incomplete blocking effect after stimulation were observed. Favorable clinical courses were associated with a faster regression of the theta waves and an early reinstitution of alpha activity. Focal signs and lateral differences were rarely hints of an increased susceptibility to attack. It is general experience that the degree of deficit in consciousness and the degree of EEG slowing, as well as the regression of the EEG changes and the recovery of consciousness, are parallel phenomena (Gastaut, 1954; Fischgold and Mathis, 1959). This observation generally refers to the suppression of consciousness during coma in which both wakefulness and conscious activity are extinguished. A separate disturbance of wakefulness and consciousness as manifested in the coma vigile of the apallic syndrome is thereby not taken into account.

The present investigation of apallic patients with an exact clinical and electroencephalographic examination of the remission stages confirms the observation which is known from other comatose states: In general, clinical improvement is associated with an acceleration in EEG activity. A close correlation between wakefulness and EEG changes, however, is not seen in any of the cases. In spite of increasing wakefulness, in the coma vigile the theta and delta waves frequently still constitute the predominating EEG activity. Only with the onset of conscious activity is it gradually accelerated and can, even after many years when no more appreciable clinical remission has taken place, further alternate with an increase in alpha activity and a regression of focal symptoms (Figs. 1 and 2). This is not surprising, since the EEG reflects the neuronal activity of the cerebral cortex to which are bound consciousness and the higher cerebral functions, but not wakefulness. Since an alpha activity may quite well predominate in the coma vigile stage (Fig. 6), there is no strong interdependence between conscious activity and rapid EEG activity. An alpha EEG may also be found in the case of suppression of both wakefulness *and* consciousness (Loeb et al., 1959; Lücking, 1972). Since the neuronal activity of the cortex and thus of the EEG is dependent on the intactness of the cortex as well as of the subcortical structures, different damage patterns of the brain and, at the same time, different clinical conditions may be associated with an identical EEG. While anoxia mainly results in cortical damage, a diffuse brain edema (posttraumatic or metabolic) rather produces damage to the cerebral white matter and, as a result of tentorial herniation, a lesion in the mesodiencephalic region. The prognostic value of the EEG in the apallic syndrome must also be seen under the following aspect: Predominating theta-delta activity which persists largely unchanged for several months during the transition to the clinical remission stage points to a significant lesion of the hemispheres. An increasing alpha activity already appearing at the beginning of remission suggests a slighter cortical involvement and a stronger subcortical lesion. Taking clinical symptomatology and development simultaneously into account, the EEG may contribute to the prognostic evaluation (Vigouroux et al., 1964). Other criteria for EEG evaluation are of relatively minor importance. An acceleration of alpha frequency within the range of 9-11/s, for example, still occurs after many years (Fig. 2) without any further clinical improvement. Focal symptoms, contralateral as well as homolateral to the site of trauma, can often be recognized only after regression of the severe general changes, and in the course of normalization above the other regions it often appears as if these signs were increasing (Fig. 7). Temporal foci often show a jumping from one side to the other and predominate in the defect stage on the side of the trauma. Only in relatively few patients are constant bitemporal foci found, which can be expected as a result of tentorial herniation of the mediobasal components of the temporal lobe. Epileptic phenomena as a result of increased cerebral susceptibility to attacks may be important only in connection with the clinical findings: From among five patients with multiply evidenced spike potentials, only two patients had suffered from one jacksonian attack and only one patient was under anticonvulsive medication. On the other hand, in three patients who had suffered from focal attacks, epileptic activity of the EEG could not be verified at any time.

Summary

The investigation involves 23 patients who developed a traumatic apallic syndrome after severe craniocerebral trauma. All patients showed a favorable course with regression of the apallic syndrome to a defect stage of differing severity. The observation time was from 4 to 6 years with regularly performed clinical examinations and repeated EEGs. Altogether, 119 EEGs were evaluated. The correlation of EEG findings with the clinical development of the apallic syndrome showed considerable individual variability in this group of patients. The degree and regression of the EEG changes were correlated with the reinstitution of conscious activity and the higher brain functions rather than with the degree of wakefulness. Severe and moderate generalized changes which persist unaltered throughout the first months, point to a lasting functional damage of the cortex. On the other hand a reappearance of alpha activity already present in the coma vigile or early remission stage points to only slight involvement of the cortex without allowing definite conclusions regarding possible lesions of the subcortical structures and the brain stem. Prognostic statements are possible only within these limitations. Focal symptoms and lateral differences reflect local damage without a strong relation to the site of the trauma. Even with consistent irritative and epileptic phenomena, the development of cerebral attacks is rarely observed.

23. Studies on Sleep During the Apallic Syndrome

B. BERGAMASCO, L. BERGAMINI, A. BRICOLO, and G. DOLCE

The presence of electroencephalographic and behavioral patterns typical of sleep in unconscious patients was established some time ago (Jouvet et al., 1961; Chatrian et al., 1963; Silverman, 1963; Hess, 1965; Bergamasco et al., 1966a, b; Bricolo, 1966; Cadilhac et al., 1966; Lepetit et al., 1966). There have also been studies on the correlation between the organization of sleep, degree of coma, and anatomic cerebral lesions (French, 1952; Jouvet et al., 1961; Silverman, 1963; Bricolo, 1966; Cadilhac et al., 1966; Lepetit et al., 1966). Finally, it has been suggested that the type of sleep organization might yield useful elements for a prognosis (Bergamasco et al., 1966a, b; Bricolo, 1966). The research carried out by Dolce and Kaemmerer (1966), Gentilomo et al. (1966), Bricolo (1966), Rosadini and Gentilomo (1967) appears particularly important, since they studied the EEG patterns of sleep in a group of comatose patients who were evolving towards the apallic syndrome. These authors reported that they had found all the various phases of physiologic sleep, noticing only a peculiar gradual recovery of each single phase, characterized by the constant delay of desynchronized sleep with REM which always reappears after the complete restructuring of synchronized sleep. These initial observations led to further research on the sleep of comatose patients and in particular in cases of prolonged comas and of apallic syndromes. These studies were undertaken during the past few years by sleep laboratories in Turin, Frankfurt, Genoa, and Verona.

Case Material and Methods

The case histories involve 46 cases of prolonged posttraumatic comas in the various stages of the apallic syndrome. In all cases we performed diurnal and nocturnal longitudinal electropolygraphic recordings, sometimes even protracted for over 24 h. Eight patients were monitored up to the favorable or unfavorable evolution of the morbid picture (i.e., until recovery or exitus). The case material also includes 18 patients in posttraumatic comas, who were monitored day and night with seriated polygraphic recordings during the acute stage. The conditions of four of these patients evolved into apallic syndromes.

The recording of the electroencephalogram was performed through platinum-gold pin electrodes inserted into the scalp of the frontal temporal, central parietal, and occipital regions of both hemispheres; the recording of eye movements, the electromyogram, and the electrocardiogram were performed through disc electrodes affixed onto the periorbital regions, the muscles of the nape, and onto the sternocleidomastoideus and the lower limbs. Respiratory movements were recorded by means of a piezoelectric transducer. Finally, the patients were observed directly, and any behavioral event was written on the EEG record. The recordings were studied, with a correlation of the various data every 20 s. Sleep was divided into five phases: "Falling-asleep" phase or Stage I; spindles phase or Stage II; the K complexes or Stage III; nonreactive phase or Stage IV; and REM or paradoxical sleep or Stage V.

Results

After gathering and comparing the data obtained by various research teams (Bergamasco et al., 1968a, b; Bricolo et al., 1967, 1968a, b; Dolce and Kaemmerer, 1966, 1967), the following conclusions were reached:

1. Sleep Patterns During the Midbrain Stage of the Apallic Syndrome

The results refer to four patients from the Bergamini-Bergamasco case histories and to five patients from the Dolce series. In two cases Bergamini-Bergamasco observed typical patterns of sleep which at first were isolated and later showed nictemeral organization and the presence of all phases of physiologic sleep (Fig. 1). The other two cases in their series revealed no polygraphic patterns of normal sleep. These cases had an unfavorable prognosis, while the two former patients reached the remission stage. Dolce, in his five cases, did not observe the typical patterns of sleep at this stage.

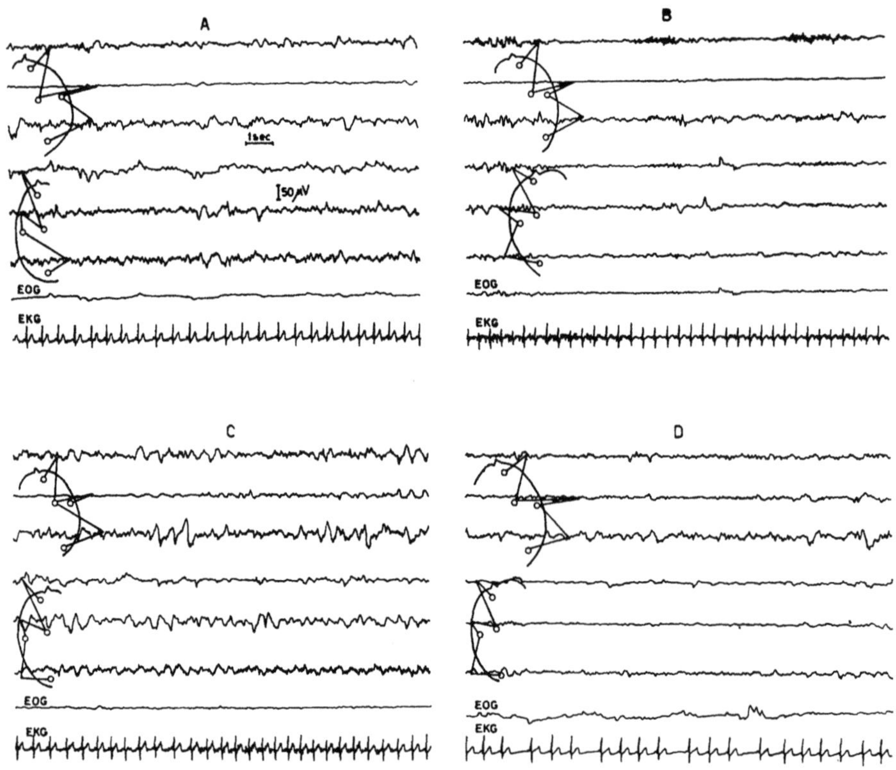

Fig. 1. EEG, EOG, and EKG of mesencephalic comatose patient (B.B., 20 years old) during the day *(A)* and during the night *(B, C, D)*. Easily distinguished normal sleep patterns in the night-time recordings: Phase II with spindles *(B)*, Phase IV with hypersynchronized slow waves *(C)*, REM phase with bursts of rapid eye movements on the EOG, desynchronized EEG, and irregularities of heart frequency *(D)*

2. Sleep Patterns During the Apallic Syndrome

Most of our research has been devoted to the sleep studies of this stage. Dolce and Kaemmerer (1967) observed patterns of typical sleep in all of their 12 cases, although with individual differences. Bricolo et al. (1967) observed sleep patterns in eight cases (Fig. 2) and no polygraphic signs of sleep in six cases (Fig. 3). Bergamasco et al. (1968a) studied 12 cases, eight with sleep patterns and 4 without. At a later data Bricolo et al. (1968a) studied a further

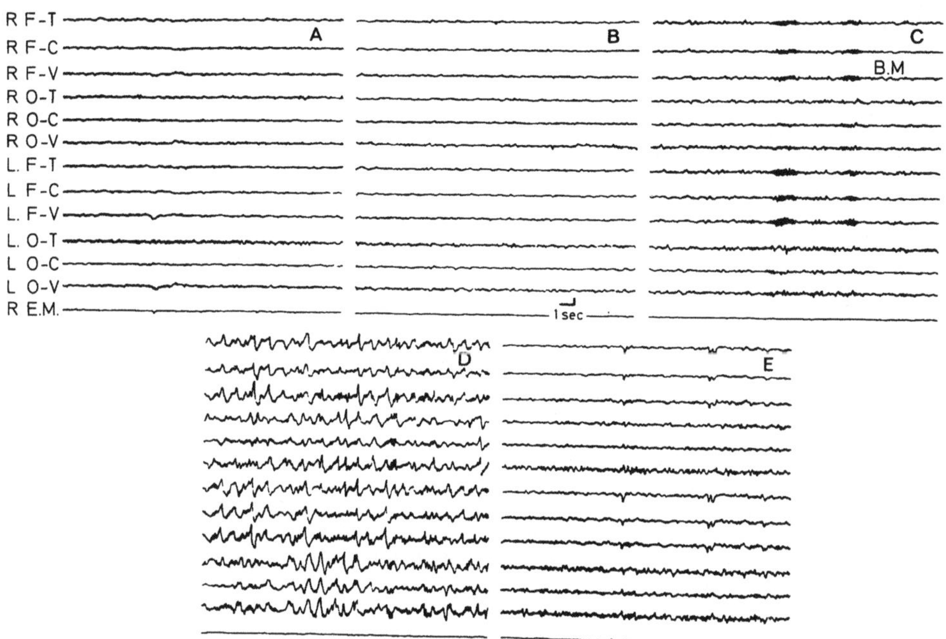

Fig. 2. Complete structure of sleep in akinetic mutism (45 days following head injury): EEG recording. *R:* right; *L:* left; *F:* frontal; *T:* temporal; *C:* central; *O:* occipital; *V:* vertex; *REM:* eye movements. *(A)* Subject's eyes are open (wakeful-like state). *(B-E)* Behaviorally asleep. EEG patterns in these conditions are typical of sleep phases I *(B)*, II *(C)*, III *(D)* and V *(E)*

series of 22 patients with similar proportions. Bergamasco et al. (1968b) and Bricolo et al. (1968b) demonstrate that the organization of sleep at the full stage of the apallic syndrome has prognostic significance. Indeed, the patients who at this stage of the apallic syndrome do not show nocturnal polygraphic patterns typical of sleep usually do not improve, while patients with a good structure of sleep from a polygraphic viewpoint usually have a favorable evolution.

3. Sleep Patterns in the Remission Stage

The recordings of Dolce and Kaemmerer show that there are no significant differences compared to the sleep of normal people, except for a gradual recovery of the paradoxical phase.

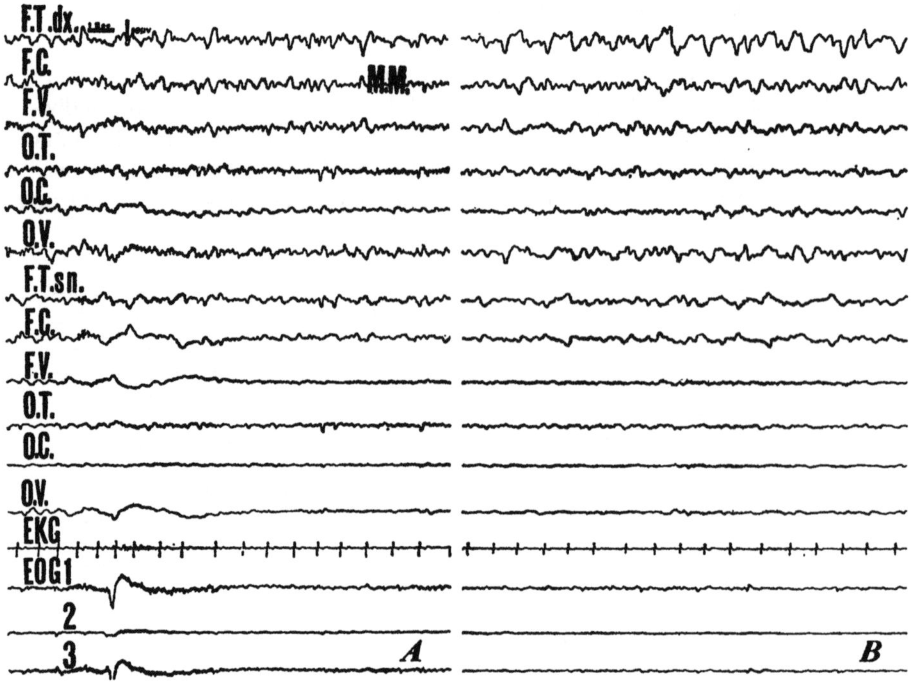

Fig. 3. M.M., 18 years old. Apallic syndrome unvaried for 12 months following severe head injury complicated by acute subdural hematoma of the left convexity. Electropolygraphic pictures during the wakefulnesslike phase *(A)* and during sleep phase *(B)* 328 days after injury. Note that EEG tracing remained extremely monotonous during duration of recording (24 h). (*F:* frontal; *T:* median temporal; *C:* central; *V:* vertex; *O:* occipital; *dx:* right; *sn:* left; *EKG:* electrocardiogramm; *EOG 1, 2, 3:* ocular movements)

Conclusions

From these summarized data, which are the result of several thousand hours of nocturnal recordings, we can draw *a posteriori* a single unequivocal conclusion: In apallic syndromes with a favorable clinical evolution, there is an early appearance of satisfactory electroencephalographic manifestations of sleep resembling in all aspects those recorded during the physiologic sleep of normal people. As a matter of fact, these sleep patterns already appear at times in the initial midbrain stage, and the basic EEG activity, EEG reactivity, and sleep organization towards a nictemeral cycle is gradual. This was described by Dolce and Kaemmerer (1967), as follows:

At the onset of the apallic stage the EEG at times reveals the first signs of reactivity: A burst of delta waves on the frontal regions following painful stimuli. The basic EEG activity accelerates progressively from 4 to 6-7 c/s. The appearance of an 8 c/s rhythm on the posterior regions (which might be early), does not correspond to an appreciable alteration of vigilance: The degree of incommunicability remains unvaried. The 8 c/s rhythm is never constant, but intermingled or alternated with diffuse slower activity. Its frequency does not increase and it does not reveal completely the effect of a block upon the opening of the eyes.

The sleep phases on the EEG are at first incomplete: During the first 4 months following the trauma, paradoxical sleep is rarely observed; the sigma rhythms, K complexes, and some periods of electrical arousal appear often on both hemispheres, in a rather asymmetric manner. Paradoxical desynchronized sleep increases progressively in time, up to 15% of the total sleep period. The phases of this sleep usually appear in one isolated episode, 3-4 h after the onset of the synchronized sleep of stage IV. The hypnogram is complete only 3-4 months after the brain injury, and thus the typical pattern described by Jouvet is missing. This researcher had described the presence in man of only slow sleep in cases of lesions of the brain stem and of only desynchronized sleep with REM in cases of severe lesions of the cerebral cortex and of the white matter. In conclusion, the adult brain, which apallic syndrome reduces to a mesencephalic level, reacquires more or less completely its upper functions, not through a new process but due to the slow reinstatement of preexisting functions. This possibility is already well demonstrated at certain stages of remission. Despite the fact that the clinical picture remains stationary, the EEG shows, through the months, a progressive evolution towards normality.

In cases where the bioelectric reorganization of nocturnal sleep does not take place or takes place to an incomplete degree, there is usually a poor clinical evolution, even if it is long lasting. This suggests greater severity of the cerebral lesions and a lack of reintegration of the higher functions of the brain, which has been reduced to mesencephalic levels.

24. Complementary Examinations of the Central Nervous System Activity in the Apallic Syndrome

S. MINGRINO

One of the most important problems in the apallic syndrome is represented by the study of the central nervous system activity, which is particularly difficult to examine during a condition of unconsciousness. The more elements of the complex clinical picture available, the more accurate the diagnostic and prognostic evaluation of the patient. These consider-actions explain the search for ever new and more sophisticated methods of investigating the functions of the central nervous system.

Three new methods of studying different aspects of brain activity in apallic patients are reported here (1) the vestibulo-ocular reflex, (2) the acoustic-stapedial and malleolar reflex, and (3) the nictemeral modifications of blood cortisol.

Physiopathologic Basis

1. Vestibulo-ocular (v-o) reflex. Nervous structures mediating the v-o reflex are located in the pons and mesencephalon (Fig. 1). Researchers have concluded that at least two path-ways of connection between vestibular and ocular nuclei exist through the posterior longi-tudinal fasciculus (f.l.m.) and the reticular substance (s.r.) (Lorente de Nò, 1933; Mingrino et al., 1966). The pathway through the f.l.m. is oligosynaptic and mediates the slow com-ponent of the v-o reflex, while the nystagmic response is elaborated in the polysynaptic pathway of the s.r. (Lorente de Nò, 1938; Szentàgothai, 1950; Mingrino et al., 1966).

These two pathways present a different resistance to trauma. In fact, it was found that in patients with acute head injuries the nystagmic response is the first to be altered in its patterns and may even disappear, while the slow response remains and is abolished only in deep coma (Mingrino et al., 1965).

2. The acoustic-stapedial and malleolar (a-s-m) reflex is mediated by nuclei of the pons; the stapedial reflex by the acoustic and facial nuclei, and the malleolar reflex by the acous-tic and motor trigeminal nuclei (Fig. 1).

3. Nictemeral rhythm of blood cortisol. The normal level of blood cortisol in man changes during the day from 4 to 15 mg/100 ml and is higher around 8 a.m. Cortisolemy depends on hypophyseal secretion of ACTH, which is controlled by the supraoptic and infundibular nuclei of the hypothalamus. Experimental investigations have demonstrated that many encephalic structures influence ACTH secretion through hypothalamic centers by stimulation or inhibition. Among these suprahypothalamic centers, the most important are the reticular substance of the mesencephalon, the cortex, and the limbic system (Mason, 1958).

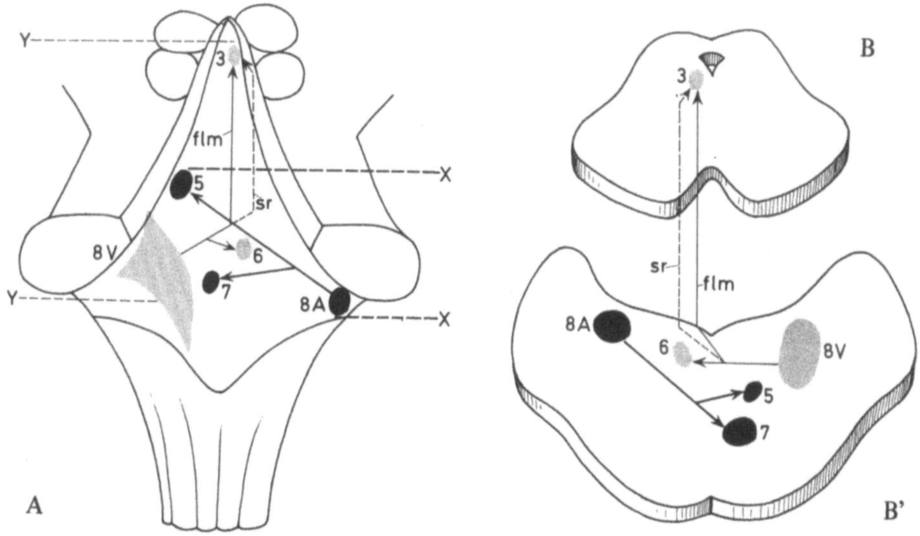

Fig. 1. *(A)* Posterior surface of the brain stem with floor of the fourth ventricle. The segment *(Y-Y)* indicates the site of structures mediating the v-o reflex; the segment *(X-X)* comprises the structures underlying the a-s-m reflex. *(B-B')* Transversal section of mesencephalon and pons respectively. *3*: oculomotor nuclei, *5*: motor trigeminal nucleus, *6*: abducens nucleus, *8 V*: vestibular nuclei, *8A*: acoustic nuclei, *flm*: posterior longitudinal fasciculus, *s.r.*: reticular substance

Material and Methods

Ten patients presenting a picture of apallic coma after head injury which had been sustained 4-8 weeks previously were selected for study. Patients with peripheral paralysis of the facial nerve, lesions of the external and middle ear, or whose X-rays showed fracture of the petrus bone, were excluded. High fever or inflammatory processes were also reasons for exclusion.

1. The v-o reflex was evoked by cold caloric stimulation, injecting 10 ml of water at 18°C into the ear canal; if this did not activate the reflex, irrigation was repeated with ice water. The patient was kept in a supine position with the head flexed forward 30 degrees and with the eyes open.

2. The a-s-m reflex was examined by recording the impedance of the ear through an electroacoustic device. By means of this apparatus the unknown impedance of the tympanic membrane is balanced and compared with a variable impedance standard. The reflex was elicited by giving the stimulating tone to the controlateral ear.

3. The nictemeral rhythm was studied by examining the variations of the blood cortisol level every 4 h, starting at 8 a.m.

Results

A. Vestibular stimulation evoked different types of ocular responses:

1. Nystagmic responses with some irregular patterns were seen in six patients. Four recovered without deficit, one patient retained a mild ataxia and another had severe neurologic and psychiatric deficits.
2. Slow responses were observed in four patients, in two of them the responses were associated with some nystagmic jerks. Only one patient from this group recovered.

B. The acoustic-malleolar and stapedial reflex was bilaterally present in all patients.

C. The study of the nictemeral blood cortisol level revealed that all of the patients showed modifications of the cortisolemy during the day. The basal level of cortisol was higher than normal in two patients. Five patients showed alterations of the circadian rhythm, as a higher value of cortisolemy occurred at different periods of the day, in the afternoon, or in the evening. Among these patients were the three who presented slow ocular deviation and two patients with nystagmic response. Three patients with normal circadian rhythms and two with altered rhythms of cortisolemy survived.

Discussion

Alterations in the v-o and a-s-m reflexes indicate a lesion in the pons or mesencephalon. The v-o reflex is particularly sensible and useful, as its response can vary according to extension of the lesions. Previous study has demonstrated that patients with acute head injuries who show nystagmus have a better prognosis than patients with slow ocular deviation (Mingrino et al., 1965). Findings in apallic paitnets do not have a clear prognostic significance. However, the small number of cases studied seems to confirm the results obtained in acute cases.

The a-s-m reflex may be present or absent, but its response is otherwise uniform. The segment of pons it explores is adjacent to nervous structures studied by the v-o reflex (Fig. 1), and it is very likely that both reflexes will be affected or spared by the trauma at the same time. Since the a-s-m is an oligosynaptic reflex and thus behaves like the oligosynaptic pathway of the v-o reflex, it is still present when associated with nystagmic or slow deviation response. In all the patients studied the reflexes of the brain stem were present, although the v-o reflex was more or less altered, implying that the reticular substance was partially damaged.

An alteration in the circadian rhythm of ACTH secretion must be interpreted as a consequence of lesions of the nervous centers that control it. Normal rhythm is maintained either in patients after prolonged bed rest or in subjects kept in darkness for a long time (Orth et al., 1967). Eik-Nes et al. (1958) found that some comatose patients presented variations of the blood concentration of cortisol after head injury or other organic lesions, but these occurred at different hours of the day without a normal rhythm. Krieger and Krieger (1966) demonstrated a significant alteration in the circadian rhythm of blood cortisol, particularly with lesions in the hypothalamus, temporal lobe, and pretectal area. Spandri et al. (1966) found that, in acute-traumatic-comatose patients, cortisolemy was uniformly elevated during the day in most of the severely affected cases, while patients with mild comas presented normal circadian rhythms. The responses to ACTH, metopiron, and L-8-V administration led to the conclusion that the hypophysis did not present significant alterations, while hypothalamic and higher nervous centers were partially damaged.

It has also been demonstrated that the circadian rhythms of sleep and ACTH secretion are closely related, and that ACTH stimulation occurs during paradoxic sleep (Weitzmann et al., 1966). It is thus understandable that alterations in sleep rhythm, with the frequent disappearance of paradoxic sleep, reported in apallic patients (Bricolo et al., 1968), may provoke alterations in the secretion rhythm of ACTH.

Conclusions

All the examinations described here contribute some information regarding the functional activity of the central nervous system in apallic patients. The v-o reflex particularly, with its different types of response, gives much detailed and original data on brain stem activity which can be useful for the prognosis.

25. Electronystagmographic Findings Following Traumatic Apallic Syndrome

E. SCHERZER and F. GERSTENBRAND

Introduction

For several reasons it appeared to be of interest to carry out electronystagmographic investigations in patients who had displayed a traumatic apallic syndrome. It is known from the clinical signs of this condition that there are functional disturbances in the optovestibular system during the traumatic apallic syndrome. So far, no reports have been published on systematic electronystagmographic examinations in such cases. It also seemed worthwhile to investigate the question of whether or not the electronystagmogram can provide an accessory parameter in evaluating the severity and prognosis of the clinical condition.

The present paper is only a preliminary report, since it is planned to continue the examinations on more patients. Despite the small number of cases studied up to now, some interesting results are already apparent, as will be shown.

Materials and Methods

Seventeen patients who developed an apallic syndrome following a craniocerebral injury were examined in this study. The accidents had occurred 2 months–6 years previously. Except for one girl, all of the patients examined were males. The age distribution ranged from 7 to 38 years. At the time of the electronystagmographic investigation three patients were in the intermediate remission phase, five patients were in the final remission phase, and nine patients had reached the definite defective state. Since electronystagmographic recordings with a Tönnies rotating chair (1932) can only be performed with the patient in a sitting position, it was not possible to carry out such examinations during the acute stage of the apallic syndrome.

With regard to the clinical signs of brain stem disturbances present at the time of these examinations, the cases were divided into three groups: cases with slight, moderate, or severe clinical signs. Similarly, the electronystagmographic abnormalities were assessed as slight, moderate, or severe. It is true that these classifications are somewhat subjective; however, errors in the results are not expected, since the clinical and electronystagmographic findings were always classified by the same investigator for each field. Moreover, the degree of severity of the electronystagmographic abnormalities was first assessed without knowledge of the clinical state.

The electronystagmographic examinations were carried out as described by R. Jung (1953). Here it proves useful to distinguish three different parts in the optovestibular investigation: (1) The search for spontaneous oculomotor phenomena, with the eyes open and closed, (2) the registration of optokinetic nystagmus by means of an optic pattern moving in the four different cardinal directions, and (3) the registration of vestibular nystagmus produced by the stimulus of rotation to the left and right.

This investigation was supported by the Scientific Fund of the General Insurance Company against Accidents, Austria.

Both spontaneous and experimental (optokinetic and labyrinthine) eye movements were recorded continuously as changes of the periorbital electric field in its vertical and horizontal planes. The optokinetic stimulation was achieved by means of parallel black and white stripes projected onto an arched (concave) screen; the vestibular stimulation was produced by rotating the patient at a constant acceleration slightly above threshold until the final velocity of 90°/s was reached, and later by stopping the patient's rotation abruptly (deceleration = negative acceleration).

Results

1. Of the 17 patients examined who had undergone a traumatic apallic syndrome, seven showed spontaneous pathologic phenomena. Two cases showed gross alternating deviations of the eyes, especially when the lids were shut, combined with ocular dysmetria. In two other gross fixational eye movements and ocular dysmetria were found without the occurrence of alternating deviations. Spontaneous nystagmus with the eyes closed was seen in three patients, swinging horizontally in two cases, and swinging upward in one case. In one patient who also showed ocular dysmetria, the vehement vestibular stimulus caused by the abrupt stopping of the rotation chair brought forth a transitory provocational nystagmus swinging upward, a phenomenon that subsided after a short while.

Slow horizontal pendular deviations of the eyes, with the lids shut, like the eye movements seen in healthy persons during fatigue and drowsiness, were registered rather frequently, viz., in nearly half the cases (8 patients). One of these showed repeated periods of slow high-amplitude pendular eye movements alternating with periods of rapid low-amplitude to-and-fro eye movements (so-called *Gegenrucke*).

2. Abnormalities of the optokinetic nystagmus were present in nine out of the 17 injured persons examined. In three cases the disturbances were seen in only one direction and in two cases they were seen in both directions in the horizontal plane. One patient displayed optokinetic abnormalities in the vertical plane, especially in the downward, but also to a slighter degree in the upward direction. Three patients had omnidirectional optokinetic disturbances which were very strongly marked. As for the severity of optokinetic abnormalities, all possible gradations–from moderate dimunition of the expected physiologic response to complete decomposition of nystagmus–were encountered.

3. Out of the 17 patients examined, 12 showed disturbances of the vestibular nystagmus when examined on the rotating chair. The most frequent abnormality of this kind was vestibular directional preponderance (6 patients). In three injured persons, considerable hypoexcitability, in two inexcitability, and in one hyperexcitability of the vestibular system were found.

The electronystagmographic findings in the above-mentioned different parts of the investigation (1-3) were established separately in each patient. On the basis of these findings, an overall evaluation was made with regard to the absence or presence of functional disturbances of the optovestibular system. In the latter cases the quantitative aspect of such abnormalities was also taken into consideration. Thus the overall electronystagmographic evaluations were classified into four different groups: normal, slightly abnormal, moderately abnormal, and severely abnormal. All 17 cases examined are incorporated in Table 1 according to the severity of the clinical signs (disturbance of brain stem functions), recovery phase of the traumatic apallic syndrome, and electronystagmographic findings.

Table 1. Survey of 17 patients who have undergone electronystagmographic examinations following traumatic apallic syndrome

Clinical recovery phase	Clinical brain stem signs slight	moderate	severe	Number of cases
Intermediate			+++	
remission phase	+++		+++	3
Final	+		+++	
remission phase	+			5
	++			
	+++			
Defective phase	N	++		
	N	++		
	N			
	+			
	+			9
	+			
	+			
Number of cases	12	2	3	17

N = Normal electronystagmogram
\+ = Slightly abnormal electronystagmogram
++ = Moderately abnormal electronystagmogram
+++ = Severely abnormal electronystagmogram

In the intermediate remission phase the electronystagmogram was severely abnormal in all three patients. In the final remission phase the electronystagmographic findings were abnormal in all five patients of this group. However, they were highly abnormal in only two cases, whereas the abnormalities were considered to be of a slight degree in two patients and of a moderate degree in one patient. In the defective state there were two moderately abnormal, four slightly abnormal, and three normal electronystagmographic recordings.

Among the 12 patients with slight clinical signs of brain stem dysfunction, three had a normal, six had a slightly abnormal, one had a moderately abnormal, and two had a severely abnormal electronystagmogram. Both cases with clinical brain stem signs of a moderate degree were in the defective stage and showed moderate electronystagmographic disturbances. The three patients with severe clinical brain stem signs had highly pathologic electronystagmograms and were in the intermediate or final remission phase.

Discussion

Abnormalities of the electronystagmogram can be interpreted and assessed only in the light of the entire clinical picture, particularly taking into consideration the otiologic findings. For instance, vestibular directional preponderance, a rather frequent abnormality, can be caused by central or peripheral lesions. Vestibular hyperexcitability and optokinetic disturbances, however, are always of central origin. But even in these cases it is not always clear from the beginning whether the disorder arises from a brain stem lesion or not. Optokinetic abnormalities are related to hemispheric or brain stem damage. In hemispheric lesions, though, there is a more rapid recovery of such disturbances. Long-standing optokinetic abnormalities are therefore always cause for suspecting lesions in brain stem structures. Only exceptionally is a given electronystagmographic disorder related to a lesion in a relatively small circumscribed area, e.g., vestibular hyperexcitability (location of lesion in the vicinity of the vestibular nuclei, i.e., part of the brain stem and cerebellum). In addition, physiologic phenomena may appear at an augmented rate. In the material studied this was particularly the case for slow horizontal pendular movements of the eyes, which must be considered as an expression of increased fatigability in posttraumatic conditions (Jung, 1953; Kornhuber, 1966; Scherzer, 1968). Successive periods of slow pendular deviations and rapid low-amplitude to-and-fro movements of the eyes are a special combination of different physiologic signs, which, in this constellation, are an important clue to considerable fluctuations in the patient's state of vigilance (Scherzer, 1968).

From what has been said, it is obviously essential that the electronystagmographic findings be integrated sensibly into the entire clinical picture. Not observing this exigency may easily give rise to incorrect interpretations. As can be gathered from Table 1, the electronystagmographic records of our patients in the intermediate remission phase were still severely pathologic. Normal findings were seen only in the defective state. Slight abnormal tracings were encountered first of all in the defective state, but sometimes even towards the end of the remission phase. Moderate pathologic findings could be seen both during the last period of the remission phase and during the definite defective state.

As for the quantitative relationship of clinical and electronystagmographic disorders, cases with pronounced clinical brain stem signs showed severely pathologic electronystagmograms. Patients with only slight clinical brain stem signs, on the other hand, had a diversity of electronystagmographic findings, whereby a correlation existed between the degree of electronystagmographic abnormality and the clinical phase in which the patient was at the time of the investigation.

Despite the small number of cases in our material, which does not allow for statistical evaluation, the trend of the electronystagmographic findings toward two dependences can be recognized: (1) dependence on the clinical recovery phase after the traumatic apallic syndrome; (2) dependence on the degree of severity of the brain stem signs as evidenced clinically without the aid of electronystagmographic examinations. Hence, it can be stated that the amount and extent of electronystagmographic disturbances are first dependent on the time factor (in the intermediate remission phase only severely pathologic tracings were found) and later, i.e., during the definite defective state, upon the clinical picture of the brain stem signs. However, toward the end of the remission phase, which is situated between the two above-mentioned stages, an interaction of (1) and (2) seems to exist.

Longitudinal surveys in individual cases (Scherzer, 1968) which do not belong to the material of this study, provide good support for these assumptions. Yet, for the actual scientific proof of the cited correlations, many more electronystagmographic examinations of patients who have passed through the clinical condition of traumatic apallic syndrome will be necessary. Only then can a definite answer be given on the value of electronystagmographic registrations in such cases.

26. Cerebral Blood Flow Reduction After Severe Head Injury and Its Relationship to the Extent of Brain Damage in Apallic Syndrome

W.-D. HEISS

In most types of coma, cerebral blood flow (CBF) is reduced (Kety, 1949). This reduction is usually accompanied and probably induced by a decrease in oxygen consumption (Lassen, 1959). Following severe head injury, cerebral circulation time (Taylor and Bell, 1966), CBF, and cerebral metabolic rate for oxygen ($CMRO_2$) are decreased (Ingvar et al., 1964; Baldy-Moulinier and Frèrebeau, 1969; Shalit et al., 1970; Meyer et al., 1970); however, an increased CBF was sometimes observed shortly after the head trauma in animal experiments (German et al., 1947; Brown and Brown, 1954) and in patients (Shalit et al., 1970). This intensified cerebral perfusion, which was not paralleld by an equally increased $CMRO_2$, suggests the presence of a luxury perfusion syndrome (Lassen, 1966). After this initial phase CBF is reduced. The present study has attempted to establish whether or not the reduction of CBF is proportional to the brain damage in patients with the apallic syndrome and whether or not the measured CBF value furnishes prognostic information.

Material and Methods

The investigations were performed in 37 patients with an apallic syndrome, which was a sequela of head trauma in 32, and caused by other brain damages in five cases (two with intracerebral hemorrhage, thrombosis of intracranial veins, asphyxia during asthmatic seizures, subacute sclerosing encephalitis). These patients with an apallic syndrome were categorized into four groups according to the clinical course and/or to the grade of recovery after long-lasting rehabilitation therapy.

Group 1: Eight patients, who died without any signs of recovery from the full apallic syndrome within a period of 1 1/2-4 months after the trauma.

Group 2: Eleven patients, whose clinical state improved slightly to a state with severe neurologic and mental deficits (six cases) or who died after slight recovery because of secondary complications (five cases).

Group 3: Eleven patients who recovered from the apallic syndrome to a state with a medium deficit. These patients were able to take care of their own personal needs, to communicate, and to walk. One of these patients died of septicemia.

Group 4: Seven patients who recovered completely or with only some minor deficits usually resulting from primary brain lesions (slight paresis of limbs, residue of aphasia, mild dementia) and whose resocialization was possible.

These 37 patients with apallic syndromes were compared with 16 patients (group 5) who suffered from severe head trauma without the development of apallic syndrome. [In six the brain was permanently and severely damaged (group 5a), ten patients recovered well or with slight neurologic deficits.] Illustrating case histories of patients of every group may be found in the original paper (Heiss et al., 1972a).

CBF was measured with a modified technique (Heiss et al., 1968) of the xenon clearance method (Lassen and Ingvar, 1963). Four to ten mci ^{133}Xenon in saline solution (1-3 ml) were injected into the internal carotid artery and the cerebral activity was recorded by means of a scintillation camera. Flow in one or both hemispheres was registered with dual ratemeter and writer. Regional cerebral blood flow (rCBF) of small areas of 12 x 12 mm was measured simultaneously by connecting the camera to a dual analog digital converter with a 1600-word memory. Activity coming from small registration areas was accumulated for short periods of time and transferred to a digital magnetic tape. During one washout study of 10-min duration, the information of 70 sampling periods was stored. The rCBF values of all the individual areas (50-100 in one hemisphere) were computed off-line and the results printed in the form of rCBF maps. A detailed description of the system used and of the important parameters (energy resolution, spatial resolution, count loss, statistical error of the results, and reliability of the measured values) may be found elsewhere (Heiss et al., 1972b).

Arterial blood pressure taken by a sphygmomanometer from the brachial artery was in the normal range and did not differ in the four groups. Arterial pCO_2 was measured in 11 patients during the blood flow studies; the values obtained were in the normal range (38.2 ± 3.6 mm Hg).

Results

Hemispheric Blood Flow

Most rCBF measurements were performed after the acute stage during a stabilized apallic syndrome or during the early stages of recovery, thereby avoiding the period of possible hyperperfusion and the influence of intracranial space-occupying lesions and edema on cerebral circulation. CBF was recorded many months after the trauma in a few patients in a state which represented the highest level of recovery. The values obtained did not differ from CBF measured in other patients of the respective groups at an earlier time after the trauma (two in group 3, two in group 4). Because of this fact, we were justified in including these patients in the study.

Repeat measurements of CBF were performed in 11 patients during the apallic syndrome and during different recovery phases. A marked clinical improvement in eight cases was accompanied by an increase in CBF in only three cases (24.6-32.9, 36.6-43.4, and 35.6-57.1 ml/100g/min); in the other five cases CBF did not change significantly (mean 26.5 and 26.6 ml/100g/min, respectively). In three patients who had a fully developed apallic syndrome with progressive impairment of the general condition, repeat measurements resulted in nearly identical values (mean 21.5 and 21.0 ml/100 g/min, respectively). These findings demonstrate that CBF does not parallel clinical improvement or impairment in most cases. Thus we feel justified in including in our study the few rCBF values which were not taken during the early stage.

In Table 1 the mean values ± S.D. of the CBF values measured in patients of the different groups are given. f represents total flow calculated as a mean with the height-over-area method and the bicompartmental analysis of the washout curves, f_G is the flow of the fast perfused compartment. Mean flow values of the groups were compared mutually using the Student's t-test and the Duncan t-test; significant differences could be found between the f of groups 1 and 2 ($t = 2.427$, $P < 0.05$), 1 and 3 ($t = 5.376, P < 0.01$), 1 and 4 ($t = 6.074, P < 0.01$), 2 and 4 ($t = 2.979, P < 0.05$), and 5a and 5b ($t = 2.679, P < 0.02$) and between the f_G of groups 1 and 2 ($t = 2.687, P < 0.02$), 1 and 3 ($t = 3.385, P < 0.01$), 1 and 4 ($t = 6.014, P < 0.01$) and 2 and 4 ($t = 2.925, P < 0.05$).

Table 1. Mean value ± S.D. of total flow and flow in gray matter in groups with apallic syndrome (1-4), in head injury patients without apallic syndromes (5a and b), and in group without cerebral lesions. F value of analysis of variance and η also given for apallic groups.

Group	Number of patients	f ml/100g.min	F	η	f_G ml/100 g.min	F	η
1	8	22.6 ± 3.1			41.3 ± 9.2		
2	11	29.1 ± 6.9			54.6 ± 11.6		
			10.224[a]	0.694		8.813[a]	0.667
3	11	34.3 ± 5.5			56.1 ± 9.6		
4	7	39.1 ± 7.0			69.5 ± 8.9		
5a	6	28.2 ± 3.6			49.0 ± 5.9		
5b	10	34.9 ± 5.4			58.7 ± 10.8		
Normal control	30	50.1 ± 5.7			81.9 ± 11.9		

[a]F (3,33; 0.001) = 6.886.

Analysis of variance (F values given in the right column of Table 1) proved the significant differences of the four groups of patients with apallic syndromes with respect to their flow values and the validity of the discriminating variables. The F values obtained are highly significant ($P < 0.001$). The increase in flow values from group 1 to group 4 permitted us to show the relationship between the category scales of the prognostic groups and the ratio scales of the CBF values with η, whose significance is indicated by the highly significant F values from the analysis of variance. This value η was significant for both flow parameters and gives a comparable estimate as to what extent recovery depends on the blood flow values.

Regional Blood Flow

In apallic patients rCBF was decreased diffusely all over the brain, showing values in the range of the hemispheric CBF (Fig. 1). In 15 cases, in which primary cerebral injury led

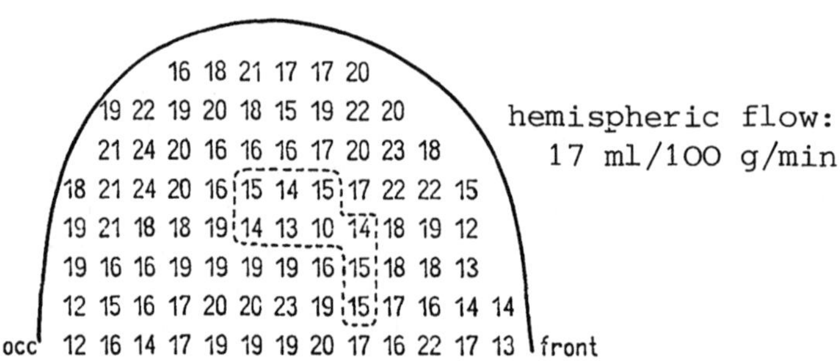

Fig. 1. rCBF map of right hemisphere in apallic patient. Flow is diffusely decreased with an area of further impaired blood supply according to primary cortical lesion in fronto-central area

to a secondary midbrain lesion and consecutively to the apallic syndrome, areas with further impaired circulation corresponding to the traumatically injured brain regions were observed. These rCBF alterations corresponded to permanent or long-lasting neurologic deficits or to pathologic anatomic findings in autopsy cases.

In the patients of group 5, in whom the brain injury was not followed by an apallic syndrome, CBF usually was also decreased (Table 1). However, in contrast to the patients with an apallic syndrome, regional differences were much more prominent and were, with the exception of two, observed in all cases regionally measured. Blood supply in these damaged areas was markedly impaired, which had a decisive effect on the hemispheric blood flow values. Usually in these regions a decrease in the relative weight of the gray matter was detectable (Fig. 2). In two patients who had suffered from subdural hematoma, regional hyperperfusion in the damaged area was observed 35 and 75 days after the trauma. Such a regional luxury perfusion was not seen in our apallic patients. In the few patients in this group who underwent repeat examinations, CBF increased with the improvement of the localized traumatic lesion.

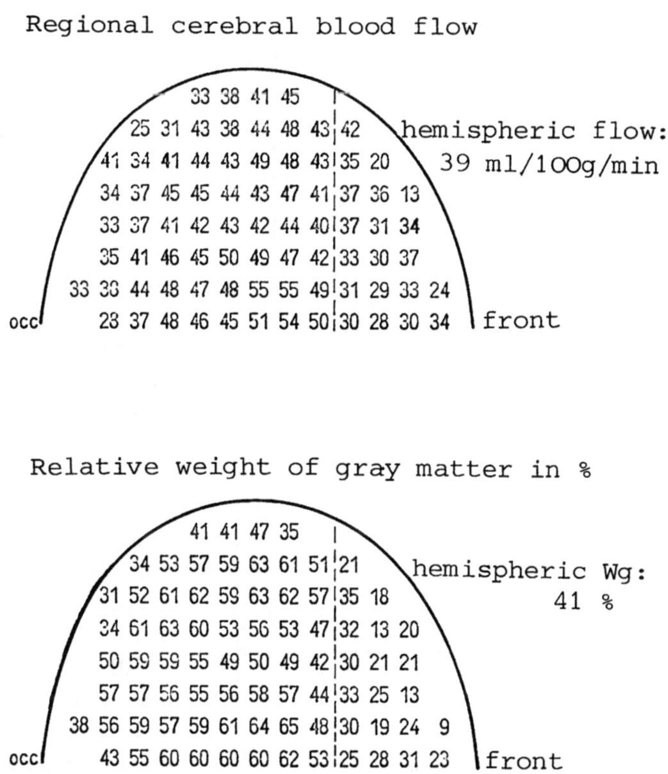

Fig. 2. rCBF and regional relative gray matter weight of right hemisphere of patient with fracture of frontal bone and contusion of frontal lobe. Flow and relative weight of gray matter are diminished in corresponding area

Correlation of CBF Values with Pathologic Findings

All eight patients in group 1, five patients in group 2 and one patient in group 3 died. In order to obtain some information on the dependence of the decrease in CBF on the anatomic lesions, an attempt was made to correlate the CBF values with the findings in the nine autopsy cases. The results are shown in Table 2. In all of these patients the CBF study was performed during the fully developed apallic syndrome. In spite of different localization and intensity of the anatomic lesions and in spite of different CBF values, the patients showed identical clinical symptoms. In order to obtain a statistical estimation of the dependency of CBF on the extent of the brain stem lesion, a Spearman rank correlation was calculated, arranging the patients according to the severity of their lesions and according to the CBF value. Both arrangements were done independently. The calculated rank correlation coefficient (r_s) between total flow and size of lesion was 0.817, between flow in gray matter and extent of lesion 0.800. Both these correlation coefficients are highly significant ($P <$ 0.01).

Table 2. Blood flow values and brain stem lesions in 9 autopsy cases with apallic syndrome (Lesion in I: floor of 3rd ventricle and/or periaqueductal gray matter, II: mesencephalic reticular formations, III: pontine reticular formations, IV: dorsolateral pontine tegmentum, V: pontine basis).

Patient	Age	Cerebral blood flow (days after accident)	f	rank	f_G	rank	Death days after accident	Rostral brain stem lesion I	II	III	IV	V	Rank
S.F.	54	50	19.5	1	28.5	2	77	+	+	+	+	+	1
K.Z.	56	35	25.4	4	50.4	5	108	+		+	+	+	2
A.F.	54	28	26.0	6	38.2	3	60		+	+	+		3
J.K.	20	85	20.0	2	27.7	1	90			+	+		4
K.P.	40	67	21.8	3	55.4	6	216			+	+	+	5
R.D.	18	90	25.7	5	46.2	4	122				+		6
F.B.	22	30	38.0	7	61.6	7	54	+[a]					7
R.H.	14	23	41.8	8	61.8	8	79					+	8
H.B.	13	60	48.2	9	65.2	9	105					+	9

[a] Hypothalamic lesion outside reticular formation.

Discussion

The high pathogenetic and prognostic importance of lesions in the rostral brain stem for patients suffering from severe posttraumatic impairment of consciousness was assumed by several authors and again stressed by Jellinger and Seitelberger (1970). Intra vitam these lesions can hardly be visualized and only indirect signs may be found by means of EEG and pneumoencephalography. The fact that the brain stem influences function, metabolism, and perfusion of the cerebral cortex (Ingvar et al., 1964; Shalit et al., 1967; Ingvar and Sourander, 1970) yields measurable parameters which indicate the extent of the brain stem lesion and give some information on the prognosis in individual cases. CBF and $CMRO_2$ were used as such parameters in patients during the acute phase after the injury, mainly as a biologic test of death of the brain (Bès et al., 1969; Baldy-Moulinier and Frèrebeau, 1969; Shalit et al., 1970; Brock et al., 1969; Brodersen, 1971).

If a patient survives the initial stage, an apallic syndrome develops in many cases which may last for several months. During this time, death may occur from late complications or secondary diseases, or the patients may show progressive improvement to different final states of recovery with or even without neurologic deficits (Gerstenbrand, 1967). Because of the uniform symptomatology of the apallic syndrome in different patients, the final outcome cannot be judged by clinical means alone. This investigation yielded some additional information through measurements of the CBF. The limited number of patients studied and the statistical fluctuation of the results do not permit us to specify a critical value of CBF above which the patient will recover completely, or a low critical level under which the patient will die. But at least a significant CBF difference between four prognostic groups, a significant dependence of the prognosis on the CBF values, and a correlation between the extent of brain stem lesion and the brain perfusion in these patients were shown.

The results presented in this study allow the conclusion that CBF measurements after the acute stage may be used to judge the extent of brain stem lesions and to predict the state of recovery the patient may reach with rehabilitation therapy. It may be assumed from the repeat and late measurements that reduction of CBF in apallic patients depends on the anatomic lesions within the brain stem. The close correlation of the size of the brain stem lesion and the reduced CBF supports this assumption. With rCBF measurements primary circumscribed cortical lesions are already detected during the apallic syndrome. These lesions cause the permanent neurologic deficits. More knowledge about them is important for the arrangement of individual rehabilitation programs for apallic as well as for other patients suffering from localized traumatic brain injury.

Summary

In 37 patients with apallic syndromes and in 16 patients suffering from sequelae of head trauma without an apallic syndrome, hemispheric and regional cerebral blood flow were measured. Using analysis of variance and t-test, significant differences of mean CBF were found between four groups of apallic patients categorized according to the clinical recovery and a significant relationship between prognosis and CBF values was demonstrated by η. In nine autopsy cases significant rank correlation was obtained between the extent of brain stem lesion and CBF reduction. The rCBF measurements revealed areas of primary cortical lesions above all in head injury patients without apallic syndromes, in whom the reduction of total CBF was often due to the circumscript lesions, whereas in apallic patients rCBF was very often reduced diffusely all over the brain. The measurement of CBF provides an important tool for the prognosis in patients with apallic syndromes and for the prediction of permanent neurologic deficits.

Acknowledgments

This investigation was supported by the Österreichischen Fonds zur Förderung der wissenschaftlichen Forschung and by the Jubiläumsstiftung der Österreichischen Nationalbank. Special thanks are due to Prof. K. Jellinger (Neurologisches Institut der Universität Wien, Director: Prof. F. Seitelberger) for providing the autopsy findings and for his help in the categorization of the anatomic brain lesions.

VI. Therapy

27. Early Treatment of the Initial Stage of the Apallic Syndrome

C. LEHMANN

The main causes of respiratory insufficiency are breathing disorders due to disturbances of the autonomic brain stem functions, which is one of the symptoms of the acute secondary midbrain syndrome caused by an intracranial space-occupying process, brain edema, and the subsequent herniation of the upper brain stem.

Insufficient spontaneous ventilation, i.e., inadequate volume, is supported by assisted ventilation. Controlled pressure equipment such as the Bird or Bennet respirators or the Dräger assistor are suitable for this purpose. In these respirators the inspiratory phase is triggered by the inspiratory suction of the patient. This equipment permits the administration of oxygen and the individual adjustment of the inspiratory suction, maximum ventilation pressure, and respiratory flow rate. If the patient ceases to breathe spontaneously an automatic change to mechanical ventilation is provided. Controlled ventilation is necessary as soon as irregular breathing occurs, i.e., breathing with decreased frequency and progressively larger apneic phases, as seen in Cheyne-Stokes respiration, with hyperventilatory gasping in the transition stage to the bulbar brain syndrome, or with complete respiratory arrest in the full stage of the bulbar brain syndrome.

In these cases, alternating pressure ventilation is to be preferred, since a flow curve composed of positive and negative pressure phases with a low mean ventilation pressure offers decisive advantages for prophylaxis and treatment of brain edema.

Controlled volume equipment such as the Dräger Spiromat and Engström respirators, which are mainly used to control ventilation, permit adjustment of the amount of ventilation, which is calculated by a nomogram. The oxygen portion of the inspired air, the respiratory rate, the maximum inspiratory and expiratory pressure, and the respiration time ratio can be selected. The Dräger Spiromat 661 permits three pulmonary distensions after every 100 respirations. These serve in the prophylaxis and treatment of atelectasis.

All newer ventilators make provisions for warming and humidifying the inspired air. The effectiveness of the ventilation must be checked by regular analysis of blood gases.

The most important drugs used for the sedation of patients with stretch cramps and respiratory depression are listed in Table 1. The duration of action of these sedatives is usually 3-6 h. In most cases administration by intramuscular injection or addition to the infusion every 6 h is adequate. Prolonged medication with the drugs mentioned may produce depression of cardiac activity and of the cardiovascular system, disorders of gastrointestinal function, hepatic damage, limitation of renal function, and drug addiction. Therefore, on principle, these drugs should only be prescribed after the effects and side effects have been considered.

In a few cases it is possible to adjust the patient simply with sedative agents to control ventilation. However, the additional muscle relaxants should only be used when absolutely

Table 1. Individual doses necessary for sedation

Age	Body weight kg	Dolantin 1 Amp. = 2ml = 100 mg	Thalamonal 1 Amp.=10 ml 25 mg DHBP, 10,5 mg Fentanyl	DHBP 1 Amp. =10 ml = 25 mg	Atosil 1 Amp. = 2 ml = 50 mg	Psyquil 1 Amp. = 1 ml = 20 mg	Valium 1 Amp. = 2 ml = 10 mg	Nembutal 50 mg/ml
6 months	7	–	0.1 ml	1.25 mg = 0.5 ml	7 mg = 0.3 ml	2.0 mg = 0.1 ml	1.5 mg = 0.3 ml	14 mg = 0.3 ml
1 year	10	15 mg = 0.3 ml	0.3 ml	1.75 mg = 0.7 ml	10 mg = 0.4 ml	3.0 mg = 0.15 ml	2 mg = 0.4 ml	15 mg = 0.3 ml
2 years	12.3	20 mg = 0.4 ml	0.4 ml	2.0 mg = 0.8 ml	15 mg = 0.6 ml	3.5 mg = 0.18 ml	2 mg = 0.4 ml	20 mg = 0.4 ml
3 years	14.1	20 mg = 0.4 ml	0.5 ml	2.25 mg = 0,9 ml	15 mg = 0.6 ml	4.0 mg = 0.2 ml	3 mg = 0.6 ml	25 mg = 0.5 ml
4 years	16.3	40 mg = 0.8 ml	0.6 ml	2.5 mg = 1.0 ml	15 mg = 0.6 ml	5.0 mg = 0.25 ml	3 mg = 0.6 ml	30 mg = 0.6 ml
5 years	19	40 mg = 0.8 ml	0.7 ml	3 mg = 1.2 ml	20 mg = 0.8 ml	6.0 mg = 0.3 ml	4 mg = 0.8 ml	35 mg = 0.7 ml
6 years	20.6	40 mg 0.8 ml	0.8 ml	3.75 mg = 1.5 ml	20 mg = 0.8 ml	6.0 mg = 0.3 ml	4 mg = 0.8 ml	40 mg = 0.8 ml
10 years	30	60 mg = 1.2 ml	1.0 ml	3.75 mg = 1.5 ml	30 mg = 1.2 ml	9.0 mg = 0.45 ml	6 mg = 1.2 ml	60 mg = 1.2 ml
14 years	40	80 mg = 1.6 ml	1.0 ml	5 mg = 2 ml	40 mg = 1.6 ml	12.0 mg = 0.6 ml	8 mg = 1.6 ml	80 mg = 1.6 ml
18 years	70	100 mg = 2 ml	1.5 ml	5 mg = 2 ml	50 mg = 2 ml	20.0 mg = 1 ml	10-15 mg =2-3 ml	250 mg = 5 ml
20-40 years	70	100 mg 2 ml	1.5-2 ml	5 mg = 2 ml	50 mg = 2 ml	20.0 mg = 1 ml	10-15 mg =2-3 ml	250 mg = 5 ml
40-55 years	70	75 mg = 1.5 ml	1.5-2 ml	5 mg = 2 ml	50 mg = 2 ml	20.0 mg = 1 ml	10-15 mg = 2-3 ml	250 mg = 5 ml
55-70 years	70	50 mg = 1 ml	1-1.5 ml	5 mg = 2 ml	50 mg = 2 ml	20.0 mg = 1 ml	10 mg = 2 ml	150 mg = 3 ml
70 years or older	70	25 mg = 0.5 ml	1.0 ml	3.75 mg = 1.5 ml	40 mg = 1.6 ml	15.0 mg = 0.75 ml	10 mg = 2 ml	100 mg = 2 ml

necessary, since experience has shown that the disturbance of relaxed patients during ventilation produces considerably more severe incidents than with assisted ventilation, which assumes an insufficient but nevertheless still present spontaneous respiration. The side effects of muscle relaxants are effects on the cardiovascular system and on intestinal peristalsis. Secondary sequelae are muscular atrophies which make the subsequent return to spontaneous breathing more difficult.

Of all the drugs which are used, Imbretil appears to be most suitable. It has the longest duration of action and it produces neither histamine release nor a limitation of peristalsis. The initial dosage of Imbretil is about 8 ml i.v. With adequate sedation, additional doses of 4 mg at intervals of from 2 to 4 h are adequate.

The *cardiovascular system*, i.e., the pulse rate and the blood pressure, must be controlled continuously. A suitable electrocardiographic oscilloscope with an acoustic monitor should be used. Patients with a midbrain syndrome have a highly labile cardiovascular system, and this may result in a dangerous decrease in blood pressure.

According to Reissigl (1965), shock is an acute hemodynamic disorder in which capillary blood flow is reduced to such an extent that tissue hypoxia associated with metabolic disorders and acidosis occurs. This leads to functional and morphologic changes in the organs. The acute cerebral ischemia which is produced by shock may cause a diminishing of the function of the cerebral cortex or even of the centers in the brain stem and constitutes the most important cause of brain edema. Thus, the most urgent task is volume substitution with plasma substitutes of plasma expanders until whole blood is available. However, one must beware particularly of indiscriminate administration if the patient shows symptoms of increased intracranial pressure or if there is a danger of pulmonary congestion.

The use of cardiovascular agents with a peripheral effect is contraindicated during the stage of vasoconstriction. Vasopressors increase peripheral resistance and enhance metabolic acidosis despite the increase in blood pressure which they produce. Substances which produce vasodilatation inhibit vasoconstriction due to sympathetic factors and improve the microcirculation and the oxygen supply to the tissue. The best-known representative of sympatholytic agents is Hydergin.

Patients with a midbrain syndrome have a tendency towards severe *hyperthermia* which should be counteracted by cooling to normal temperatures. Damage to brain stem centers responsible for temperature regulation causes peripheral vasoconstriction and thus produces interference with heat loss, giving rise to an increase in the temperature of the body nucleus. Controlled hypothermia decreases the oxygen consumption, lowers the energy requirement, decreases tachypnea, and constitutes a good prophylaxis against peripheral cardiovascular failure.

A combination of physical and pharmacologic measures permits high body temperatures to be reduced to normal within a few hours and maintains them in this range. We use icebags, prescribe antipyretic agents and wet compresses on the lower part of the legs, Hydergin or neuroleptic agents for peripheral vasodilatation, and eliminate shivering with the phenothiazine derivative Atosil.

Dehydration for prophylaxis and treatment of brain edema should be carried out only after the diagnosis has been established, since the decrease in brain volume which it produces may favor expansion of the existing hematoma. Substances which act by increasing the intravascular osmotic pressure and thereby eliminate edematous fluid from the tissues are useful in the treatment of brain edema. Because of the severe rebound effect, urea should only be used during surgery, if at all. In contrast to this, the hexahydroxy alcohol mannitol has this disadvantage only to a minimal degree. It is used in a dosage of 1 g/kg body weight. Administration requires an indwelling catheter for regular measurement of the urine output. In patients with anuria, the use of mannitol is not only ineffective but even dangerous since, particularly in patients with heart failure, it may produce pulmonary edema due to the rapid increase in the intravascular fluid volume. The use of the cell-sealing carbonic anhydrase inhibitor Diamox and of the hexahydric alcohol sorbitol, whose osmotherapeutic effect is achieved by restricted tubular reabsorption, offers additional possibilities for prophylaxis and treatment of brain edema.

Incorrect regulations of respiration produce *disorders of acid-base equilibrium*, the extent of which is determined by blood gas analysis. Hypoventilation produces respiratory acidosis; hyperventilation produces respiratory alkalosis. Metabolic factors may increase these irritations, but they can also mask them. Crises due to respiratory factors can be eliminated by changing the respiratory and ventilatory magnitudes, by tracheotomy and adequate ventilation on the one hand, and on the other hand by limiting the respiratory minute volume.

Metabolic acid-base shifts existing alone or with other factors are compensated for by the administration of suitable buffer and electrolyte solutions or by the administration of weak acids. Patients with metabolic acidosis receive sodium bicarbonate and tris buffer and, under certain circumstances, also sodium or potassium lactate. One-molar solutions are administered according to the following formula: Excess negative base x body weight in kg x 0.3. More infrequent metabolic alkalosis can be corrected by the administration of acid valencies. Mild disorders are compensated for by 1-molar potassium chloride or lysine hydrochloride solutions, severe conditions with 0.1 N hydrochloric acid.

In unconscious patients the *prophylaxis and treatment of infection* is of the utmost importance. Due to the increased loss of resistance of the whole body, secondary infections can be avoided only with difficulty and only for a limited period of time. The most threatening complication is pneumonia, to which patients with insufficient respiration and patients with controlled ventilation are particularly exposed. Tracheotomy facilitates ventilation and cleansing of the bronchial system, but it also represents an additional source of infection since the physiologic conditions of respiration are eliminated and mucosal and cartilaginous defects of the tracheal wall cannot be avoided. Prolonged indwelling catheters and the loss of the physiologic intestinal flora result in an increase in urinary tract infections and enteritis.

The resistance of the individual types of bacteria which frequently occur and the problem of hospitalization which is thus produced require a careful selection of drugs. The optimum dosage should be combined with a maximum bactericidal defect and with minimum toxicity. Laboratory examination of the tracheal secretions, urine and feces, three times a week with the respective sensitivity studies, are absolutely essential prerequisites for effective treatment. We prefer the broad spectrum antibiotics cephalothin and cephaloridin which can be recommended because of their low toxicity and the resulting maximum dosage possibilities.

The nasogastric tube feeding outline presented in Table 2 is an example of hypercaloric nutrition for patients with an acute midbrain syndrome, and for patients in the full stage of the apallic syndrome. Stardit, which we use, has major advantages because of its tolerance and the ready solubility in relatively small amounts of water. During the first few days the patient is fed parenterally in order to prevent symptoms of subileus. We start oral feeding on the 5th day which, by the 8th day, consists of 4000-5000 calories administered in a fluid volume of 2500 ml. In nearly all cases the food is administered by stomach tubes which are reinserted for each feeding to avoid ulceration, gastritis, and parotitis.

Nursing care and physiotherapeutic treatment should be carried out by competent and specially trained personnel, as prophylaxis of infections and preventive measures against inactivity contractures and decubitus ulcers are almost exclusively their responsibility.

Summary

Early treatment of the acute midbrain syndrome covers the initial symptom complex of the apallic syndrome, which is dominated by unconsciousness, stretch position with stretch

Table 2a. Caloric composition of some food concentrates. Caloric content % of dry substance

	Stardit	Biosorbin	Braun's Oral	Sonana
Protein	23.5%	19.0%	21.4%	25.0%
Carbohydrate	66.5%	61.0%	56.0%	50.0%
Fat	3.5%	12.0%	13.0%	14.0%
Water	2.5%	4.0%	4.0%	
Minerals	4.0%	3.0%	4.0%	5.0%
Daily ration	5 x 160 g	5 x 100 g	5 x 100 g	5 x 100 g
Calories per daily ration	3000	2200	2250	2190
Calories per 100 g	375	440	450	438

Table 2b. Example of an intragastric feeding plan

1st to 4th day	5th day	6th day	7th day	8th day
parenteral feeding (550 to 2000 ml)			4 a.m. 80 g Stardit to which 150 ml water is added /150 ml beer	5 a.m. 160 g Stardit to which 500 ml of water is added 200 ml beer
	10 a.m. 200 ml tea unsweetened	10 a.m. 200 ml tea sweetened 100 ml gruel	10 a.m. 80 g Stardit to which 150 ml water is added/150 ml broth	10 a.m. 160 g Stardit to which 300 ml of water is added 200 ml broth
	4 p.m. 200 ml tea unsweetened	4 p.m. 200 ml tea sweetened 100 ml broth	4 p.m. 80 g Stardit to which 150 ml water is added 150 ml fruit juice	3 p.m. 160 g Stardit to which 300 ml of water is added 200 ml fruit juice
	10 p.m. 200 ml tea unsweetened supplemented by 1000-1200 ml of i.v. fluids	10 p.m. 100 ml tea sweetened 100 ml broth supplemented by 1000 ml of i.v. fluids	10 p.m. 80 g Stardit to which 150 ml water is added 150 ml beer supplemented by 750-1000 ml of i.v. fluids	8 p.m. 160 g Stardit to which 300 ml of water is added 200 ml beer *Midnight:* 160 g Stardit to which 500 ml of water is added/200 ml beer

cramps of all extremities, increased muscle tone and disorders of autonomic functions of the brain stem. The aim of treatment is to prevent the development of an apallic syndrome.

Preservation of the vital functions, i.e., respiration, blood circulation, and temperature regulation of the body, must be regarded as the first and most important measure. Stretch cramps require corresponding sedation or relaxation.

Disturbances of the acid-base equilibrium and electrolyte balance produced by a disorder of the vital functions must be eliminated.

These immediate measures are followed by prophylaxis of infection, prescription of sensible hypercaloric nutrition, and prevention of contractures from inactivity and decubitus ulcers.

Immediately after treatment is begun, even unconscious patients with adequate ventilation should be intubated to avoid aspiration or to relieve it by suction to ensure an adequate oxygen supply.

28. The Medical Therapy of the Apallic Syndrome *

A. BRICOLO

The treatment of the full stage of the apallic syndrome, which can at times be very protracted, is based on several factors: An appropriate and intense psychomotor rehabilitation (Gerstenbrand, 1968a), a special hypercaloric diet, and the choice of a drug therapy which will induce and maintain the best possible conditions for the resumption of cerebral functions. Drugs which may be useful in the therapy of the protracted stages of coma are summarized in Table 1.

Table 1. Drugs used in the therapy of protracted stages of coma

Psychoanaleptic drugs	
Sympathomimetic amines	Amphetamine Methamphetamine
Antidepressants	Tricyclics Monoamine oxydase (MAO) inhibitors
Neurotransmitters	L-dopa
Neurometabolic regulators Neurotrophics	Laevoglutamine GABA DMAE Centrophenoxine Pyrithioxine Vitamins Nucleotides Phospholipids
Psychotogenic drugs	Lysergic acid Diethylamide (LSD) Mescaline
Cerebral vasodilator drugs	
Anabolizers	
Muscle relaxants	

Psychoanaleptic Drugs

Psychoanaleptics and psychotonics are a group of heterogeneous psychotropic drugs. Although their structures can differ widely, they all act as stimulants of the central nervous

* Supported in part by the Marastoni Foundation.

system (CNS) and usually improve vigilance and psychomotor activities without, however, altering the patient's adherence to reality.

The drugs do not always have the same activating effects on all nervous functions. In the same manner, the neuropsychologic and neurochemical action mechanisms of some of them are not entirely clear. Among these drugs are compounds which act mainly on vigilance, such as the sympathomimetic amines, or on the tone of depressed moods, such as the antidepressants. Finally, other drugs produce secondary or inconstant indirect psychoanaleptic effects. The latter compounds have not yet found a definite place in psychopharmacology. This heterogeneous group includes neurotransmitters, neurotrophics, and neurometabolic regulators which have recently been introduced into clinical practice.

The effect of sympathomimetic amines generally resembles the response to stimulation of adrenergic nerves, but there are often differences in the details and in the intensity of action of the drugs. Several of these compounds have such a profound effect on the CNS that they are of value in specific clinical conditions (Goodman and Gilman, 1970; Model, 1970). Amphetamine is one of the most potent sympathomimetic amines with respect to stimulation of the CNS. Methamphetamine has more pronounced central effects than amphetamine and is accompanied by less prominent peripheral action.

The results obtained in patients treated with these drugs are alertness, decreased sense of fatigue, increased initiative and ability to concentrate, euphoria, increase in motor and speech activities, but with the number of errors not necessarily decreased. There may be undesirable side effects such as anxiety, tremors, confusion, agitation, disphoria, hyperpyrexia, arterial hypertension, delirium, arrhythmia, etc. (Weiss and Laties, 1962; Welch, 1966). At present most researchers deny any practical usefulness of these drugs in the psychiatric field. However, as far as we are concerned, amphetamines may be extremely useful in certain stages of the psychomotor rehabilitation of apallic patients. We must recall here that psycho-organic syndromes often seem to have a great tolerance for these drugs, together with clearly favorable clinical results (Lasagna and Epstein, 1969).

Antidepressants. The tricyclic group (imipramine: Tofranil and amitriptyline: Adepril) represent the drug of choice in any mild-to-moderate depression. Amitriptyline is the most indicated one if a more intense sedative effect is desired. The monoamine oxidase (MAO) inhibitors (isocarboxazid: Marplan; nialamide: Niamid) comprise a heterogeneous group of drugs that have in common the ability to block oxidative deamination of naturally existing amines. Because their effectiveness in mental depression and phobic anxiety states is relatively slight and their toxicity relatively high, they must be reserved mainly for patients who are refractory to other treatment. Antidepressant drugs are often required during certain stages of the evolution of a posttraumatic coma, when there are predominant symptoms of psychomotor inhibition, as well as during the remission stages of an apallic syndrome when accompanied by depression of any kind.

Neurotransmitters. It has been demonstrated that dopamine plays an important role as a physiologic neurotransmitter or neuromodulator (Hornykiewicz, 1966; McLennan and York, 1967). The beneficial action of its precursor, L-dopa, on parkinsonian symptomatology seems to depend on reintegration of the dopaminergic action in the corpus striatum and in the substantia nigra, which is normally deficient in this type of patient (Klawans, 1968).

Experiments on animals have made available neuropharmacologic, neurophysiologic, and biochemical elements which prove that dopamine plays an important role in the organization of the sleep-wakefulness cycle (Jouvet, 1969). L-dopa produces EEG and behavioral patterns of arousal (Monnier and Tissot, 1958; Mantegazzini and Ferrara, 1960; Harner and Dorman, 1969), neutralizes the hypnogenic effect of 5-hydroxytryptophane (McGeer et al., 1963), reinstates the sleep of reserpine-induced insomnia (Matsumoto and Jouvet, 1964), and eliminates the inhibitory effects of fatigue on paradoxical sleep (Matsumoto et al., 1968).

It should be noted here that direct application with the iontophoretic method of dopamine on the neurons of the cat's caudate nucleus has shown this compound to have an inhibitory action (McLennan and York, 1967) and that the caudate nucleus and the putamen usually have inhibitory effects on the activity of cortical neurons. L-dopa will produce a striking state of excitement in a cat pretreated with an inhibitor of monoamine oxidase (Reis et al., 1970) and a behavior similar to sham rage that counteracts the depressant action of reserpine (Blaschko and Chrusciel, 1960), which reduces the level of dopamine in the striatum. L-dopa in parkinsonians induces modifications in nocturnal sleep patterns (Wyatt et al., 1970) and, from personal research, an increase in the spindling and paradoxical sleep with regularization of the nictemeral cycle (Bricolo et al., 1970a and b).

All these data led us to consider dopamine as a neurotransmitter with a final "activating" effect on the subcortical mechanism responsible for consciousness, behavior, and regulation of motor activity. On these bases, we tested the effects of this therapy on a group of patients in a protracted comatose state. The only previous therapeutic study had been carried out in Vienna by Gerstenbrand (personal communication), who had used intravenous dopa at a maximum dosage of 75 mg, without obtaining any positive results.

We treated a group of 36 patients with oral L-dopa at an average dosage of 4 g/day, continued over long periods of time. Eight patients were in the full stage of an apallic syndrome, 12 were in the transition stage, ten were recovering from an acute midbrain syndrome, and six were in the initial stage of remission.

The evolution of this group was definitely more favorable compared with the group before the introduction of L-dopa. Among the various symptoms, those more positively influenced were akinesia, seborrhea, and the vigilance level. The neurologic residual sequelae, on the other hand, did not seem to decrease. All of the apallic syndromes thus treated, except for one, were followed by a more or less complete stage of clinical remission. The duration of the initial coma was also considerably reduced (Bricolo and Dalle Ore, 1970; Bricolo and Formenton, 1971).

Hypothetically, the mechanism of the positive action of L-dopa on the apallic syndrome might consist of the reintegration of aminergic activities of the midbrain structures, especially at the pons level.

Metabolic Regulators and Neurotrophics. Glutamic acid and l-glutamine account for about one-half of the total nonprotein nitrogen in the human brain. They play a role in some important cerebral metabolic processes (Meister, 1957). L-glutamine is actively absorbed by the intestinal mucous and can easily overcome the blood-brain barrier (Waelsch, 1955). Le Beau et al. (1962) were the first researchers to use it in neurosurgery for the treatment of consciousness impairment secondary to head injuries. They also used it postoperatively, with encouraging results. In our own experience, l-glutamine used in high doses, either orally or endovenously, proved quite useful in speeding improvement during the arousal phase of acute coma as well as during the remission period of the apallic syndrome.

The best results are obtained by combining l-glutamine and pyridoxine with α-aminobutyric acid (Acutil-Gaba). Gamma-aminobutyric acid (GABA), the precise role of which is still under discussion, is a physiologic component of the brain (Krnijevic, 1970). This substrate for the oxidative metabolism of the central cortex is derived from glutamic acid in the presence of the active forms of pyridoxine. It has been studied as a possible modulator of the excitatory state of the central neurons.

Dimethylamino ethanol (DMAE) was considered by Pfeiffer et al. (1957) to be a precursor or cerebral acetylcholine. Thuillier et al. (1959) combined some of its derivate esters with auxine (vegetable growth factors) and obtained some compounds with particular psychoanaleptic effects. Its prototype, centrophenoxine (Lucidril), favors some of the effects of adrenaline in the experimental animal; it elicits the cerebral disinhibition of acetylcholine and reduces the sedative effects of reserpine. It also has normalizing effects on the affected values of arterial pressure, of body temperature, and of diuresis.

Gerstenbrand et al. (1963a) have a particularly interesting theory: They believe that the basic substance of Lucidril might interfere with the metabolism of catecholamine in the sense of a specific action on dopamine. This drug has been widely used, with good results, in posttraumatic psycho-organic syndromes, in atherosclerotic dementia, in confusional states, in Huntington's chorea, in oligophrenias, and in parkinsonism (Delay and Deniker, 1961; Michon et al., 1961;and numerous others). With reference to its action on unconsciousness, very good results have been reported, especially by French researchers (Coirault and Deligne, 1960; Delay et al., 1960; Pelage et al., 1960; Thuillier et al., 1960; and others). There have been reports of very good and sometimes even spectacular results. This disagrees in part with Italian researchers, who appear far less enthusiastic (Bozza-Marrubini and Rossanda, 1961).

Gerstenbrand et al. (1963a) performed a careful study of the effects of this drug on a group of patients with acute and chronic consciousness impairment. They obtained favorable results in partial apallic syndromes and negative results in complete apallic syndromes. Our own experience also proves that the drug does not alter positively the consciousness level in protracted and stabilized unconsciousness, while it has given encouraging results in light comas, in remission stages, and in psycho-organic syndromes with a tendency toward somnolence.

Pyrithioxine (Encefabol), derived from pyridoxine and devoid of vitaminic properties, is a substance which has many and varied influences on the CNS, by interfering with the cerebral metabolism in a way which is not yet completely understood. It acts on the blood-brain barrier and determines a sharp increase in the transport of glucose to the brain (Quadbeck et al., 1962; Becker and Hoyer, 1966). There has been wide clinical experimentation with this drug, especially in Spain and Germany. These experiments yield satisfactory results for several neurologic diseases (organic psychosyndromes, neurasthenic syndromes, and chronic alcoholism, retarded psychomotor development in childhood, etc.). It causes an increase in the psychomotor functional efficiency without, however, producing central stimulatory effects such as those obtained with amphetamines, nor does it have tranquilizing or hypnotic sedative effects. These characteristics, together with the total lack of toxicity and absence of undesirable side effects, make pyrithioxine one of the drugs with good possibilities of being useful in the treatment of the apallic syndrome. Our experience in this field is similar to Gerstenbrand's (1967), who observed greater speed in the remission of apallic syndromes in his patients.

Vitamins are necessary for a normal metabolism. Man is incapable of synthesizing them in his body, and they must be supplied abundantly in the diet. The increased needs of the unconscious patient make it necessary to administer a daily supplement of the B complex, i.e.: thiamine (B_1), riboflavin (B_2), nicotinamide and pyrodoxine (B_6), folic acid and cyanocobalamine (B_{12}); of ascorbic acid (vitamin C); of vitamin D; and of vitamin E.

It must be borne in mind that the use of high doses of vitamin compounds, which many researchers advise and use in the treatment of many neurologic diseases caused by degenerative or involutive lesions, has given such poor results that a specific therapeutic effect on the brain tissues can be positively excluded.

Nucleosides, nucleotides (ADP, ATP, UTP) and nucleic acids (ARN, ADN, etc.) have been used in fatigue as well as on the vigilance levels by several authors. These compounds favor the utilization of glucose at cerebral and peripheral levels. Some of these compounds, like ARN, are involved in the processes of learning and memorizing.

Phospholipids (Tricortin) have been widely used in the treatment of postcomatose and postcontusive cerebral syndromes. This drug is used in an effort to correct the metabolic imbalance of the brain caused by the injury to carbohydrate, protein, and lipid metabolism (Curri et al., 1964; Ishii et al., 1966).

Some Japanese researchers have recently introduced citicholine (Nicholin) in the control of many cerebral disorders. This compound is the essential substratum for the synthesis of lecithin and has an activating action on the ascending reticular function. Researchers who have used the compound in posttraumatic unconsciousness are unanimous in stating that it has an arousal effect (Yasuda and Namba, 1970).

Psychotogenic Drugs

These compounds, also known as psychomimetics, hallucinogenics, and psychedelics (LSD, mescaline), belong to various chemical categories. Their mechanism of action is as yet unknown, but they produce changes in mood, affectivity, ideation, and perception. They often determine sharp changes in the critico-ideative processes and dissociative syndromes. These are extremely powerful drugs which exert a strong influence on the CNS. Their action, if not properly controlled, can be extremely dangerous when used by inexperienced persons. These drugs are widely used today without any control and represent the most worrisome and negative side of modern psychopharmacology (Valzelli, 1970).

The present-day use of psychodysleptics must be severely restricted to special, highly specialized psychiatric situations (Shepherd et al., 1968), since their moderate usefulness is counterbalanced by the grave dangers which might ensue. We believe that these drugs might be tested—at least "experimentally"—in the study of the apallic syndrome, and especially in those cases which have been diagnosed as irreversible.

Cerebral Vasodilator Drugs

Among the numerous vasodilators, only some can really improve cerebral circulatory conditions in man. Modern cerebral pharmacodynamics (Gottstein, 1966; Geraud et al., 1965) show that some compounds have positive vasodilating effects accompanied by a sharp increase of cerebral oxygen. These drugs are papaverine, isolated from the alkaloids of opium, and Hydergine, a combination of the hydrogenated alkaloids of ergot and cyclandelate (Ciclospasmol).

Hydergine has proven to be an especially useful compound in the treatment of atherosclerotic and traumatic encephalopathies. It increases the cerebral blood flow as well as the utilization of oxygen by the brain, and it intensifies the metabolism of the sympathoblast.

Anabolizers

Following major head injuries and during protracted encephalopathy there is a profound catabolic state, leading to a widespread loss of tissue, wasting of muscles, shrinkage of the vital organs, and loss of depot fat. If large amounts of proteins can be fed to the patient, the negative balance of nitrogen can be reduced, but it is usually difficult to counter the catabolic process.

Androgens and anabolic steroids reduce the negative balance and may convert it into a positive one. Their effects depend on protein and total caloric intakes (Fruehan and Frawley, 1963). The compounds introduced (Dianabol, Durabolin, Winstrol, and Orgabolin) should have a considerable anabolic effect and a relatively lower androgenic effect than testosterone and its close relatives. Their administration in protracted posttraumatic comas is extremely useful and masculinization slowly subsides.

Cobamide (Indusil, Anabasi) has recently been introduced in clinical practice as an anabolic agent. This coenzyme, physiologically present in the body of mammals, stimulates cellular protein synthesis and also indirectly conditions the utilization of glucides and lipids and is devoid of undesirable side effects (Shinton, 1966). Our experience with this compound in protracted unconsciousness proves that its anabolizing effects are less constant and positive than those of steroids, while we confirm the absolute lack of undesirable side effects.

Muscle Relaxants

The treatment of hypertone, of rigidity, and of muscular spasticity in the apallic patient is extremely important. Indeed, a successful treatment with muscle relaxants is often the cause of the patient's recovery.

Pharmacology offers numerous compounds which decrease muscle tone by acting on the various levels of the nervous system (mephenesin, methocarbamol, carisoprodol, meprobamate, diazepam, chlorpromazine, etc.). The choice of the most suitable drug for each single case should be made on the basis of the clinical and electromyographic examinations of the kind of hypertone. This will permit the most favorable conditions for an efficient physiokinesic therapeutic treatment.

Comments

The treatment at the different stages of the apallic syndrome is complex and is based on an appropriate and intense psychomotor rehabilitation (Gerstenbrand, 1968a, b), as well as on the correct choice of drugs which will induce and maintain the conditions most favorable to the recovery of cerebral functions. The compounds which might somehow be useful at the apallic stage are listed in Table 1. This list, even though summarized, shows that it might be necessary to use compounds which differ widely among themselves not only in their chemical structures but in their clinical effects as well.

Since an ideal medication which can compensate for the function of the destroyed nervous cells has not yet been found, pharmacology must avail itself primarily of compounds with a nonspecific pharmacodynamic action. Consequently, it is often impossible to influence one single cerebral function. This is the case, for instance, with psychoanaleptics, and particularly with sympathomimetic amines, which have an excitant action not only on the highest nervous structures but also on the entire body. Apallic patients, especially in the early stages of their evolution, have qualitative and quantitative decreases in sleep (Bricolo et al., 1968a, b), as well as severe muscular hypertones. These factors in themselves contraindicate the use of stimulants. Indiscriminate administration of psychotonic amines or of other compounds which increase the level of wakefulness can be a serious therapeutic error in the majority of apallic patients. They are often already spontaneously in the strange situation of being completely devoid of activity and consciousness, while manifesting very high levels of wakefulness. To load these patients with stimulating drugs might further deteriorate their altered condition as well as increase their muscular rigidity, which is already quite severe.

To date there are not very many therapeutic possibilities of influencing positively and lastingly the levels or contents of consciousness with psychotic compounds. Koestler (1967), in a recent discussion on the subject, reported that it is fundamentally wrong to expect these drugs to enrich the mind, to introduce something that is not already there. According to Koestler, psychopharmacology can add nothing to mental faculties. It can, at best, eliminate obstacles or blocks which will not let it function properly, improving the coordination among preexisting circuits.

The pharmacotherapy of the apallic syndrome, when it is established according to these principles, should prefer compounds which activate directly or indirectly the cerebral metabolism and favor the transmission of nervous impulses at a synaptic level.

29. Problems of Tracheotomy in Patients with the Apallic Syndrome

A. BERGER

During the treatment of severely injured patients, especially in cases of severe cerebral traumas, it is extremely important to provide for sufficient oxygenation and to have a secure way to the trachea, because there is very often a need for long lasting assisted ventilation, and one is confronted with a time limitation in performing the nasal tracheal intubation. Treatment of the severely injured patient consists of two important points: (1) The first is to have a good and very easy access to the trachea for the necessary assisted ventilation. Especially in brain-damaged patients it is necessary to avoid the stimuli caused by the clinical stresses of the tracheotomy. (2) The second point is to have rehabilitation in mind and therefore avoid the typical posttracheotomy failures. Follow-up studies (Hohage, 1966; Kucher et al., 1967) have demonstrated the relatively high frequency of early and late complications after a classic tracheotomy. The frequency of bleeding after erosion was 2%, and severe tracheal stenosis could be found in 5.2% of the cases. Other authors (Otteni and Gauthier-Lafaye, 1969; Berger et al., 1970a, b) reported similar results. This follow-up study brought us to the question of whether it is possible to change some technical parts of a tracheotomy and thereby achieve better results and avoid primary and late complications.

Method

The new method should meet the following criteria:

1. The frequency of bleeding after erosions should be lowered.
2. Infection in the immediate vicinity of the tracheotomy and later trachealstenosis should be avoided.
3. Handling and care of the tracheotomy should be easier and more secure.
4. The tracheotomy should be prepared for the problems of long-term assisted ventilation.

With all of the above-mentioned points in mind, we perform our principally transisthmian tracheotomy, so that the trachea is opened by a longitudinal incision. A skin mucosal tunnel is prepared which lasts for the entire duration of the tracheotomy. The closure of the tracheotomy is not accomplished through wound healing, but is performed with a local skin flap.

Technique of Operation

1. Tracheotomy. During general anesthesia with a tube in place, the skin incision is made as with a Kocher incision. The plathysma is incised and the subfascial venae are ligated. The longitudinal short muscles of the neck are divided at the median line. The isthmus of the thyroid gland is divided into two pieces, and under careful protection of the tunica adventitia tracheae (Fuchsig, 1960) the tracheal wall is freed. The trachea is incised longitudinally between the second and fifth cartilage. The skin flaps of the incision are sutured to the tracheal wall with six to eight sutures (chromic catgut) (Fig. 1a, b). A secure coverage of the greater arteries and veins of the neck and the veins of the fascia is then performed, thus avoiding the danger of bleeding and of an infection from the stoma into the neck tissue.

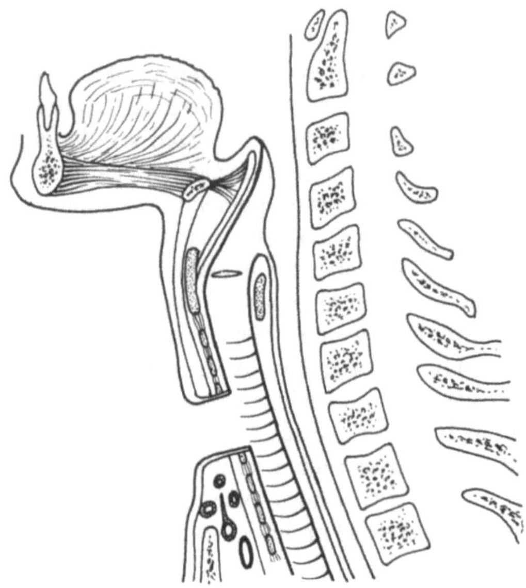

Fig. 1. (a) "Skin-tube" tracheotomy. Skin flaps sutured to the anterior tracheal wall (schema). (b) "Skin-tube" tracheotomy, schema, cross section

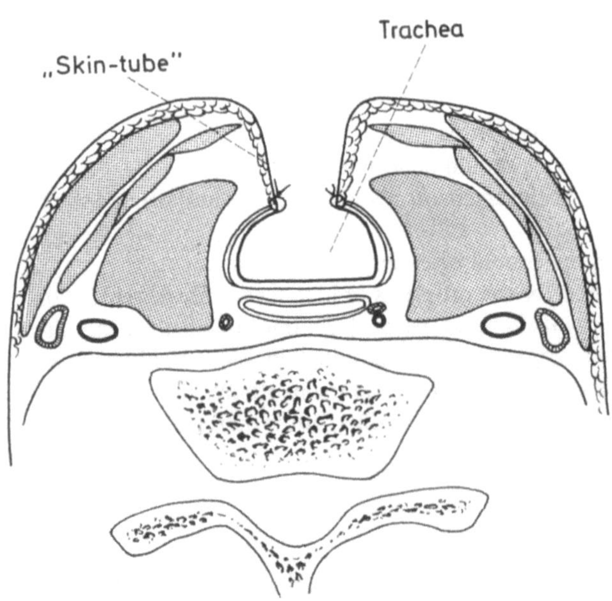

Fig. 1b

2. Plastic Surgical Closure of the Tracheotoma. If there is no longer a need for a tracheotomy after examination of the trachea through X-ray, tracheoscopy, and respiratory examinations, the trachea can be closed with a local skin flap ("swinging door") (Fig. 2). If the examinations do not show a severe stenosis, i.e., a stenosis greater than one-third the diameter, the skin tunnel is circumcised 12 mm from the stoma and a pedicle flap is attached to the tracheal wall. The skin dermis flap is then sutured to the opposite side of the tracheotoma under moderate tension. Air tightness is checked, and the tracheotoma is closed without tension. The straight muscles of the neck are then freed and sutured together in the median line. With this method a scar adhesion to the skin and tracheal wall can be avoided. A drainage is made before closure of the skin. The patient receives antibiotics for 5 days postoperatively. Before the patient can go back to a rehabilitation center, an X-ray control of the trachea is performed.

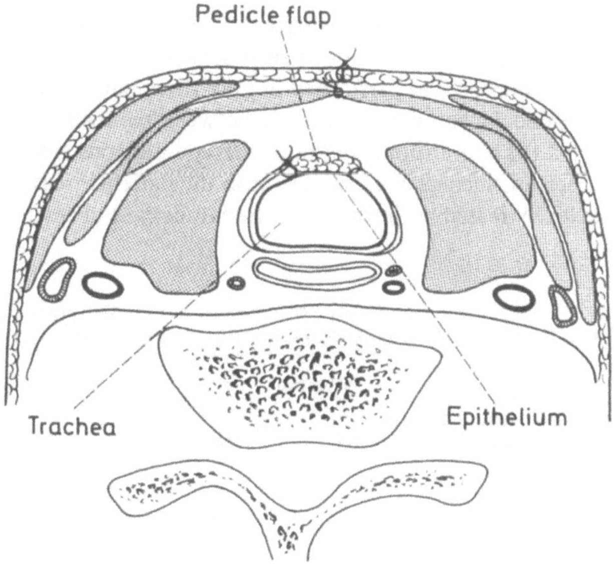

Fig. 2. Active closure of the "skin-tube" tracheotomy (cross section)

Results

Since mid-1966 we have treated 228 patients with this method. Most of the patients had a severe head injury or suffered from tetanus, myasthenia or intoxication. The ages of the patients varied from 6 to 69 years. Sixty-six patients are still alive, thus allowing a survey of the trachea in these patients to be made. Twenty-six patients had undergone assisted ventilation between the 1st and the 35th day. The duration of the tracheotomies was between 3 and 116 days (Berger et al., 1970b). In none of these patients did we see any bleeding from an erosion, or any orificial infections. Out of these 66 patients an operative closure with a flap was made in 51 cases, whereas 15 patients had a healing of the tracheotomy by granulation. Therefore, it was possible to compare these two groups. The result of this study is that the primary complications are obviously not different in the two groups, but that the frequency of the tracheal stenosis is significantly different between the group in which the tracheotomy was closed with a flap and the one in which the tracheotomy was closed by normal wound healing. The results of our "skin-tube" tracheotomy can be seen in Table 1.

Table 1. Comparison of number of cases of tracheal stenosis in skin tube tracheotomies with flap closure vs. spontaneous closure

	Number	0	1/3	1/2	2/3
"Skin-tube" tracheotomy with flap closure	51	38	10	2	1
"Skin-tube" tracheotomy with spontaneous closure by granulation	15	6	4	3	2

The cosmetic results were satisfactory. The scars are mostly tender and small, and in most cases adhesions could not be seen between the tracheal wall and the skin. A second cosmetic operation was performed in only three patients because of the thickness of the scar. In Table 2 a comparison is made between the tracheotomy with active closure of the stoma and the conventional method with spontaneous closure of the stoma; significantly fewer cases of tracheal stenosis appear in the patients treated with the former method than in those treated with the conventional method of tracheotomy.

Table 2. Comparison of number of cases of tracheal stenosis in tracheotomies with flap closure vs. spontaneous closure

	Number	0	1/3	1/2	2/3
"Skin-tube" tracheotomy with flap closure	51	38	10	2	1
Tracheotomy wound technique with spontaneous closure	82	27	24	20	11

With these results in mind we can conclude that the criteria can be met with this operation. The bleeding after erosion of an artery and the orificial infection could be avoided. The frequency of the tracheal stenosis later is decreased in spite of the fact that the duration of the canulement did not show any correlation with the frequency of the stenosis. Stenosis of the trachea can also be seen more often if the patient is older. This kind of tracheotomy immediately after the operation presented no problems for the nurses. Changing the tubes is possible any time without special training. The cleansing of the trachea, which is absolutely necessary with severely brain-damaged patients, is easily accomplished. In addition, there is no severe mechanical stress on the stoma, which is an important part of the treatment and rehabilitation of patients during the apallic syndrome. For rehabilitation, closure by a plastic procedure represents the treatment of choice. Cosmetic results are satisfactory.

A plastic surgical closure of the tracheotomy is especially useful in tracheotomies of long duration and with patients requiring long-lasting assisted ventilation.

Summary

A new method for a tracheotomy in severely injured patients is reported. The concept consists of two parts. The tracheotomy is performed using a skin tube and therefore creating a real stoma during the whole time of intubation. The tracheotomy is then closed by a local skin flap. The frequency of erosions, infections and also posttracheotomy tracheal stenosis could be significantly lowered.

30. Utilization of the Tonus Regulating Reflexes in the Rehabilitation of the Apallic Syndrome

U. SEIFERT-MIELKE

It is unfortunate that one customarily identifies and analogizes the phylogenetic phases of development of man with his ontogenesis, i.e., assuming in the case of a "disintegration" or a destruction of the brain that the ontogenetic "levels" of cerebral function are identical with phylogenetic "phases." This view is controversial. In psychiatry, correspondingly, a demented person does not sink to the level of a dog or, finally, to that of a reptile. Even under the conditions of dementia he possesses specifically human characteristics which, together with the remaining mental activity, do not allow him as an individual to exist at another phylogenetic level. Basically, this is also true for the motoric functional levels. The specific form of the tonicity pattern in man is always apparent and thus produces a state which is peculiar to man and which only appears in cases of cerebral destruction. Therefore, we assume that the exercises leading to a redistribution of tonicity and to the restitution of functions and, finally, of performances, are essentially bound to the simultaneous integration of reflex chains at a higher level, and particularly at the level of the cerebral cortex of man (Müller, 1968).

Magnus and de Kleijn (1912, 1930) described reflexes in animals which are bound to certain positions and movements of the body and which ensure the animal's standard position in space. A group of such reflexes appears at a certain stage of the child's physiologic development, but then, in the course of the maturation of the brain, they are inhibited or suppressed (Schaltenbrandt, 1925). However, if they are maintained for a longer period of time, or reappear at a later stage, conclusions on disorders of certain pathways or centers of the brain can be drawn (Kretschmer, 1953; Pia, 1957; Poeck and Hubach, 1963). Another group of reflexes can only be demonstrated under pathologic conditions.

Reflexes of Posture

(Peiper, 1949; Gottschlick, 1955; Müller, 1968; Moro, 1920).

The following reflexes of posture were first described by Magnus and de Kleijn (1930).

1. The tonic labyrinthine reflex: Obtained by tonus reflexes starting from the labyrinth. In the prone position they cause an increase in the flexor tonus; in the dorsal position they cause an increase in the extensor tonus. When the child is being pulled up by his arms, the head drops backward with the vertebral column being stretched so that neither raising of the head nor sitting is possible.

2. The asymmetric tonic cervical reflex ("fencing position"): An increase in the tonus of the extensors of the limbs on the same side as the chin when the head is turned aside

and simultaneous increase in the tonus of the flexors of the limbs on the same side as the skull when the head is turned aside. Thus, optically controlled grasping, playing, and independent eating and drinking are impossible.

3. The symmetric tonic cervical reflex: Stretching of arms and simultaneous flexing of legs as well as raising of the head. In the case of a passive flexing of the head in a dorsal position, flexing of arms and stretching of legs.

4. Positive and negative supporting reaction.

5. The tonic grasping reflex of hands and feet.

6. The Moro reflex.

Reflexes of Position

(Peiper, 1949; Pia, 1957; Müller, 1968).

1. The labyrinthine reflex on the head (Landau's reflex)
2. The labyrinthine reflexes of the head on the body, of the body on the head, and of the body on the body

Since the tonicity pattern in decerebrated persons depends on the position of the head in space (otoconial reflex–tonic labyrinthine reflexes on the limbs) relative to the position of the head to the body (symmetric or asymmetric tonic cervical reflex), the child is fixed in an abnormal position. Therefore, the principles of treatment are based on the following factors (Bobath, 1949, 1964; Bobath and Bobath, 1950; Müller, 1964):

1. Inhibition of the abnormal tonic reflex action; it helps to normalize and stabilize the muscular tonus.
2. Establishment of pathways of the higher coordinated labyrinthine reactions in their regular successive phases of development. This is done on the basis of the normalized muscular tonus.

Such treatment is possible due to the fact that one and the same stimulus within one and the same reflexogenic zone of a certain reflex can cause inverse reflex responses, i.e., stimulation during flexing can produce extension or vice versa (reflex inversion according to Sherrington, 1898). According to Uexkuell, the explanation is given by the fact that in primitive forms of motion the afferent input into the central nervous system is always led into the elongated muscles and that the retracted muscles are always in the state of central inhibition. This caused Magnus (1924) to formulate his well-known interconnection law:

> The central nervous system reflects at any time the condition of the musculature of the body. The condition of the muscles of the whole body, their retraction or contraction, their elongation and relaxation determine at any time the distribution of excitatory or inhibitory processes within the central nervous system.

Correspondingly, the condition of the muscles determines the flux of stimulation or inhibition from the central nervous system. This means that the proprioceptors of the muscles control their own central nervous system. It is therefore possible to influence and control the state of the central nervous system from the periphery, i.e., from the proprioceptors of the muscles. The (passive) change of the abnormal attitude and the alteration of the condition of the muscles must necessarily lead to a redistribution of excitatory and inhibitory processes within the central nervous system. In this way it is possible to interrupt reflex chains which are unfavorable to the tonus and open up new pathways for these chains.

At first, *reflex inhibitive* positions are brought about, i.e., positions representing a complete inversion of the abnormal positions (e.g., head in intermediate position, flexed forward, arms crossed over the chest, vertebral column flexed, legs flexed, abducted, if necessary). All originally contracted muscles are thus elongated and the stimulation flows into the now extended muscles. Since the reactivation of the postural and equilibrium reactions integrated at a higher level is the only possibility to ensure a stable, normal tonus, exercise of these reflexes must follow. Constant repetition ensures success, particularly since the synaptic transmission along certain chains is made easier by the previous activity in these connections. This is especially the case with synergies belonging to phylogenetically established chains–for instance, the postural and labyrinthine reactions.

These statements are illustrated by data from the record of patient Maret G. (record No. 68/70).

Born on the expected date; labor was induced according to schedule. Weight:3.900 g, length: 56 cm. At the beginning, development was normal. During an infection at the age of 8 months, hyperpyretic temperatures up to 42.5°C with disorientation and tonic-clonic spasms were observed.

Findings upon admission: Coma vigile; unmodulated hoarse crying; spastic tetraparesis; fencing position on both sides (Fig. 1), opisthotonos with the head dropping backward when the child was pulled up (Fig. 2); bending-extended position of the limbs with midposition of the head; when touched at any place, sudden extension spasms with cloni; in prone position, all limbs and the head were flexed; however, the latter was not turned aside; positive Marinescu on both sides. The EEG indicated a diffuse cerebral lesion without focus. The

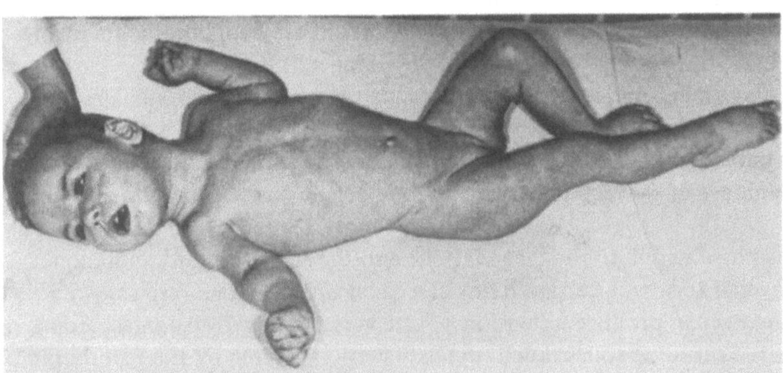

Fig. 1

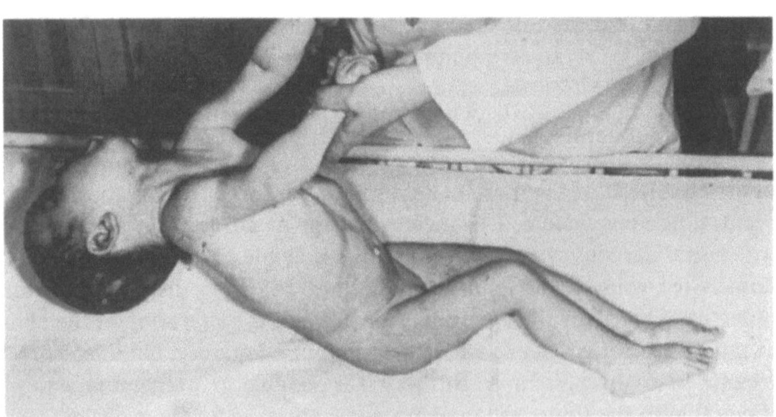

Fig. 2

PEG (4 months after the infection) showed coarse atrophies of cerebrum and cerebellum, arachnitic adhesion on the basic cisternae, cisterna magna, and convexity. Carotid angiography showed subdural, mainly frontoparietal effusions on both sides with blocking of discharging veins and circulatory bypass via the central veins; axial compression.

Decompression was achieved by fenestration of both capsular layers. A second operation with removal of both capsular layers followed after 1 month because of recidivation of subdural hematoma. The rehabilitation was subsequently intensified. Parallel to the improvement of the tonic conditions (tetraparesis now clearly improved, Landau I positive for a short period), higher performance levels were developed after a short period. The child can focus, smiles, reacts adequately to optical and acoustic stimuli, recognizes people, and eats and drinks spontaneously.

Summary

The characteristic reflexes of position and posture, described in animals, appear as well in specific stages of development of a child, or persist or reappear during disturbances of analogous brain centers or cerebral tracts. Since the tonus pattern of decerebrates in general depends on the position of the head in relation to the body, the patient is usually in an abnormal position. Therefore, during rehabilitation, the abnormal tonus reflex activity is first inhibited by adequate exercise, and on the basis of the muscle tonus, returned to normalcy. Thus, the way is prepared for more coordinated position and equilibrium reactions. While specific tonus patterns are established, a higher level of the brain's efficiency develops simultaneously.

31. The Rehabilitation of the Apallic Syndrome During the Phase of the Reintegration of the Higher Function Stages

R.A. DIETZE

In the following, an attempt is made to report on the measures promoting the reintegration of higher functional stages during the apallic syndrome, starting with the functional phase at the pons level, based on a knowledge of the remission stages and of the functional ontogenetic development.

Even while the patient is still in the phase of the acute midbrain syndrome, a rehabilitation program should be initiated–apart from the actual treatment–together with anesthesists and the bordering special disciplines. In general, acute midbrain syndromes last for periods of up to 2 weeks; remission frequently takes place surprisingly quickly, assisted by light, pain, and sound stimuli in rapid succession. These are the first stimuli which introduce remission. At the beginning of coma vigile, stimulation should be continued with great intensity. It has been shown that the patient reacts with an increased respiration to affective stimuli such as maternal attention to a newborn child. However, at this stage there are no other reactions.

The emotional stimuli at this stage include caressing sounds, caressing, and cradling the body, or, with older patients, of the head. At this stage care must still be taken to prevent contractions conditioned by the position; the patient does not move yet, sucking and swallowing still fail to take place, and special feeding is necessary.

With every application of the feeding tube, the release of primitive oral patterns must be tested. If these are present, the functional level of an infant has been reached, and food may be given with the bottle. Only then will oral gripping ensue as an automatic mechanism, but manual grasping does not yet take place. At this stage the establishment of contacts must be intensified; the patient already begins to concentrate and to grasp at everything offered; the eye-mouth coordination is intact. This phase is characterized by a motor agitation with an as yet holokinetic motor pattern (Lesny, 1965).

This agitation has a nuance of anxiety, attention must be more intense than before, and patients frequently calm down and appear to become more attentive when addressed by certain people. Optical stimuli induce mouth reactions but are not recognized. It appears that this process can be shortened by obtaining toys familiar to the patient from early childhood–particularly in the case of children–even if these toys are greatly worn. It is noted that, even more than the visual image, the *smell* of the familiar object and the haptic impression of the familiar shape stand in the foreground (Fig. 1).

It is possible that the acoustic and osmic, as well as the haptic perceptive qualities, set in much sooner than the primary optic perceptive faculties. At this point the time has arrived for offering the patient food of markedly varied tastes, in order to reanimate the eating stereotype.

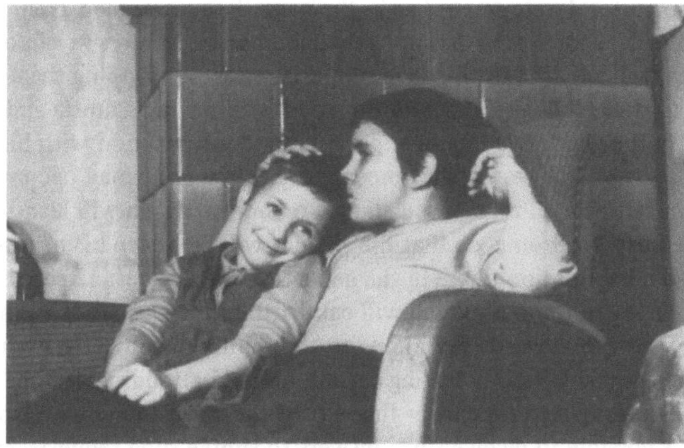

Fig. 1. Orientation attempts with aid of osmic analyzer

The haptic afferent stimulation is soon followed by the subsequent manual grasping reaction. Motor development is now in the monokinetic phase. The patient grasps at everything within his reach and puts it into his mouth, as the eye-hand-mouth coordination is intact. This stage requires increased attention on the part of those looking after the patient, who might swallow needles, soap, chemicals, etc. Similarly, there is an automatic biting reaction, with tearing and biting of bedclothes. It is recommended that a rubber wedge for sucking and biting be placed in the patient's hand and that he be clothed in a one-piece combination pyjama or nightdress. This spasmodic gripping and biting may still exist paroxysmally after reintegraion of the highest functional stages and is then felt by patients as a compulsion. For example, a girl, treated by us for many years, announced the setting in of snapping or biting paroxysms during anticipation. It is interesting to note that, in view of the cerebral functions that have been reintegrated in the meantime, the mechanism may be interrupted by the transformation of the inhibiting coercion into a purposeful action—e.g., eating bread, which was then successfully done by the girl herself.

The first contact sounds are observed in the phase of paroxysmal biting. These begin with a low whimpering and at times loud screaming, such as that of an infant. Smiles are never observed. Here as well, aversion comes before advertence (D. Müller, 1968). When the low whimpering begins it is accompanied by symptoms of fear and aversion. It is important at this time that the patient be calmed acoustically and haptically; this can frequently be done merely by a calming sound. The patient is now obviously attempting—by producing searching sounds—to assure himself of the presence of those attending to him. Optic agnosia as well as amnestic disturbances make him aware of his helplessness, so that he behaves like a young animal or infant by producing searching sounds and waiting for a guiding sound, as observed and described by Lorenz (1961) in the rearing of a young gray goose. This behavior also continues up to maximal remission phases. Thus, for example, a girl could only be left alone, provided that vocal contact was maintained with her. If this was not done, the child would hastily follow and forcefully clutch and bite the withdrawing person. Once vocal contact has been established, the closest relatives should be allowed to talk intensely, and to play phonograph records. The goal in this connection is the creation of "reminiscence islands"—this time only by the acoustic analyzer—thereby preparing for the language remission.

The motor development has in the meantime proceeded from cranial to caudal and the patient, insofar as he has not remained paretic as a result of corresponding local brain injuries, will advance to the dromokinetic phase by skipping the cratikinetic phase. He will begin to walk, but is still greatly impeded by his optic agnosia and will not find his way about in the ward. Even in an experimental confrontation with his familiar environment at home he will be helplessly agnostic, even though he may become intensely excited by familiar but not yet recognized sounds or smells, which will lead to a relapse into the Klüver-Bucy syndrome, so that the patient will bite even his nearest relatives.

The rehabilitation phase in the acoustic sphere is best effected with the aid of well-known nursery rhymes, which will call forth grunting sounds to the melody, partly containing individual words pertaining to the rhyme or song. These rhymes or songs may also acquire a signal value, by letting certain defined attending persons sing certain defined songs. The language appears in the text of the song, thereby improving modulation.

It is possible to receive sung answers to simple sung requests, even though at first they may be restricted to "yes" and "no" in various modulations. At the beginning the patient is greatly exhausted by the singing of the song, so that even during the singing he will begin to snap for air. Language will set in unexpectedly, with a starting echolalia. The impulse will still be obstructed in relation to the readiness for linguistic expression. At the same time, phenomena of unrestrained impulses of the orbital brain may be observed, such as lewd expressions and sexual actions. These expressions may subsequently also be felt as coercions and be improved by cortical inhibitions such as counting the lewd expressions (such as "foul sow," etc.). The girl concerned frequently apologized even in anticipation of these coercive verbal expressions. During this phase there are frequent moments of fondling and seeking physical proximity, with a beginning differentiation. It will be observed that this seeking is very largely steered by the sense of smell. The snapping of the Klüver-Bucy syndrome passes into an intense sniffing and smelling phase, in particular the hair of attending persons and the sniffing of all objects within reach.

Optical agnosia still prevails and causes the main difficulties in the course of the further rehabilitation. With an almost intact acoustic orientation accompanied by a sense of smell, the patient again becomes capable of learning, which we were able to prove by experiments. Optically, there is also a partial stimulation of the primary field of perception, so that various objects are avoided and obstacles may be evaded.

The optical agnosia is many-sided and consists in the first place of an object agnosia and prosopagnosia as well as a simultan agnosia (Pötzl, 1928; Gloning and others). In our case history, the optical orientation was improved only in the course of the systematic new learning of the letters of the alphabet (Fig. 2a-d); agraphia and alexia gradually receded in the course of practicing the recognition of the letters with the aid of a primer which the girl had already used in the first class at school. Reading ability greatly helped in orientation. All objects were then consolidated in the mind in a combination of acoustic, haptic, and osmatic presentation and their definition made with the aid of letters. The concept "door," for instance, was practiced by letting the patient feel, knock on, smell the door—by smell orientation in the space on both sides of the door—slam the door, feel the draught of air, and go in and out of the door. The concept was then fixed through the medium of letters, and there was certainly an optical island of reminiscence. It also happened that, in the girl's independent search for the door, a cupboard door would be opened and she would want to go into the cupboard, but then the narrowness and also the smell would cause her to note the error, which resulted in affective excitement and relapse into the Klüver-Bucy syndrome.

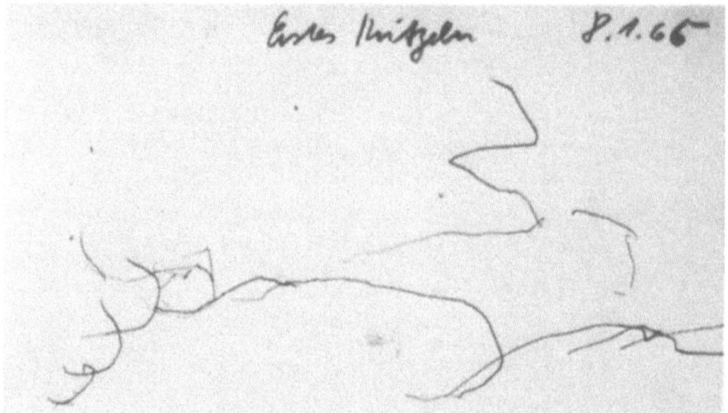

Fig. 2a

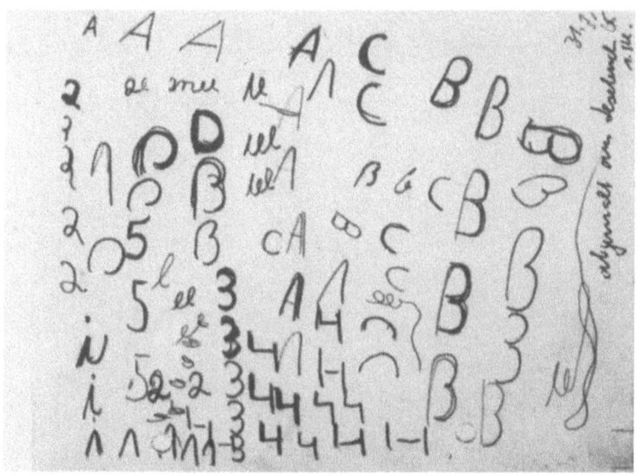

Fig. 2b

Fig. 2. Restoration of writing capability and ability to recognize writing. (a) First scribbling 3 months after beginning of disease. (b) Letters and figures are copied, partly distorted, still without recognition. (c) Recognition of written signs and attempts to establish written contacts with the environment with aid of selection of letters from alphabet chart. (d) Seven months after first writing attempts. Correct writing, with the exception of several spelling mistakes. Letter reveals full restoration of personality and patient's own judgement of agnosia vestiges

Despite rehabilitation of this subject over a period of years, a prosopagnosia and geographical agnosia, as well as difficulties in the recognition of properties of material still persist up to the present time. This is coupled with a particular weakness of memory. Haptic recognition was applied from the start in order to promote optical recognition: The child was sent to a course in ceramics, with excellent results (Fig. 3). She can recognize ceramics without hearing the sound of the material. The recognition of other materials was not practiced as intenselx, since they were not suited to figurative shaping. The girl finished an extended polytechnical 12-class school with standards equal to those required by the upper 4th grade of the former type of high or grammar school, and a professional education as a librarian.

This long process occurred in only one case with the delayed reintegration of the highest functional levels; in all other cases the return of functions began with the start of affective responsiveness. However, in some cases the ability to eat was not yet restored. As soon as this mechanism is again intact, however, very good prospects are offered for

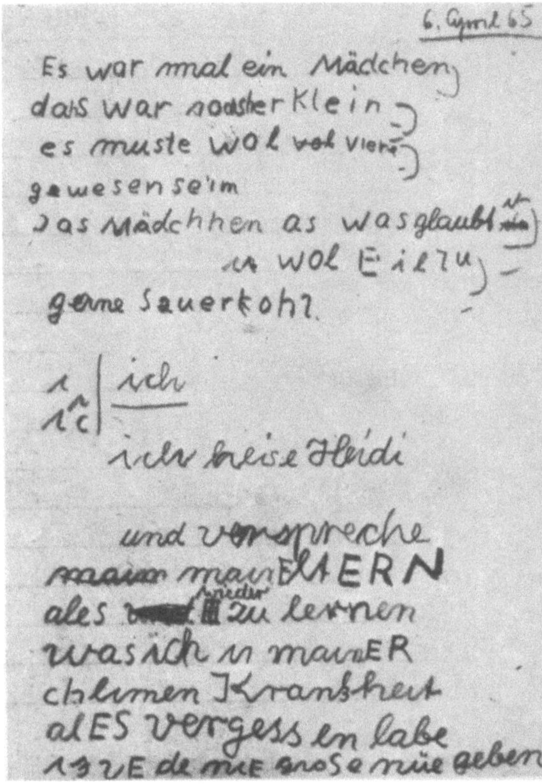

6. April 65

Es war mal ein Mädchen
dass war sodster Klein
es muste wol vol viere
gewesen seim
Das Mädchhen as was glaubt
... wol Eilzu
gerne Sauerkohl.

i | ich
ic |

ich heise Heidi

und verspreche
mauELtERN
ales wieder zu lernen
wasich in mauER
chlimen Kranbheit
alES vergess en labe
13 vE de mie grose müe geben

Fig. 2c

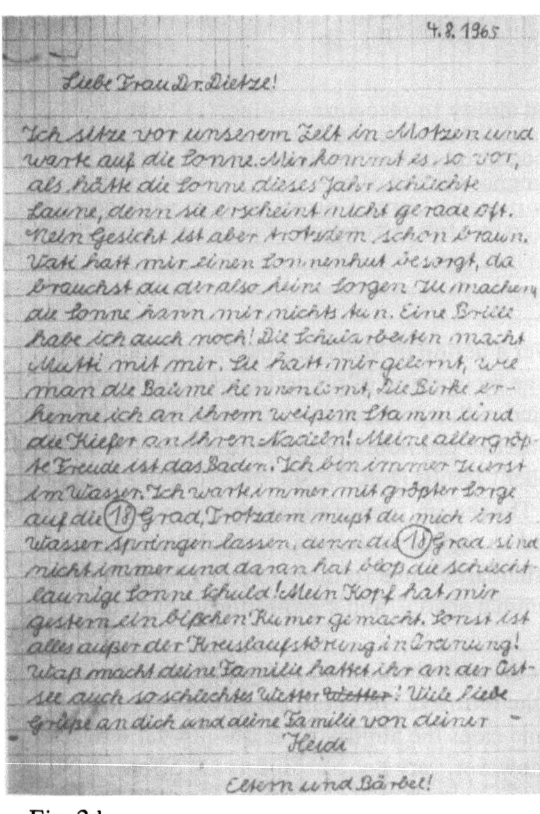

4. 8. 1965

Liebe Frau Dr. Dietze!

Ich sitze vor unserem Zelt in Motzen und wart auf die Sonne. Mir kommt es so vor, als hätte die Sonne dieses Jahr schlechte Laune, denn sie erscheint nicht gerade oft. Mein Gesicht ist aber trotzdem schon braun. Vati hatt mir einen Sonnenhut besorgt, da brauchst du dir also keine Sorgen zu machen, die Sonne kann mir nichts tun. Eine Brille habe ich auch noch! Die Schularbeiten macht Mutti mit mir. Sie hatt mir gelernt, wie man die Bäume kennenlernt. Die Birke erkenne ich an ihrem weißem Stamm und die Kiefer an ihren Nadeln! Meine allergrößte Freude ist das Baden. Ich bin immer zuerst im Wasser. Ich warte immer mit größter Sorge auf die (18) Grad. Trotzdem mußt du mich ins Wasser springen lassen, denn die (18) Grad sind nicht immer und daran hat bloß die schlechtlaunige Sonne Schuld! Mein Kopf hat mir gestern ein bißchen Kummer gemacht. Sonst ist alles außer der Kreislaufstörung in Ordnung! Was macht deine Familie hattet ihr an der Ostsee auch so schlechtes Wetter? Viele liebe Grüße an dich und deine Familie von deiner

Heidi

Eltern und Bärbel!

Fig. 2d

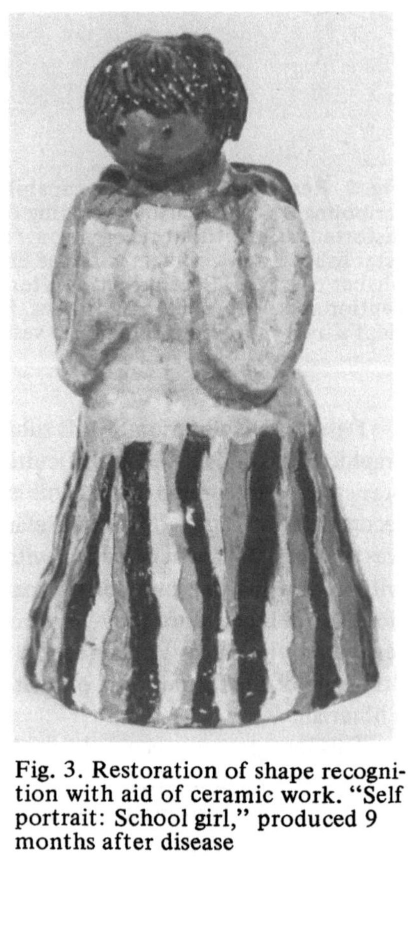

Fig. 3. Restoration of shape recognition with aid of ceramic work. "Self portrait: School girl," produced 9 months after disease

rehabilitation if the right starting point is found. This generally lies in affectively colored reminiscence images from childhood, or, in the case of children, from the 3rd year of life—the time of the earliest memory formation and impressions (D. Müller, 1968) brought about by various stimuli.

In summary, it can be stated that the rehabilitation phase begins with the transition of the acute mesencephalon syndrome to the coma vigile and is continued in consideration of ontogenetically known levels of achievement, with key stimuli from early childhood, with their affective nuances playing an important part. The phase of contact establishment during the coma vigile phase will pass into the phase of resocialization, which may last for a few days or even several years, depending on the discernible pathologic deficiencies of the brain.

During rehabilitation, the damaged analyzing ability of the brain shows on one hand a pseudocompensation in the process of cognition, such as a marked development of the sense of smell and the faculty of acoustic differentiation, and, on the other hand, a support of remission by means of reminiscence formation with the aid of sounds, smells, and images from early childhood, since these engrams can be best recalled, presumably because of their affective nature.

There are also transitory stages free of defects and even intermittent apallic syndromes such as the author observed in the radiation of a pons tumor (Dietze et al., 1968). On the basis of the experiences collected in the course of many years of endeavor for rehabilitation after an apallic syndrome caused by a sudden interruption of the connections between pons and cortex, it may be stated that the final result of the treatment cannot be predicted for weeks or even months. There are no remission trends and thus hardly any rehabilitation chances for apallic syndromes brought about by tissue damage between the cortex and the pons, such as demyelination processes, in which a progression to a mesencephalon syndrome and final bulbar brain syndrome can be clearly traced.

32. The Rehabilitation of Patients with Apallic Syndrome in the Therapeutic Community

F. GERSTENBRAND and C.H. LÜCKING

One of the main principles in the rehabilitation of apallic patients is that rehabilitation has to be started in every case as soon as possible. More precisely, the rehabilitation of an apallic syndrome has to be started in the acute phase of a severe brain damage which corresponds to the acute midbrain syndrome. During this phase, which was termed "preparatory phase" (Gerstenbrand, 1968), all precautions should be taken to provide the most favorable basis for the actual rehabilitation. The main precautions taken should concentrate on the prevention of cachexia, decubitus, contraction of joints, and periarticular ossifications. Thus a favorable basis for rehabilitation could be obtained. In this phase the application of hypercaloric nutrition and a special physicotherapy using the tonus-regulating reflexes are of special importance. While the enormous consumption of energy is compensated by the hypercaloric nutrition, the physicotherapy effects an indirect training of the motoric functions and causes a simultaneous activation of the reticular system leading to a reactivation of vigilance.

In the following stage, i.e. the stage of active rehabilitation, the patient has to be transferred to a special rehabilitation unit. At the time of transfer, the apallic patient should be in a good general condition with a stabilized feeding regimen. No complications with tracheostoma should aggravate the first phase of remission, which is the beginning of contact with the surroundings. Patients in a full state of an apallic syndrome should be transferred to a rehabilitation unit only if the results of the check-up examination (EEG, PEG, xenography, EMG) show signs of a good prognosis. The problem of taking care of those patients with an apallic syndrome showing no signs of a remission and from whom no remission can be expected, is not yet solved. For the aftercare of those patients, the installation of a special unit which can meet the requirements for treatment of these severest cases must be suggested. If apallic patients are transferred to a unit not suitable for their care, most of them will die within a short time despite modern medical treatment. According to our experience, a rehabilitation unit for patients with severe brain damage should consist of 18-20 patients of both sexes selected independently of the degree of the brain damage and its etiology. Patients with an apallic syndrome can be added to such a group. All patients live in a large family in a community area, complete with sleeping, living, working, and gymnastic rooms. A rehabilitation center may consist of several such units. Every rehabilitation unit has to be cared for by a staff comprised of specially trained medical and nursing personnel. The medical staff includes, besides neuropsychiatrists, one or two psychologists, one orthopedist, a neurosurgeon, an otolaryngologist, and an ophthalmologist. Of special importance is the close cooperation with an anesthesiologist of the intensive care unit. In the ward staff are included a logopedist, physiotherapists, social workers, occupational therapists, and a vocational guide.

Every rehabilitation unit is divided into subgroups: the mobilization group and the special therapeutic or achievement group (*Leistungsgruppe*). After transfer, the new patient, irrespectively of the severity of his brain damage, enters the mobilization group consisting of maximally five patients in close spatial contact with the patients of the other subgroup. The new patient transferred to the mobilization group of the rehabilitation unit is evaluated for brain damage by clinical examination and other diagnostic procedures such as EEG, EMG, X-ray of the skull and the cervical spine, pneumencephalography, and laboratory tests. Moreover a battery of psychological tests is carried out to obtain a performance profile. This profile demonstrates various concentration, and motor and speech functions. Based on the results of all the examinations, an individual rehabilitation program is designed. The program also considers the individual's social and professional status.

After transfer each patient is incorporated in the mobilization group. For adaptation to the new environment, no more than 2 weeks are usually necessary. The check-up mentioned above is carried out after the time of adaptation. The examinations have to be performed as carefully as possible. In some cases the pneumencephalography can be postponed to a later date especially when this examination was already performed during the period in the intensive care unit. In the beginning of treatment at the rehabilitation unit, the maintenance of hypercaloric nutrition has to be strictly observed. Sometimes the nutrition regimen is only possible with a combination of parenteral nutrition and tube feeding. This regimen, however, should be gradually replaced by spoon-feeding. For this purpose the oral reflexes can be utilized. The progressing remission, especially the entrance into the Klüver-Bucy phase, supports this development. The pseudobulbar paralytic symptomatology in cases with anoxic brain damage mostly disturbs oral feeding.

In the rehabilitation period in which the remission state of an apallic patient is comparable to optic dominance of the 3-month-old-child (Müller, 1968), the mother role of the attendant nurses is of great importance to the resumption of contact with the outside world. This also applies to the remission of speech ability. Naturally it is necessary in this state of rehabilitation to continue all the intensive care measures such as control of electrolytes, caring of decubitus, prevention of secondary peripheral nerve lesions as well as the application of special physiotherapy (tonus regulating reflexes) with increasing use of the active physiotherapeutic methods. The logopedist should start as soon as possible with exercises. Before beginning with verbal contact it is advantageous to teach the apallic patient a code-system (twinkling of eyes, etc.) with the help of which he is able to answer.

Equivalent to the mother role of the nurses, especially to that of the head nurse of the unit, the physicians (mainly the head of the department) have to assume the position of the father in the social relations of the patient. Praise and admonition as well as constant encouragement and exhortation are necessary.

In the rehabilitation unit those patients who have already achieved an improved state or who are suffering from a lesser form of cerebral damage may be called upon to help in the general care of the apallic patients. Likewise, their spontaneous offers of help should be encouraged. These patients can assist the nurses in feeding and can do other simple services in the care of the severe cases, as well as give assistance to the logopedist and physiotherapist. Moreover they are establishing a verbal contact with their "fellow-sufferer" and are exerting themselves in a cordial way for the severely injured.

At the end of the Klüver-Bucy phase, the apallic patient who is already out of bed may be introduced to the achievement group in the workroom, at first just to be present during the common singing and reading exercises or to watch television. After a time of adaptation the recovering apallic patient may participate in the exercises, and while his remission is progressing he will become a full member of the achievement group. The time which a patient has to remain in the mobilization group depends on the severity of the brain damage and the arising complications. It varies from a few weeks to several months. In rare cases it is even necessary to interrupt the rehabilitation and to transfer the patient to a nursing home, a decision causing a lot of problems in every case.

In the achievement group the rules and functions of the therapeutic community are fully applied. As a result of the different grades of the brain damage of the group members and the variety of their cerebral failures, and because of the introduction of new patients who are at the beginning of their remission course, an "ordering of achievement" arises which places "achievement demands" upon individual patients. The patient who is not yet very active is cared for by one who is already in an advanced state of remission and thereby receives an increased impulse for activity. Noting the difference in the recovered disturbed brain functions and comparing one's own improvement to the others seems to be an incentive to the patients. Compensatory actions between the single members of the community develop. A patient unable to walk by himself will be supported by a partially recovered stroke patient. In this system, the number of paramedical persons is at the same time increased, thus providing assistance to the members of the mobilization group.

Productivity of the single patient is stimulated by group dynamics, as each patient wants to do better than the other. Performance differences provide incentive and oblige the more disabled patients to increase their efforts in order to attain the standards set by their fellow patients. Besides individual production, there is a "collective compulsion" to produce. The group incentive must be directed not only toward achievement demands and achievement results, but also above all toward a positive cohesion within the group, which expresses itself through reciprocal aid and support. According to his premorbid personality and depending on the grade of his cerebral damage, every patient is entrusted with certain tasks within the group community. Subgroups are formed, based on the clinical picture and professional interests. Patients of other rehabilitation units of the rehabilitation center can be added to special subgroups. The achievement group has a fixed daily program which is determined by the patients themselves. It contains the schedule for the physiotherapy, for the training of the higher brain functions as well as for the spare time and regulates the events of the day for the whole group. One of the patients should be responsible for the adherence to the daily program and also for the positive incentive in the group. He should also act as a speaker for the whole group. For this important task a patient should be chosen who is at an advanced stage of rehabilitation and who appears to be particularly suited for it.

Between the entire rehabilitation group and the staff team, a dynamic relationship should be created. The responsibility for this may be shared by the head of the unit and by the head nurse. The various roles in the staff team have to be balanced. Inconsistency immediately leads to group unrest which has a negative effect upon the readiness to produce achievements. Every week the status and progress of each patient is evaluated in regular staff sessions. Regular checks such as EEGs, laboratory tests, psychologic testing for the performance profile and other examinations are made. With a consequent establishment of continually revised programs, the achievement demands are directed for the whole group.

A further factor in the group dynamics is added by the necessary inclusion of relatives and personal friends as well as friends of the professional milieu. Relatives and friends should be acquainted with the type of brain damage and with the expected change in the personality of the patient. It is necessary to explain to them as much as possible in order to produce a positive influence on the injured. The cooperation of relatives and friends is particularly important in the case of an apallic syndrome. In a further state of remission the method of bifocal group therapy can be used.

In the rehabilitation of the apallic patients, the therapeutic community creates a useful framework and may be regarded, especially for those cases of severe brain damage, as a provisional social environment that prepares the patient for the reintegration into normal society.

33. The Orthopedic Treatment of Patients with Apallic Syndrome

K. ZHUBER, M. SALZER, and F. GERSTENBRAND

Most patients with an apallic syndrome show a characteristic disorder of motor functions which is manifested in an increase of muscle tone and a disorder of body posture, corresponding to the midbrain posture. The upper extremities are thus adducted in the shoulder and flexed in the elbow, while the hand is in a fist position. The lower extremities show a slight flexion of the hip and knee joint, as well as plantar flexion of the feet. But sometimes variations are found that are caused by a lateralization of the midbrain lesion. This again causes an asymmetric posture of the joints, whereby the hip joints are not only flexed but also adducted in one joint and abducted in the other.

These changes of posture are maintained by a centrally regulated increase of muscle tonus. Without treatment a prolongation of these postural anomalies will cause contracture of muscles and a "freezing" of the joints in this position. In the first phase, passive joint movements are still possible; but after shrinking and shortening of the muscles and ligaments, myogenic and subsequent arthrogenic contracture will result. The severity of such an increase of the muscle tone could be observed in one of our patients, who developed a bilateral luxation of the hip as a consequence of the adduction spasm.

A further complication of the apallic syndrome is the development of new bone tissue around the large joints, termed as periarticular ossification. Only a few reports are available concerning periarticular ossifications in connection with the apallic syndrome (Jeannopoulous et al., 1961; Gerstenbrand et al., 1970a), while numerous authors have reported on this problem in association with traumatic spinal cord lesions (Abrahamson, 1948; Armstrong-Ressy et al., 1959; Damansky, 1961; Déjérine and Ceillier, 1918; Liberson, 1953; McNeur, 1954; Miller and O'Neill, 1949; Hardy and Dickson, 1963). But periarticular ossifications were also observed in several other neurologic diseases, such as myelitis (Damansky, 1961), central hemiplegia (Irving and Le Brun, 1954), brain tumor, and meningitis (Lorber, 1953), as well as poliomyelitis (Costello and Brown, 1951; Freiberg, 1952). In the latter, ossifications were also described in the metacorpophalangeal joints. Ossifications of this kind are rarely seen following extensive burns (Johnson, 1957; Evans and Smith, 1959).

Orthopedic Therapy

Therapeutic measures in treatment of the apallic syndrome are initially concentrated on the immediate preservation of life. Even at the earliest stage the orthopedist has to be consulted. The prevention of decubitus ulceration and joint contracture is of greatest importance during the intensive therapy period, and depends on a disciplined routine of nursing management, which includes turning the patient at regular intervals of 4 h. During the initial stage, i.e., the phase of the acute midbrain syndrome, the patient reacts to the slightest external stimuli with stretch cramps and an emergency reaction which stresses his circulatory and metabolic system. Early attempts at passive joint movements are rejected by the patient's vegetative lability. Passive joint movement should be started and later intensified, only after subsidence of the acute disinhibition of the muscle tone. Before that, special physical therapy has to be commenced by using the tonus-regulating reflexes. In the subsequent course of the remission stage, physical treatment gains in importance.

If, in spite of these measures, joint contractures develop, different orthopedic measures must be undertaken. In addition, it is of the greatest significance to consider the patient's general condition as well as his trophic situation. Premature active orthopedic treatment using casts or bandages, may lead to formation of decubital ulcers on the extremities. They will cause unfavorable healing tendencies and retard the course of remission.

Treatment with Casts

The utilization of removable casts enables one to keep an extremity in a certain passive position. Early in the course of the apallic syndrome this aid may be used as a prophylaxis in joints prone to contracture in order to prevent a malposition. In addition, already existing contractures may still be treated in this manner. A succession of casts are used. The procedure is as follows: A joint inclined to contract is passively extended after which a temporary cast is applied. After an interval of several days this procedure is repeated until correction is achieved. Finally, during mobilization of a patient, these casts may be used for keeping joints within the allowable maximum flexion and extension. Applications of this kind require little effort and since they can be removed, the casts will not interfere with the patient's nursing care. Even physical therapy may be continued without interruption. Pressure points must be watched carefully since decubital ulcers may develop. Cast treatment will be unnecessary after the patient has regained active muscle function.

Wedging

Existing myogenic contractures or already developed arthrogenic contractures on a single joint, may be treated with a wedged cast. Initially a circular cast is applied around the joint to be treated. Transsection of the cast and the maximum possible extension of the joint follow. Then the cast is fixed in this position. Within a few days the contracted tissue will adapt to the temporary extension, after which the above procedure may be repeated.

Redressment

In some rare cases of an apallic syndrome, redressment may offer a further possibility of mobilizing a joint fixed in a malposition through a forced joint movement under narcosis.

Gentle handling is most important to avoid fractures of the usually porous bones. The corrected joint is again kept in casts of plaster.

Tenotomy

Tenotomy may be undertaken if it is impossible to correct a myogenic contracture with one of the above-mentioned methods. Here the tendinous part of the shortened muscle is transsected in a Z-shape. After the joint position is corrected, the incised portions of the tendons is adapted and the extremities fixed in a cast. This procedure is especially suited at the knee joint and the Achilles tendon.

Periarticular Ossification

Periarticular ossification may present a therapeutically difficult problem, and this complication is therefore given special attention. In more than 10% of patients with an apallic syndrome, periarticular ossification may develop. Etiologically diverse factors have been made responsible for this; however, none have given a satisfactory explanation.

The most frequent site of ossifications is the elbow, followed by the hip and knee joint. The shoulder is hardly ever affected, and we have never observed changes of other joints.

Clinical manifestations of ossifications are first apparent through limitation of movement of the affected joints. Palpation of the region of the joint reveals firm to bony resistances, clearly demarcated against the surrounding tissue. This is connected with limited ability of movement and atrophy of the muscle. Besides the new bone formation, muscle contracture will mean additional enhancement of the motion disability.

The extent of new bone formation may vary greatly, from small osteophytes that cause only a moderate degree of limitation of movement, to bone bridges which encase a joint and cause complete stiffness. Real osseous ankylosis occurs only rarely.

Changes are radiographically seldom apparent before the 4th week of onset of the disease (Hardy and Dickson, 1963). First, vague and cloudy inhomogeneous shadows are found which gradually gain in density. Further in the course of the disease, the initially diffuse outline will become distinct from the surrounding tissue until finally the bone bridges are radiographically recognizable as highly differentiated bone. Cessation of new bone formation is best seen in serial radiographs. If no further enlargement of the bone bridges with regard to their extension is observed, the end of the ossifying process may be assumed. This process usually takes 7-8 months (Miller and O'Neill, 1949; Hardy and Dickson, 1963).

Morphology

Principally, all tissue originating from the mesenchyma may be drawn into the ossifying process. The transformation takes place first in the periarticular tissue and later in the neighboring muscles. The joint capsule stays unaltered for some time and shows only degenerative changes. In persistent periarticular ankylosis of the joint, all structures of the joint, including the cartilage, are drawn into the ossifying process. The newly formed tissue finally shows all characteristics of a highly differentiated bone (osteons, blood-building tissue, yellow marrow) (Déjérine et al., 1919).

Indications for Operation

The timing of operation of periarticular ossifications is important. Removal of bone too early may result in a recurrence of ossification even though the operation seems at first satisfactory. The functional ability of the muscular system controlling the joint is of significance. Meticulous topographic knowledge of the ossifications and their relation to vessels and nerves is a prerequisite of any operation of this kind. Finally, the active restoral of function of the extremity being treated must be reasonably related to the extent of the operation to be performed. The goal of treatment of patients with apallic syndrome as compared to patients suffering from spinal cord lesions should not only be in the improvement of the position but also in the regaining of active mobility of a joint.

Operative Therapy of Periarticular Ossification

A radical excision of the bone bridges, independent of the affected joints and the extent of the ossification, is the goal of treatment. This is especially important at the cartilage-bone border. Intraoperative, after the new bone is chiseled off, joint movement must be extensively free. Preparation of the elbow joint may cause trouble because of the sheathed-in arteria cubitalis or nervus ulnaris. In the knee joint great care must be taken to avoid damage to the remnants of the collateral ligaments because their debilitation may cause joint instability. The removal of bone bridges surrounding the hip joint may bring difficulties, for this joint may be completely enveloped by ossified tissue.

Results of Operated Periarticular Ossifications

Surgical experiences of apallic syndrome patients with periarticular ossifications are absolutely encouraging when the operative indication was strictly performed and the operation properly timed. Best results and greatest increase of mobility were attained after removal of bone bridges of the elbow joint (authors' experiences from 6 operated joints) (Fig. 1a, b). The range of motion attained primarily after operation was maintained for 6 years. Operative intervention, other than exact joint rectification, such as plastic operation of the elbow joint, are of no value and must be looked upon as overtreatment. Operative interventions on hip joints with great hindrance of mobility may achieve significant results, even though they are technically difficult (three operated hips). Especially in bi-

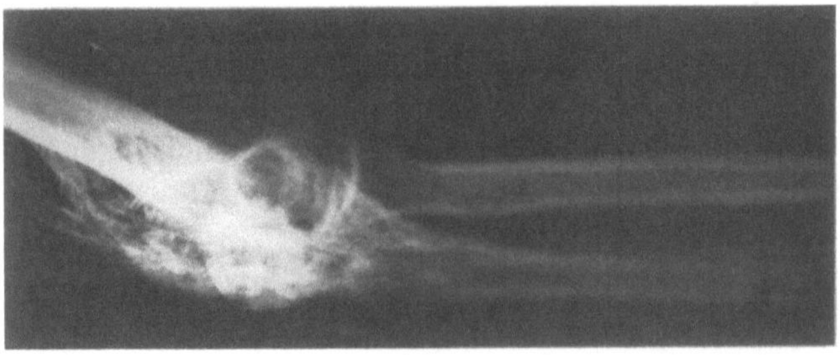

Fig. 1a

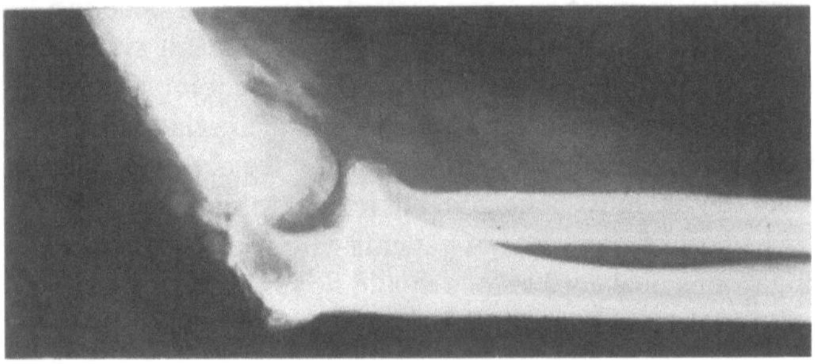

Fig. 1b

Fig. 1. Traumatic apallic syndrome, periarticular ossifications, left elbow with marked formation of bone bridges, dorsal. Patient P.C. male, 40 years old. (a) Before operation, (b) 5 months after operation. Corresponding to operative report joint capsule was mostly unaltered, ulnar nerve sheathed by bone tissue

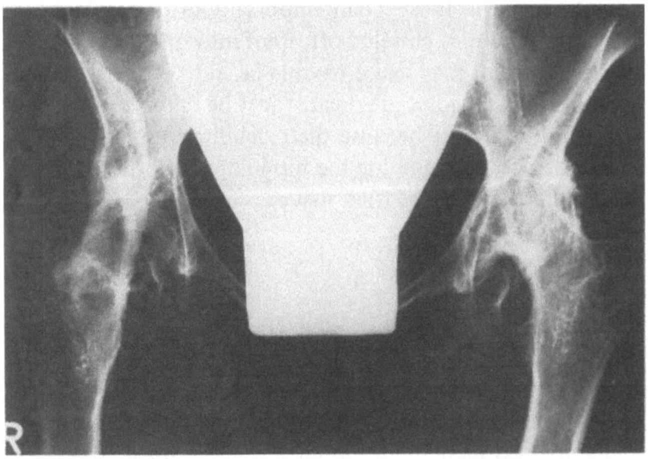

Fig. 2a

Fig. 2. Apallic syndrome as sequela of massive hemorrhage of corpus callosum; periarticular ossification of both hip joints with total ankylosis. Patient E.M., female, 24 years old. (a) Before operation, (b) 2 months after resection of femur head and collum, left side, with satisfactory function, moderate recidivism

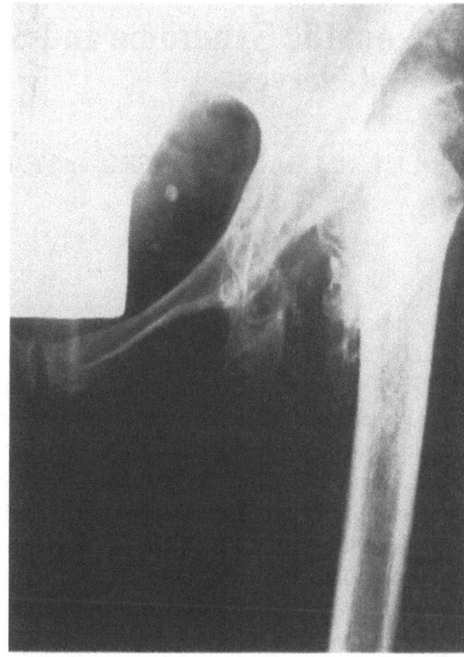

Fig. 2b. (Legend see p. 212)

lateral ankylosis (Fig. 2a, b), surgical treatment will facilitate the patient's ability to walk and sit. Regarding postoperative results, the knee joint is the least amenable; the only indication for operating is bilateral involvement (three operated joints). All operative interventions will only then give satisfactory results if intensive and long-term physical exercise can be guaranteed. Physical exercise should be commenced a few days after operation and possibly be carried on for several months.

34. The Apallic Syndrome and Secondary Lesions of Peripheral Nerves

B. MAMOLI, E. SLUGA, H. ZACHERL, and F. GERSTENBRAND

Secondary lesions of certain peripheral nerves may occur in cases involving long-term unconsciousness due to cerebral damage (Gerstenbrand et al., 1971; Laederich and Bernard-Pichon, 1935; Mertens, 1961; Olsen, 1956; Tönnis, 1958); they are also found in bedridden patients (Mumenthaler and Schliack, 1965; Woltman, 1930) and under certain conditions of treatment and occupational exposure (Carr, 1957; Gerhard, cited in Mumenthaler and Schliack; Laederich and Bernard-Pichon, 1935; Sprofkin, 1958; Wilhelm, 1970). The number of patients displaying an apallic syndrome with concomitant secondary lesions of peripheral nerves is increasing. Although holistic treatment, preventive measures, attention to bedding, prophylactic measures against decubital ulcerations, and persistent physical therapy are a constituent part of modern intensive care (Krenn, 1972) secondary peripheral nerve lesions may still be observed in patients with apallic syndrome.

Clinical Data

In the past nine years (1964-1972), at the Department of Rehabilitation of the Neurological University Hospital in Vienna, 27 out of 94 patients with an apallic syndrome revealed definite damage of one or more peripheral nerves. The patients came from the intensive care units of both surgical clinics of the University of Vienna and from other surgical departments. Exact data about the time of occurrence of these nerve lesions are usually not available, because the clinical symptoms are masked by the unconsciousness, immobility, and poor general condition of the patient. Furthermore, the attending physician pays most of his attention to the function of the vital organ systems. Whenever such patients enter the phase of remission and rehabilitation, neurologic complications arising from secondary lesions attract his full attention and invariably present obstacles to rehabilitation measures. However, it is possible that in some cases the peripheral nerve lesion may already have existed some time prior to the full development of the clinical symptoms.

The localization of the secondary peripheral nerve lesions in 27 patients is shown in Table 1. According to our practical experience, local pressure is of primary importance. This is consistent with the fact that almost exclusively anatomically exposed peripheral nerves are involved. Among the patients observed, no polyneuritic symptoms were found. The following additional factors have to be included in our considerations: metabolic disturbances, endotoxins, hyperergic reactions, hypoxia during the acute phase of the apallic syndrome, anemia, and pronounced deficits in metabolic energy carriers during the long period of parenteral alimentation (Gerstenbrand and Galanti, 1972). Even loss of weight is hazardous during peroneal paralysis (Sprofkin, 1958).

Table 1. Localization of the secondary peripheral nerve lesions in 27 patients with apallic syndrome

Nerve	Left	Right	Bilateral	Isolated
Peroneus	14	10	5	5
Ulnaris	9	8	2	1
Tibialis	5	6	2	–
Medianus	4	3	1	–
Ischiadicus	5	1	1	4
Radialis	3	1	–	2

As a result of rehabilitative measures, a good prognosis can usually be given. In 21 of our 27 cases complete restitution or at least a significant improvement was observed. In six cases the lesion stayed unchanged. Two patients died and could not be reviewed. Prevention and treatment of secondary peripheral nerve lesions are of equal importance. First of all, the patients' bedding needs continuous attention by the nursing staff. Repeated and rhythmic changes of position, special stuffing and mattress covers, physical therapy with passive movements of the limbs, and use of tonus regulating reflex therapy are other recommended measures.

A high caloric and balanced diet is also required. Immediately after identification of the peripheral nerve lesion, high doses of vitamin B and electric stimulation should be administered. Sometimes it is necessary to operate and remove periarticular ossifications (Gerstenbrand et al., 1970a) or other compressive pathologic structures (Mumenthaler and Schliack, 1965; Wilhelm, 1970).

Examinations, Etiology

Muscular atrophy and lesions affecting peripheral nerves as a consequence of extended comas are well-known phenomena. However, the type of damage to the nervous and muscular structures involved and its etiology have not yet been adequately explained. In order to continue our initial study (Gerstenbrand et al., 1971), additional electrophysiologic and neuropathologic tests have been carried out.

A. Results of Electrophysiologic Examinations

Electromyography was performed on a total of 27 clinically inconspicuous muscles of nine patients suffering from an apallic syndrome of traumatic origin. The muscles involved were: the m. tibialis anterior, the m. biceps brachii, the m. triceps brachii, or the m. deltoides. The electromyogram using unipolar coaxial needle electrodes revealed fibrillation potentials and monophasic positive potentials in a patchlike distribution pattern on the m. tibialis anterior (patient 3 in Table 2) and on the m. biceps brachii (patient 2 in Table 2).

The average duration of the potentials of motor units in these two patients remained in the normal range. Maximum voluntary intention always resulted in full interference pattern. In another two patients (patients 8 and 9 in Table 2), the electromyogram showed potentials of short duration, low amplitude, and polyphasic form indicating a myogenic lesion. In patients 1 and 7 (Table 2) doublets and triplets were observed on the m. triceps brachii and the m. biceps brachii; these manifestations were nonspecific signs of a metabolic disorder (Steinbrecher, 1962), even though the electrolyte values in the serum remained normal.

Table 2. Maximum motor NCV in m/sec

Case no.	age	Ulnaris n=50		Medianus n=50		Tibialis n=44		Pernoneus n=47		Ulnaris sensory NCV n=60	
		left	right	left	right	left	right	left	right	left	right
1 S.H.	30		*32 a*			*n.c.*	*41*	*n.c.*	*49 a*		
2 Z.S.	31		*45 a*	65	*69 a*	*n.c.*		*n.c.*			
3 X.E.	11		75						*49*		87
4 H.A.	39	69		64		46		52		73	
5 B.E.	30		73		58		*45 a*				
6 C.P.	40	*55 a*									
7 B.F.	32		62				52		51	65	
8 W.J.	36			61				56			
9 S.J.	27	52		60		44		47	53	62	
10 D.M.	58					46	44	*n.c.*	*n.c.*		

NCV = Nerve conduction velocity; a = split potential; n.c. = non-conductive; n = patient's lower limit of the normal range (Method: Hodes et al., 1948).
Italics refer to the NCV of nerves with clinical symptoms.

Using the method of Hodes et al. (1948), maximum motor nerve conduction velocities (NCV) were recorded for 13 paretic and 30 clinically normal nerves. At the time the NCV was recorded, serum electrolyte values were normal in all instances. In three cases pathologic values were recorded for the paretic nerves, i.e., twice for the ulnar nerve (32 ms and 45 ms, lower limit of the normal range: 48 ms) and once for the tibial nerve (41 ms, lower limit of the normal range: 44 ms). In four cases the potentials were split and a normal maximum motor NCV was registered. The splitting of the potentials was interpreted as a lesion affecting those fibers not conducting maximally. Because of the nonexcitability of six nerves their NCV could not be measured. This was the case in two patients (patients 1 and 2 in Table 2) where both the tibial and the peroneal nerves were affected on the same side; thus a lesion above the bifurcation of the sciatic nerve had to be assumed. The other case involved a patient (patient 10 in Table 2) with an isolated bilateral paresis–clinically manifest–of the peroneal nerve. In the clinically inconspicuous nerves the nerve conduction remained within the normal range and showed a normal form of evoked muscle potentials. In four patients (patients 3, 4, 7 and 9, Table 2) the sensory NCV of the ulnar nerve was measured using the method of Buchthal (1966) (Buchthal and Rosenfalck, 1966); the values recorded were within the normal range (patients' normal range: 60-90 ms).

The most interesting phenomenon observed during the electrophysiologic examination is the electromyographic evidence of fibrillations, doublets, triplets and of motor unit potentials of short duration, low amplitude and of poliphase form in some clinically inconspicuous muscles, with the maximum motor NCV remaining within the normal range. Considering the results of the biopsy, this appears to indicate a neurogenic subclinical disorder.

No conclusions about the etiology of peripheral lesions may be drawn on the basis of our electrophysiologic examinations. Some references are made in the literature to the impact on the NCV of various individual factors which may cause peripheral lesions within the apallic syndrome. The views about the effect of electrolyte shifts on the motor NCV differ. Simpson (1958) pointed out that physiologic electrolyte shifts do not result in any changes in the motor NCV. Chaumont et al. (1964) expressed a diametrically opposed opinion. Mattson and Lecoq (1968) determined motor NCV in 25 patients who had been fasting for 14-28 days. The NCV values recorded before and after fasting did not result in any significant differences. Only in two instances, the distal latency period of the peroneal nerve was slightly extended. However, Mattson's study does not preclude the possibility that nutritional deficiencies or a catabolic metabolism—as it is found in patients with an apallic syndrome—might produce a lower NCV after a period of several months. The publication of Simpson (1958) was the only one available on the subject of the effect of insufficient oxygen saturation on NCV. Simpson states that a patient with an arterial oxygen saturation of 85% was found to have a NCV of 39.3 ms in the ulnar nerve. The last and probably still the most important causative factor is external pressure. Bentley and Schlapp pointed out in 1943 that the most prominent effect of pressure is most likely hypoxia.

Animal experiments as well as clinical studies were carried out on the NCV during pressure paralysis. It was determined that a distinct drop in NCV or even a complete loss of conductivity may occur (Gilliatt and Thomas, 1960; Meyer and Denny-Brown, 1964). A study of the literature shows that a distinct reduction of maximum motor NCV or a loss of conductivity of a nerve during the apallic syndrome may be ascribed to external pressure and concomitant local hypoxia. The formation of these lesions may be encouraged if the external pressure is exerted on nerves previously damaged due to metabolic disorders.

B. Nerve and Muscle Biopsies

These were performed in a total of seven cases for which the clinical data is depicted in Table 3. The nerve biopsies were all taken from cutaneous branches of the sensory sural nerve. In three instances the muscle biopsies were taken from the proximal m. quadriceps femoris and in four cases from the distal m. peroneus brevis. The tissues were prepared for light microscopy; parts of three nerves were also arranged for examination by electron microscopy.

1. Nerve Biopsies: In all seven cases pathologic changes in the nature of degeneration of individual fibers were observed. These changes involved myelinated fibers mostly of large diameter. The pathologic changes were always widely distributed (Figs. 1, 2).

The number of nerve fibers affected differed. In two cases only a few, in four instances (Fig. 1) several, and in one instance numerous fibers were involved. Whenever there were nerves with considerable fiber lesions, different fascia were affected to different degrees.

Table 3. Nerve and muscle biopsies

Case no.	Age	Clinical data		Biopsy performed after trauma	Nerve biopsy	Muscle biopsy
		Apallic syndrome	Peripheral nerve lesion			
1 H.A.	39	Full stage 2 months remission stage 3 months defect stage severe	Not differentiable	6 months	Some disseminated degeneration of individual large medullated fibers, late stage of degeneration,regeneration	Proximal muscle: diffuse slight atrophy, some inflammatory infiltrates
2 D.R.	16	Full stage	Not differentiable	3 months	Isolated disseminated degeneration of individual medullated fibers, recent degenerative process	Distal muscle: neurogenic disseminated atrophy, slight diffuse atrophy
3 X.E.	11	Full stage 9 months remission stage	Doubtful lesion of n. peroneus right, n. ulnaris	4 months	Isolated disseminated degeneration of individual fibers, late phase of degeneration, small cicatrization	Distal muscle: neurogenic disseminated atrophy and slight diffuse atrophy
4 A.B.	11	Full stage	Doubtful lesion of the n. ischiadicus and ulnaris bilateral	12 months	Numerous degenerative medullated fibers, current degenerative process fascia affected to different degrees	Proximal muscle: moderate diffuse atrophy
5 Z.S.	31	Full stage 8 months remission stage severe	n.peroneus and and tibialis left n. ulnaris and med.right	13 months	Much disseminated degeneration of large medullated fibers, recent degeneration	Distal muscle: neurogenic grouped atrophy and moderate diffuse atrophy
6 H.G.	17	Full stage 2 months remission stage	n. peroneus bilateral	8 months	Some disseminated degeneration of large medullated fibers, recent processes next to older ones	Proximal muscle: slight diffuse atrophy and some inflammatory infiltrates
7 D.M.	58	Full stage 3 months remission stage	n. peroneus bilateral	5 months	Some disseminated degeneration of large medullated fibers, recent degeneration	Distal muscle: neurogenic grouped atrophy and slight diffuse atrophy

Fig. 1. Nerve biopsy. Several degenerations of individual large diameter myelinated fibers, recent *(a)* next to older *(b)* signs of degeneration. SBB x 40. (Case No. 1)

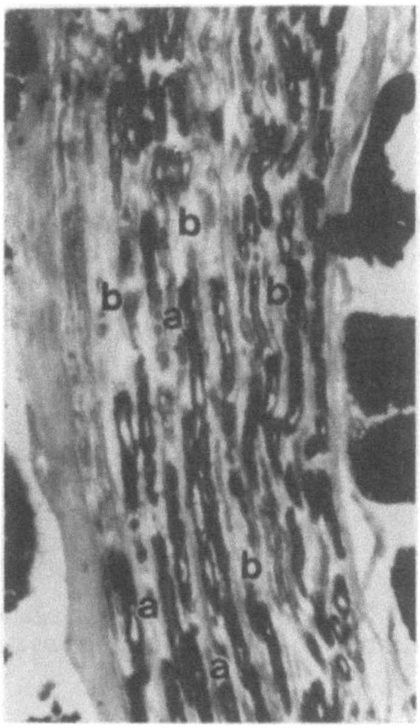

The degenerative changes of the individual nerve fibers were of a uniform nature but differed as to the stage reached. Thus, in five nerves recent fiber degeneration (Fig. 2-3) was observed. In one case the recent changes had occurred in addition to already completed processes; two nerves (one with only a few, one with several fiber lesions) revealed late stages of degeneration.

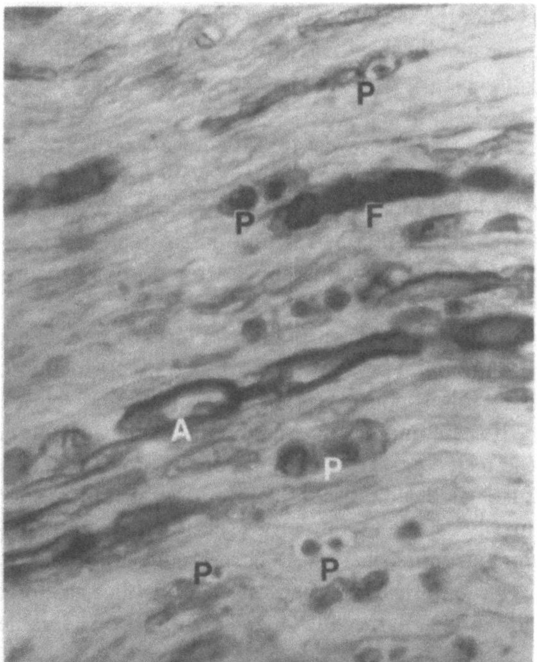

Fig. 2. Nerve biopsy, fascia section. Recent degenerations (axonal type) of myelinated fibers. Swelling *(A)* and fragmentation *(F)* of axon and myelin sheaths. Degeneration products of various sizes *(P)*. SBB x 40. (Case No. 4)

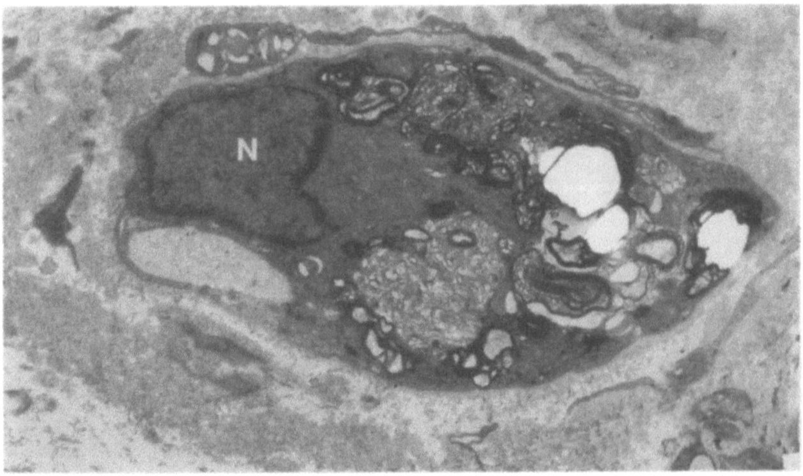

Fig. 3. Nerve biopsy, section. Degeneration of individual fiber with axon and myelin sheath disintegration. *N* = nucleus of Schwann's cell. EM magnification: x 6000. (Case No. 7)

The type of fiber degeneration was determined under the optical microscope according to swelling and fragmentation of the axon and of the myelin sheath (Fig. 2) as well as from the occurrence of fragmentation and degeneration products such as the accumulations of myelin material of varying sizes (Fig. 2). The later stages of degeneration are accompanied by a growth of the endoneurium. Depending on the extent of the nerve fiber degeneration, small cicatrical areas without fibers remained. No vascular changes were observed.

Under the electron microscope, three of the nerves disclosed disintegration of the axon and the myelin sheath structures of the nerve fibers. No selective demyelination was observed. One nerve in a late stage of the process revealed Büngner bands, indicating regeneration.

These findings reveal that the degeneration of individual fibers conforms to those from axonal lesions with a subsequent Wallerian syndrome. These studies of nerve biopsies have revealed that in all investigated cases of an apallic syndrome, peripheral nerve damage was involved. These lesions correspond to an axonal neuropathy of the myelinated fiber lesion type and are accompanied by scattered involvement of the fibers that may be slight to severe in degree.

2. Muscle Biopsies: In all cases investigated, changes were found to have taken place. In the proximal part of the muscles only slight to moderately diffuse narrowing of the fibers without considerable changes in the nuclei or the fiber diameters had occurred. In two of these muscles scattered perivascular inflammatory infiltrates were found. However, in the tested parts of the m. peroneus brevis other changes were noticed in addition to the diffuse narrowed muscle fibers. In two instances there were differences in the diameter, primarily caused by numerous scattered atrophic muscle fibers. Upon closer examination, several atrophic fibers were occasionally found next to each other.

Two biopsies, however, revealed distinct groups of atrophic muscle fibers in addition to the diffuse narrowing (Fig. 4), with a considerable increase in the number of nuclei and

Fig. 4. Muscle biopsy. Neurogenic atrophy with atrophic groups of fibers. HE x 40. (Case No. 5)

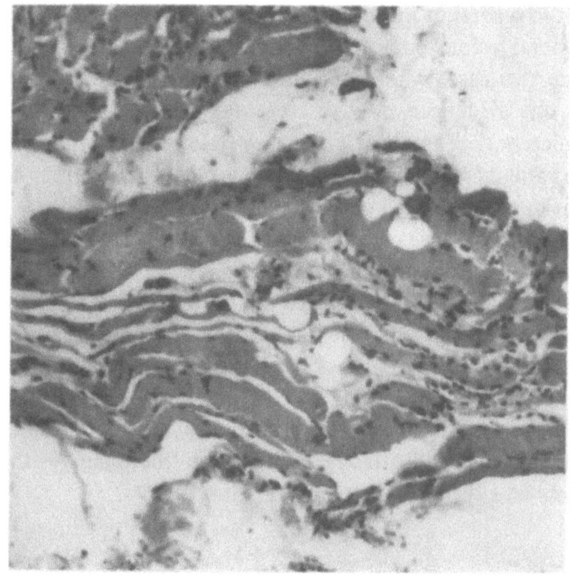

frequently with noticeable narrowing of the fibers, as well as with an occasional loss in striation. Undoubtedly, the grouping of atrophied muscle fibers corresponds to an equivalent neurogenic pattern. However, the diffuse slight narrowing of muscle fibers and considerable irregularity in their diameters were changes which at first sight signified a myopathic syndrome; only after the group patterns had been discerned was a neurogenic atrophy considered.

Taken by itself, the tissue syndrome with diffuse narrowing of the muscle fibers conforms to a bland, moderate, diffuse muscular atrophy similar to that occurring in the wake of inactivity, malnutrition or cachexia. Our studies of muscle biopsies thus demonstrate that in patients with an apallic syndrome we find a *general, moderate* loss of muscle tissue parenchyma, associated in certain regions with signs of neurogenic atrophy. In our patients these regions were found in the distal parts of the muscles investigated. The neurogenic signs may be slight to moderately severe in degree and start with a pseudomyopathic syndrome of disseminated fiber atrophies, followed later by a change to a typical, disseminated, focal fiber group atrophy.

If we take the results of the nerve and muscle biopsies together, the disseminated complete degeneration of individual fibers and the varying degrees of degeneration of the peripheral nerves explain the neurogenic lesion and the differing degree to which it is reflected in the musculature. Agreement between the extent of the nerve lesion and that of the neurogenic muscular atrophy, however, was not always present in our own investigation (viz. Table 2). This might be due to the type of nerve investigated which is sensory in nature. The possibly different effect of sensory and motor nerves could be subject to discussion. The predominant effect exerted on the distal muscles would agree with the primarily distal distribution of neuropathic processes.

In correlating the results of the nerve and muscle biopsies with the clinical data, we find that all cases with clinically manifest peripheral lesions disclose complete fiber degneration either in several or in numerous instances. Among the cases with doubtful diagnosis of peripheral lesions one revealed severe neural damage and one only discrete involvement. Of the two cases where peripheral lesions were inconspicuous from the clinical point of view, one evidenced only discrete damage. In the other, only a few nerve fibers were completely degenerated. These correlations show that the nerves of clinically inconspicuous patients also demonstrate changes and that rather numerous nerve fiber lesions are found in patients with clinical symptoms.

Even though we cannot reduce from the case material a direct linear relationship between the number of nerve fibers affected and the manifestation of clinical symptoms (as might be expected), the impression persists that discrete nerve fiber lesions result in no clinical manifestations whereas peripheral clinical manifestations always result from a more extensive range of lesions. Thus in axonal neuropathy within the apallic syndrome we have to differentiate between clinically latent and clinically evident processes.

The correlation between duration, severity, and remission of the apallic syndrome are shown in Table 3. Both cases with nerve fiber changes that had already run their course were in an advanced stage of remission.

Discussion

Do the changes in the neuromuscular structures analyzed indicate etiologic factors? The type of neural damage shown does not provide any specific pathogenetic indications. Many causes are known for axonal myelinated fiber lesions of the wallerian type, but the distribution of damage revealed in our study precludes occlusion of the vessel supplying the nerve, a cause which seldom plays a part in peripheral nerve damage. Deficient blood supply with a particular impact on large myelinated nerve fibers may also be a cause; however, in its initial phases hypoxia—according to the degree of its severity—causes demyelination and only with increasing severity do we observe axonal lesions (Chopra and Hurwitz, 1967; Eames and Lange, 1967). In the cases investigated demyelination never occurred; even though the individual nerves revealed only very discrete damage, this factor cannot be termed a primary cause.

Pressure lesions are also frequently discussed and this phenomenon is not precluded by the pattern of damage evidenced. Thomas and Fullerton (1963) described myelinated fiber changes with diameter reduction, particularly of the large diameter regions which are caused by pressure lesions of the carpal tunnel syndrome. However, in pressure lesions in which both mechanical and ischemic factors are involved, demyelination occurs (Steinbrecher, 1962) in many instances. This was proved experimentally with tourniquet tests (Dyck, 1969).

These considerations make pressure lesions an unlikely cause of the observed discrete symptoms of neuropathy which disclose only axonal lesions and are always scattered. On the other hand, such pressure lesions may be an accidental factor in those syndromes which demonstrate numerous complete disintegrations of myelinated fibers in a rather diffuse distribution. No evidence exists for electrolyte changes being involved in the formation of axonal nerve fiber lesions.

There still remains the problem of the catabolic metabolism within the apallic syndrome which may possibly affect the large myelinated fibers since the latter are very sensitive to metabolic factors. We know from the analysis of polyneuropathies that axonal neuropathies of the myelinated fiber lesion type are frequently encountered in deficiency neuropathy or in complex metabolic disorders (Erbslöh and Abel, 1970; Sluga, 1974).

Therefore we would like to discuss the assumption that as a consequence of protracted coma with its general changes, particularly in catabolic metabolism a secondary neuropathic process develops. This process has a slight to moderate effect on the large myelinated fibers and remains on the subclinical level. Accidental factors may superimpose a marked neuropathic syndrome on this slight or moderate neural damage that apparently occurs in many and possibly in all cases, and leads finally to clinical deficiencies. Among these additional factors, pressure lesions might take first place.

Mertens (1961) described a neuropathic process in protracted coma as a disseminated neuropathy with CO intoxication; he also pointed out latent or subclinical changes and observed patch-shaped medullary failures and serous exudations. These changes do not occur in the neuropathic process of the apallic syndrome. The muscular changes are, on one hand, the direct consequence of the neurogenic lesions and, on the other, correspond to a nonspecific diffuse atrophic process of moderate severity. Diffuse, bland muscular atrophy has been described as the response pattern to inanition, malnutrition, old age, cachexia, inactivity, or consumptive diseases (Adams et al., 1962). It is likely that in the apallic syndrome it is also linked to inactivity or to reduced alimentation.

In a comprehensive study of changes due to old age or cachexia, Tomlinson et al. (1969) have described the particular features of the various stages of neurogenic atrophy in diffusely atrophic muscular tissue. Such changes were also observed by these authors in some cases of cranial traumata or cerebral disorders. The correlation with cachexia in the incidence of combined diffuse and circumscribed changes should be emphasized.

Conclusions

In patients suffering from an apallic syndrome we encounter secondary peripheral nerve failures which are particularly troublesome in rehabilitation and may complicate and prolong therapy. Electrophysiologic and bioptic tissue examinations resulted in the following findings about the course and type of peripheral nerve and muscle changes within apallic syndromes of traumatic origin:

1. Neural changes occurred even in patients without clinical symptoms and revealed patch-shaped signs of denervation whereas normal motor maximum nerve conduction velocities were maintained. At the same time, a few degenerative processes occurred in individual myelinated nerve fibers together with disseminated neurogenic muscular atrophy.

2. In doubtful or clinically manifest peripheral failures, the number of degenerating myelinated fibers increased and the neurogenic muscular atrophy occurred in distinct groups. In definite clinical symptoms the maximum motor NCV was reduced or the potentials were split while the maximum motor NCV was maintained (unless a complete loss of conductivity had set in).

3. The degeneration of individual fibers is caused by axonal lesions; the *type* of peripheral neural changes always corresponded to axonal neuropathy of the myelinated fiber type, a change that also corresponds to the extent to which the NCV is reduced. The type of muscular changes agreed with that of denervation atrophy and moderate nonspecific diffuse atrophy. The latter is known to be the consequence of inactivity, deficient nutrition, or cachexia.

4. According to the course, the type, and the distribution of the neural and muscular changes described, pathogenetic factors were discussed. For the discrete lesions, metabolic factors were assumed to be responsible whereas for the more severe neural changes the additon of accidental factors, particularly pressure lesions, were considered.

Summary

Based on these findings and the clinical experience, it may be stated that patients suffering from an apallic syndrome reveal changes in their peripheral nerves and the corresponding muscles. These changes may remain subclinical or lead to clinical manifestations, i.e., functional failure of peripheral nerves. Whereas the subclinical processes appear to be related to the general consequences of prolonged coma–perhaps with metabolic factors involved–additional damage is assumed to be responsible for the changes leading to clinical manifestations. External compression is assumed to be the predominant additional cause.

35. Social Problems of the Apallic Syndrome

U.H. PETERS

The systematic collection of experiences with the apallic syndrome is still relatively recent. But there are already visible outlines of the social problems. In my experience the problems differ greatly depending on the severity of the case, less severe cases occurring where remission is possible. More severe cases will have to remain institutionalized for ever or else receive constant care when released to their families due to their inability to develop any self-activity.

Children and adolescents make up the majority of less severe cases. Rehabilitation can quite often proceed so far that residual intellectual consequences are hardly noticeable. These patients usually have a family to care for them, but their position in the family is changed. Since most apallic syndromes are caused by accidents the parents may develop guilt feelings because they often think that the accident was their fault. This situation can have advantages as well as disadvantages for the child.

In one of my cases an accident occurred when a mother had left her 9-year-old child alone for a short time. When her child was released from the hospital a few months after the accident, the mother gave up her teaching profession and devoted all her time to her son. A program of rehabilitation was arranged to exercise all day long what faculties the child had retained. Calisthenics, swimming, instruction, dancing, and singing alternated constantly. The mother succeeded in getting her child accepted in a high school in spite of an I.Q. that had been lowered to 89 by somatopsychic disturbances and low spontaneous impulses.

Thus the child obtained the highest level of training to a large extent because of the mother's guilt feelings. Because of the concentrated rehabilitation activities, the mother neglected her other children who became extremely jealous of the "apallic" child. The child depended more and more upon the mother who was his only connection with the social environment. He could not stand up to the other children in school without his mother's help. Finally difficulties in the marriage developed when the father felt neglected.

A certain number of rehabilitation centers are available for children. However, more consideration should be given to the particular patterns of children's disturbances. Adults, young or old, on the other hand, are often rudely exposed to the forces of "open" society. The most advantageous position they can assume is at the social periphery. This position does, however, provide them with a satisfying life provided they resign themselves to their loss of status in society.

The problems created by patients with severe and very severe defects are considerably more difficult. After a long time (possibly 1-3 years) of intensive and expensive effort in an intensive care ward or in a therapeutic institution, a decision about the future of the patient will have to be made since it is obvious that the treatment will not result in any further improvement. But everyone working in this field knows that a transfer to one of the large psychiatric hospitals or a release to the family may result in the death of such patients after 1-3 weeks. The treatment team thus experiences disappointment and depression, realizing that the years of intensive effort and personal involvement were in vain.

In more favorable cases, the life of the patient is preserved but many of the relearned abilities are lost again since they cannot be stimulated sufficiently.

There has been only one prominent patient with an apallic syndrome: the Russian physicist Lew Landau. On the way to his institute in Moscow he was involved in an accident which was reported at great length in the newspapers. Clinical death occurred 4 times, but Khrushchev is supposed to have said, "This man must not die." His life was therefore preserved by uninterrupted reanimation measures. During a later phase Landau was awarded the Nobel Prize–but for work he had done prior to the accident. The brain damage had made the restoration of his intellectual productivity, even to a very modest extent, impossible.

The question has to be raised as to the extent of the problem caused by the apallic syndrome, both in medicine and in society. We can see from older case material on various subjects, even in often merely anecdotal descriptions, that apallic syndrome–which can now be recognized easily due to present knowledge–was being described. We can assume from this fact that such cases have been observed from time to time at least since the turn of the century. But they probably also occurred before that time. It is the modern reanimation departments, however, which have brought about an increase in the number of these cases. This is also where we find the most intensively felt reactions to the phenomenon of the apallic syndrome. The reactions range from gentle, scientific interest to unveiled hostility. The expression that the apallic syndrome is a *danaum fatale mumus* of modern medicine is often heard. In this metaphor modern science is represented by the Greeks who fill a beautiful horse with beneficial cargo. The besieged Trojans threatened by disaster stand for modern society which fears great damage from this gift. Hostile reactions are felt most strongly in the intensive care wards, where unfavorable cases die either early or after long and intensive effort while favorable cases are soon transferred to other institutions.

In order to obtain a general view of the magnitude of the problem, we must ask how many patients have already been accommodated in such institutions on a permanent basis. Gerstenbrand mentioned that he knew personally about 300 patients with an apallic syndrome. The author has examined about 50 such patients. By sending a questionnaire to all institutions suitable for the accommodation of apallic patients during the remission phase, we have tried to conduct a general survey to obtain information on the extent of the problem today. Only 40% of the questionnaires were returned–many with the remark that no such patients were in the institution. Some questionnaires contained descriptions of patients whose illnesses were obviously not apallic syndromes. An evaluation in terms of figures is therefore not possible. Personal inquiries made it clear that the apallic syndrome and its remission phase in particular are not sufficiently understood in these institutions. Again and again the author has come across case histories that were easily recognizable as apallic syndromes, but which were placed in other diagnostic categories. During our efforts to investigate the social problems by following up individual cases, we came to realize that many different medical disciplines claim authority. The interdisciplinary character of apallic syndrome often results in cases ending up between disciplines and being passed on from one institution to the other. This work is an attempt to contribute to improving the social problems by explaining the apallic syndrome.

36. A Rating Sheet to Monitor Apallic Syndrome Patients

F. GERSTENBRAND, F. LACKNER, and C.H. LÜCKING

Following emergency therapy of cases with severe brain injury, subsequent neurologic monitoring is most important. The prime goal is to reveal early the symptoms of life-threatening severe brain stem lesions which appear as sequelae of intracranial hematoma or diffuse cerebral edema. It is also important to recognize the development of an apallic symptomatology as well as to monitor its further course, particularly the onset of remission.

Intracranial hematoma as well as diffused brain edema cause mass displacement because of supratentorial increased volume and mass movement followed by tentorial and foraminal herniation with incarceration of midbrain and bulbar brain. Patients with traumatic primary brain stem lesions seldom survive. Usually death occurs at the site of the accident (Peters, 1966; Jellinger, 1966; etc.).

Early recognition of midbrain herniation is important because it is an early sign of supratentorial increased pressure. Continuous monitoring is vital (1) because it is undetermined how the symptoms will arise, (2) because upcoming complications can be recognized in time, and (3) signs of remission will be discovered. Thus, a rating of clinical symptoms is a precondition for the revelation and further course of secondary brain stem damage. This proposition is also applicable to other cerebral pathologic processes such as hypoxic brain damage, brain abscesses, or brain tumors which are accompanied by brain edema, mass movement, incarceration, and release midbrain and/or apallic syndrome.

Since in many intensive care units only non-neurologist surgeons or anesthesiologists are normally present, it will only be possible for them to check and register the decisive clinical criteria of a nascent cerebral complication developing toward an apallic syndrome. The proposed rating sheet is designed to help the on-call doctor of an ICU in doing so.

Based on experience with a large number of patients, criteria of secondary brain stem lesion and of apallic syndrome of other origin can be easily determined and predicted. There is an acute phase as well as a chronic course leading to apallic symptomatology. The following is an example of how to use this rating sheet, outlining the course of one case of brain injury in which a midbrain syndrome occurred followed by an apallic syndrome (Table 1):

An 18-year-old male was admitted to the emergency room of the Surgical Clinic after he had fallen off his motorbike. Results of clinical investigation: unconscious when brought to the hospital, divergent position of eyeballs, narrow equal pupillas, reaction to light diminished. Flexion stretch position of extremities, synergistic flexion stretch cramps to pain stimulation, increased tendon reflexes, positive Babinski sign, increased respiratory rate. Shock stage, fracture of base of skull, angiography of carotid artery N.A.D. – 20 h after accident comatose, stretch synergisms of all extremities, pupillas enlarged, divergent eyeballs, fast respiratory rate (machinelike), increased blood pressure. Two days after trauma increasing stretch synergisms of both extremities and trunk, cramps requiring sedation and controlled ventilation. After 3 days transient spontaneous breathing, but again strong cramps. On the 6th day artificial ventilation again terminated, incipient symptoms of transition stage to traumatic apallic syndrome (stretch synergism diminished, chewing automatisms, snout reflex, respiratory rate increased, etc.). Pulse rate, temperature, and blood pressure increased.

Table 1. Sample neurologic rating sheet with typical brain injury case

Patient's name A.L.	age 18 years							I.C.U.		B 200
Time of accident	8/21/68		4.20 p.m.							
Time of check										
Month	VIII			IX				X	II	
Day	21		26	1	4	9	25	5	3	16
Hour	17	20	18	9	9	9	16	9	10	9
Day of hospitalization	1		6	12	15	20	36	46	159	172
I State of consciousness										
A Diminution of vigilance	3	4	4	3	3	3	4	3	3	0
B Special type of disturbance of vigilance	0	0	0	4	3	2	0	2	1	0
II State of reaction										
A Reaction to environment	5	5	5	5	5	5	5	5	5	4
B Reaction to pain stimuli	3	4	4	3	2	2	4	2	2	2
III Optomotoric signs										
A Size of pupilla	2	3	1	0	0	3	1	3	0	0
B Reaction to light	2	3	1	1	1	1	2	1	1	1
C Cilio spinal reflex	2	3	2	1	1	0	1	1	0	0
D Corneal reflex	0	0	0	0	0	0	0	0	0	0
E Position of eyeballs	1	2	1	1	1	1	2	2	1	1
F Deviation of eyeballs	0	0	0	0	0	0	0	0	0	0
G Movement of eyeballs	4	4	3	2	1	1	4	1	1	1
H Oculocephalic reflex	2	3	2	1	1	1	1	1	0	0
IV Chewing and pharyngeal muscles										
A Chewing muscles	1	2	2	2	2	2	2	2	2	1
B Pharyngeal muscles	1	1	1	1	1	1	1	1	1	2
V Motor functions of trunk and extremities										
A Posture	2	5	4	2	2	2	5	2	2	2
B Spontaneous synergisms	3	5	0	0	0	0	5	0	0	0
C Tonus	2	3	2	2	2	2	3	2	2	2
D Tendon reflexes	2	2	2	2	2	2	3	2	2	1
E Pyramid signs	2	2	2	2	2	2	2	2	2	1
VI Autonomous functions										
A Respiration	1	2	1	1	0	0	2	1	0	0
B Temperature	1	2	1	1	1	1	2	0	1	1
C Pulse rate	1	2	1	1	1	1	2	1	0	0
D Blood pressure	1	2	2	2	0	2	2	0	0	0
E Signs of shock	1	0	0	0	0	0	0	0	0	0
VII Primitive pattern										
A Chewing automatism	0	0	2	3	3	3	0	3	2	1
B Snout reflex	0	0	1	2	2	2	0	2	1	1
C Oral fixation mechanism	0	0	0	2	2	2	0	2	1	1
D Chin reflexes	0	0	0	1	2	3	0	2	3	2
E Grasp reflex	0	0	0	3	3	2	0	3	2	2
F Grasp toward something	0	0	0	0	0	0	0	0	0	2
G Postural reflexes	0	0	0	1	2	1	0	1	1	0
H Fixed postural pattern	0	0	0	0	1	1	0	1	1	1
VIII Affection and emotion										
A Affective emotional reaction	3	3	3	3	3	3	3	3	2	2
B Type of affective, emotional disturbance	0	0	0	0	0	0	0	0	5	4
IX Cerebral symptomatology										
A Unilateral	0	0	0	0	11	11	0	11	21	21

On 8th day parasomnic phase. On the 12th day symptoms comparable to akinetic mutism with temporary opening of the eyes, flexion of other extremities, escape reflex of legs, intensified motoric primitive pattern, autonomic functions disinhibit symptoms. Slight signs of left-side hemiparesis. On the 19th day full state of traumatic apallic syndrome with coma vigile, sleep-wake regulation timed by exhaustion, flexion stretch position of all extremities, extensive primitive patterns, posture reflexes, autonomous functions unstable. On the 36th day pneumonia; hours later, again coma. In addition, the remaining symptoms of full state of acute midbrain syndrome with spontaneous stretch synergisms, primitive pattern ceased, again controlled ventilation. Two days later symptoms of transition stage to traumatic apallic syndrome. On the 46th day again the full state of traumatic apallic syndrome. Within the following 4 months, repeated occurrences of pneumonia with subsequent full state of acute midbrain syndrome recurring to full state of traumatic apallic syndrome within several days. After 159 days onset of state of remission, decreasing coma vigile, and day-night sleep-wake regulation, primitive emotional reactions. On the 172nd day optic fixation and following, grasping toward objects decreased, but directed defending movements. After short-lasting regression to full state of traumatic apallic syndrome along with fever and septic condition caused by piodermia fast remission and stabilization. Further remission within the next few months passing through Klüver-Bucy and Korsakoff phases terminating in severe defect stage with brain stem and cerebral symptoms.

The sheet contains nine categories and subgroups. The first six categories deal mainly with acute midbrain complications of cerebral trauma and its remission. The next three categories include the transition stage to chronic brain stem lesion and hemispheric components. The extent of damage within the single categories is expressed by increasing numbers on the score. The increasing or decreasing numbers relate to progressing brain stem lesion or remission respectively. Within some categories, however, we could not stick to the principle of increasing numbers for increasingly grave symptoms. To avoid further diversion but to monitor important data and symptoms, the subgroups for position of eyeballs, swallowing, respiration, and fixed postural pattern–less grave symptoms–had to be given higher numbers.

Within the main symptoms the disposition of the development is not impeded on the sheet. The clinical deterioration within the first six categories can be ascribed to increasing numbers whereas in the additional three categories all scores except for subgroups "affective, emotional" remain zero.

The deterioration of severe clinical symptoms depending on induced sedation appears in increasing scores and has to be marked *M*; *r* for right, *l* for left, *a* for above, and *b* for below should be indicated to reveal the exact location of the symptom.

Summary: A neurologic rating sheet is proposed, which should help particularly non-neurologists to monitor neurologic features and thus reveal upcoming complications in time as well as to discover signs of remission. The sheet is described and outlined along with a typical case of brain injury. However, this monitoring can also be used for midbrain lesion of various etiologies such as hypoxia or edema.

Classification of Symptoms for Neurologic Rating Sheet

I. State of consciousness
A Diminuation of vigilance
0 None, or passed
1 Benumbed
2 Somnolent
3 Soporous
4 Coma

B Special type of disturbance of vigilance
0 None, or passed
1 Coma vigile, sleep-wake regulation timed day-night
2 Coma vigile, sleep-wake regulation timed by exhaustion
3 Short lasting opening of eyes
4 Parasomnic state

II. State of reaction
A Reaction toward environment
0 Normal
1 Talking
2 Obeying to simple commands
3 Turning towards
4 Optic following
5 Missing

B Reaction to painful stimuli
0 Normal
1 Retarded directed defending movement
2 Diminished undirected defending movement
3 Flex-stretch synergism
4 Stretch synergism, all extremities
5 Stretch synergism diminished
6 Missing

III. Optomotoric signs
A Size of pupilla
0 Normal
1 Reduced
2 Narrow
3 Wide (above average)
4 Wide
5 Maximal wide

B Reaction to light
0 Normal
1 Retarded
2 Sluggish
3 Little
4 Missing

C Ciliospinal reflex
0 Normal, not to be released
1 Little
2 Distinctly
3 Diminished
4 Missing

D Corneal reflex
0 Normal
1 Diminished
2 Missing

E Position of eyeballs
0 Normal
1 Slightly divergent
2 Distinctly divergent
3 Convergent

F Deviation of eyeballs
0 None
1 Tendency to deviation
2 Constant deviation
3 Deviation of eyeballs and head
4 Skew deviation

G Movement of eyeballs
0 Normal
1 Saccadic
2 Oscillating
3 Dysconjugated
4 Missing (eyeballs fixed)

H Oculocephalic reflex
0 Normal (not to be released)
1 Can be released weakly
2 Can be released distinctly
3 Diminished
4 Missing (eyeballs fixed)

IV. Chewing and Pharyngeal muscles
A Chewing muscles
0 Normal masseter reflex and tonus
1 Increased masseter reflex and tonus
2 Passing of increased masseter reflex and tonus
3 Missing masseter reflex and tonus

B Pharyngeal muscles
0 Undisturbed swallowing
1 Not checkable
2 Disturbed swallowing

V. Motor functions of trunk and extremities
A Posture
0 Normal
1 Stretching of lower extremities
2 Flexion of upper, stretching of lower extremities
3 Unilateral flexion with contralateral stretching
4 Stretching of all extremities
5 Stretching of extremities and trunk
6 Diminished stretching
7 Incipient atonic posture
8 Atonic posture

B Spontaneous synergisms
0 None
1 Stereotype trundling and rolling movements
2 Stretching of legs
3 Flexion stretch synergisms
4 Stretch synergisms of all extremities
5 Stretch synergisms of all extremities and trunk
6 Stretch synergisms passing
7 Stretch synergisms passed

C Tonus
0 Normal
1 Increased lower extremities
2 Increased on upper and lower extremities
3 Tonus decreased
4 Atonic

D Tendon-reflexes
0 Normal
1 Increased
2 Markedly increased
3 Diminished
4 Missing

E Pyramid signs
0 None
1 Can be released little
2 Distinctly

3 Diminished
4 Cannot be released

VI. Autonomous functions
A Respiration
0 Normal
1 Increased rate
2 Machinelike
3 Assisted respiration
4 Gasping
5 No spontaneous respiration

B Temperature
0 Normal
1 Raised
2 Hyperthermia
3 Hyperthermia decreasing
4 Spontaneous hypothermia

C Pulse rate
0 Normal
1 Increased
2 Tachycardia
3 Tachycardia decreasing
4 Spontaneous bradycardia

D Blood pressure
0 Normal
1 Lower
2 Raised
3 Hypertensive
4 Passing hypertension
5 Fall in blood pressure

E Signs of shock
0 None
1 Slight
2 Mean
3 Grave

VII. Primitive patterns
A Chewing automatism
0 None
1 Upon stimulation
2 Minor
3 Distinct

B Snout reflex
0 None
1 Released only little
2 Released distinctly

C Oral fixation mechanisms
0 Cannot be released
1 Release optical and upon touch
2 Only upon touch

D Chin reflexes
0 None
1 Released only little
2 Release distinctly
3 Can be released from remote sites

E Grasp reflex
0 None
1 Phasic
2 Tonic and phasic
3 Tonic

F Grasp toward something
0 None
1 Little
2 Distinctly

G Postural reflexes
0 None
1 Little
2 Distinctly

H Fixed postural pattern
0 None
1 Flexion stretch position
2 Magnus-De Kleyn position
3 Flexion of all extremities
4 Stretch of all extremities

VIII. Affection and emotion
A Affective emotional reaction
0 None
1 Decreased
2 Increased
3 Missing

B Special type of affective emotional disturbance
0 None
1 Overshooting joy
2 Excessive crying
3 Excessive anger
4 Primitive fright

IX. Cerebral symptomatology
A Unilateral
0 None
1 Little
2 Distinct

Bibliography

Abrahamson, A.S.: Bone disturbances in injuries to the spinal cord and cauda equina (paraplegia). J. Bone Jt Surg. **30-A**, 982 (1948).
Adams, J.H.: Central pontine myelinolysis. In: Proc. IV. Int. Congr. Neuropath., Vol.III. Stuttgart: Thieme 1962, pp. 303–308.
Adams, R.D., Foley, J.M.: Neurological disorders associated with liver disease. Res. Publ. Ass. nerv. ment. Dis. **32**, 198–237 (1953).
Adams, R.D., Victor, M., Mancall, E.L.: Central pontine myelinolysis. Arch. Neurol. Psychiat. (Chicago) **81**, 154–172 (1959).
Adams, R.D., Denny-Brown, D., Pearson, C.M.: Diseases of Muscles. New York: Harper, 1962.
Addison, T.: A Collection of the Collected Works of T. Addison. Wilks and Dadly (eds). London: New Sydenham Society, 1968.
Adebahr, G.: Gehirnverletzungen nach wochenlanger posttraumatischer Bewußtlosigkeit. Dtsch. Z. ges. gerichtl. Med. **49**, 680–684 (1959).
Adebahr, G.: Erfahrung über zentraltraumatische Gehirnnekrosen aus gerichtsmedizinischem Untersuchungsgut. Klin. Wschr. **41**, 732–733 (1963a).
Adebahr, G.: Zur Genese traumatischer Pallidum-, Balken- und Marknekrosen. Dtsch. med. Wschr. **88**, 2097–2103 (1963b).
Adebahr, G., Schewe, G.: Beobachtungen über die Relationen von Primär- und Sekundärschäden am Gehirn infolge Hirndrucks in Abhängigkeit von der Zeit. Dtsch. Z. ges. gerichtl. Med. **59**, 119–124 (1967).
Agrest, A., Roehr, E., Ruiz-Guinazu, A.: Acid based quilibrium in the cerebrospinal fluid and arterial blood in mental insufficiency. Klin. Wschr. **40**, 1045 (1962).
Ajuriaguerra, D.E., Hécaen, H., Lagani, E., Sadoni, R.: Maladie de Schilder-Foix; étude anatomoclinique d'un cas. Presse méd. **61**, 1756–1759 (1953).
Alajouanine, T.: Les altérations des états de conscience causées par les désordres neurologiques. In: Premier Congr. Internat. des Sciences Neurologiques, Brussels: Acta med. belg. , 19–41 (1957).
Albert, E.: Wechselwirkung zwischen Gehirn und Leber. In: III. Colloquium der Gesellschaft für Physiologische Chemie, April 1952, Mosbach/Baden. Berlin–Göttingen–Heidelberg: Springer, 1952, pp. 129–148.
Amann, E., Gerstenbrand, F., Jellinger, K.: Schwerer Hirnschaden (apallisches Syndrom) nach Herzstillstand bei einem Kleinkind. Pädiat. Pädol. **6**, 121–134 (1971).
Amorim, M.: Consideracores em Torno Dos Corpos Extranhos No Quobo Ocular. Bahia Med. **5**, 488–490 (1934a).
Amorim, M.: Das Vorkommen kristallischer Lipoide in den Körnchenzellen und deren histochemische Unterscheidung. Z. ges. Neurol. Psychiat. **151**, 171–191 (1934b).
Amstrong-Ressy, C.T., Weiss, A.A., Ebel, A.: Results of surgical treatment of extraosseous ossification in paraplegia. N. Y. St. J. Med. **59**, 548 (1959).
Arfel, G.: Stimulation visuels et silence cérébrale. Electroenceph. clin. Neurophysiol. **23**, 172–175 (1967).
Ashbury, A.K.: Ischaemic disorders of peripheral nerves. In: Handbook of Clinical Neurology, Vol. II. Amsterdam: Elsevier, 1970, pp. 154–164.
Ayd, Jr., F.J.: A survey of drug-induced extrapyramidal reactions. J. Amer. med. Ass. **175**, 1054–1060 (1961).
Bailey, P.: Presidential address: Concerning the localization of consciousness. Trans. Amer. neurol. Ass. 1–12 (1955).
Baldy-Moulinier, M., Frerebau, P.: Cerebral blood flow in cases of coma following severe

head injury, In: Cerebral Blood Flow. Brock, M., Fieschi, C., Ingvar, D.H., Lassen, N.A., Schürmann, K. (eds.). Berlin–Heidelberg-New York: Springer, 1969, pp. 216–218.
Bard, P., Macht, M.B.: The behaviour of chronically decerebrate cats. In: Neurological Bases of Behaviour. Bard, P. (ed.). Ciba Foundation Symposium 1958, pp. 55–75.
Bard, P., Rioch, D.Mc.K.: A study of four cats deprived of neocortex and additional portions of the forebrain. John Hopk. Hosp. Bull. **60**, 73–157 (1937).
Bas, H.: Das traumatische apallische Syndrom als Durchgangssyndrom. Med. Wschr. **18**, 835–837 (1970).
Batini, C., Moruzzi, G., Palestini, M., Rossi, G.F., Zanchetti, A.: Persistent patterns of wakefulness in the pretrigeminal midpontine preparation. Science **128**, 30–32 (1958).
Batini, C., Moruzzi, G., Palestini, M., Rossi, G.F., Zanchetti, A.: Effects of complete pontine transactions on the sleep-wakefulness rhythm: the midpontine pretrigeminal preparation. Arch. ital. Biol. **97**, 1–12 (1959); **102**, 547–566 (1964).
Batsel, H.L.: Electroencephalographic synchronization and desynchronization in the chronic "cerveau isolés" of the dog. Electroencephal. clin. Neurophysiol. **12**, 421–430 (1960).
Batsel, H.L.: Spontaneous desynchronization in the chronic cat "cerveau isolés". Arch. ital. Biol. **102**, 547–566 (1964).
Bazzet, H.C., Penfield, W.G.: A study of the sherringtonian decerebrate animal in the chronic as well as in the acute condition. Brain **45**, 185–265 (1922).
Becker, K., Hoyer, S.: Hirnstoffwechseluntersuchungen unter der Behandlung mit Pyrithioin. Dtsch. Z. Nervenheilk. **188**, 200–204 (1966).
Benini, A., Krayenbuhl, H.: L'idrocefalo occulto sintomatico degli adulti. Nuova Syndrome Clinica. Gazz. sanit. (Milano) **40**, 4–5; 145–154 (1970).
Bente, D.: Vigilanz, dissoziative Vigilanzverschiebung und Insuffizienz des Vigilitätstonus. In: Begleitwirkungen und Mißerfolge der Psychiatrischen Pharmakotherapie. Kranz, H., Heinrich, K. (eds.). Stuttgart: Thieme, 1964, pp. 13–28.
Bentley, F.H., Schlapp, W.: The affects of pressure on conduction in peripheral nerves. J. Physiol. (Lond.) **102**, 72 (1943).
Bergamasco, B., Bergamini, L., Doriguzzi, T., Sacerdote, I.: Il ciclio nictemerale del coma. Possibilità prognostiche. Riv. Pat. nerv. ment. **87**, 312–318 (1966a).
Bergamasco, B., Doriguzzi, T., Sacerdote, I., Chiono, C.: Registrazioni poligraphiche notturne in soggetti in coma posttraumatico. Boll. Soc. ital. Biol. sper. **43**, 322–323 (1966b).
Bergamasco, B., Bergamini, L., Doriguzzi, T.: Clinical value of the sleep electroencephalographic patterns in posttraumatic coma. Acta neurol. scand. **44**, 495–511 (1968a).
Bergamasco, B., Bergamini, L., Doriguzzi, T., Fabiani, D.: Sleep EEG graphic patterns as a prognostic criterion in posttraumatic coma. Electroenceph. clin. Neurophysiol. **24**, 374–377 (1968b).
Bergamini, L., Bergamasco, B.: Cortical Evoked Potentials in Man. Springfield/Ill.: Thomas, 1967.
Bergamini, L., Inghirami, L.: Cenni di fisiopatologia e clinica del coma nel cranioleso. Boll. Soc. piemart. Chir. **64**, 42–51 (1962).
Berger, A., Dinstl., K., Keminger, K., Steinbreithner, K.: Vermeidung von Tracheotomieschäden durch geänderte Operationstaktik. Langenbecks Arch. klin. Chir., Kongreßband (1970a).
Berger, A., Kucher, R., Lechner, G., Steinbreithner, K.: Die „eingenähte" Tracheotomie. Prakt. Anaesth. **284** (1970b).
Bes, A., Arbus, L., Lazorthes, Y., Delpla, M., Marc Vergne, J.P.: Hemodynamic and metabolic studies in "coma dépassé". A search for a biological test of death of the brain. In: Cerebral Blood Flow. Brock, M., Fieschi, C., Ingvar, D.H., Lassen, N.A., Schürmann, K. (eds.). Berlin–Heidelberg–New York: Springer, 1966, pp. 213–215.
Bierwisch, M.: Strukturalismus. Geschichte, Probleme und Methoden. Kursbuch V. Frankfurt: Suhrkamp, 1966, pp. 177–252.
Blaschko, H., Chrusciel, T.L.: The decarboxylation of amino acids related to tyroxine and their awakening action in reserpine treated mice. J. Physiol. (Lond.) **151**, 272–275 (1960).
Bleuler, E.: Lehrbuch der Psychiatrie, 11th ed. Berlin–Heidelberg–New York: Springer, 1969.

Bobath, B.: The importance of reduction of muscle tone and control of mass reflex action in the treatment of spasticity. Occup. Ther. **27**, 371–381 (1949).
Bobath, K.: Die Neuropathologie der cerebralen Kinderlähmung unter besonderer Berücksichtigung der Stellung und der Haltung der Wirbelsäule. In: Neurologie der Wirbelsäule und des Rückenmarks im Kindesalter. Müller, D. (ed.). Jena: G. Fischer, 1964.
Bobath, K., Bobath, B.: Spastic paralysis-treatment by the use of reflex inhibition. Brit. J. phys. Med. **13**, 121–129 (1950).
Böcker, F.: Eine Methode zur genaueren Erfassung von Bewußtseinstrübungen und Durchgangssyndromen. Schweiz. Arch.,Neurol. Psychiat. **88**, 332–338 (1961).
Böcker, F., Kinzel, W.: Durchführung und Auswertung des Syndromtests zur Bestimmung der Schwere von Funktionspsychosen. Ärztl. Gespr. **11**, 51–60 (1969).
Boeters, U.: Die Bedeutung von Antriebsstörungen beim posttraumatischen apallischen Syndrom und seinen Folgezuständen. Nervenarzt **40**, 268–272 (1969).
Boeters, U., Grahmann, H.: Zur Frage der Demenz als Folge langfristiger Psychopharmakotherapie. Int. Pharmacopsychiat. **2**, 71–77 (1969).
Boeters, U., Korenke, H.D.: Apallisches Syndrom nach Revaczinationsenzephalitis. Basel: Karger, 1972.
Boeters, U., Reimer, F.: Gibt es zerebrale Komplikationen nach Pockenschutzimpfung? Nervenarzt **41**, 223–226 (1970).
Bogaert, L. van: Une leucoencéphalite subaigre. J. Neurol. Neurosurg. Psychiat. 101–120 (1965).
Bogaert, L. van, Scholz, W.: Klinischer genealogischer und pathologisch-anatomischer Beitrag zur Kenntnis der familiären diffusen Sklerose. Z. ges. Neurol. Psychiat. **141**, 510–541 (1932).
Bonhoeffer, K.: Symptomatische Psychosen im Gefolge von akuten Infektionen und inneren Erkrankungen. Leipzig–Vienna: Deuticke, 1910.
Born, E., Binder, H.: Über eine unter dem Bild des apallischen Syndroms verlaufende heredo-degenerative Erkrankung. Psychiat. et Neurol. (Basel) **144**, 195–317 (1962).
Bottermann, P., Schwarz, K., Kollmannsberger, A., Kopetz, K.: Zur klinischen Diagnostik von Inselzelladenomen. Klinische Erfahrungen und diagnostisches Vorgehen beim organischen Hyperinsulinismus. Med. Klin. **64**, 479 (1969).
Bottermann, P., Dieterle, P., Schwarz, K., Scriba, P.C., Souvatzoglou, P.C.: Zum Mechanismus der Addison-Hypoglykämie. Med. Klin. **64**, 500–502 (1969).
Bozzamarrubini, M., Rossanda, M.: Anestesia e rianimazione nella chirurgia e nella traumatologia del sistema nervoso centrale. In: Relazione al XIV Congr. Soc. ital. Anest. Turin, Italy, 1961.
Bremer, F.: Cerveau "isolé" et physiologie du sommeil. C.R. Soc. Biol. (Paris) **118**, 1235–1241 (1935).
Bremer, F., Stoupel, N.: Facilitation et inhibition des potentiels évoqués coticaux dans l'éveil cérébral. Arch. int. Physiol. **67**, 240–275 (1959).
Breuer, M., Kaufmann, W., Tiefensee, K.: XIV. Spontanhypoglykämien bei Inselzelladenom. Med. Welt **34**, 1001–1002 (1965).
Bricolo, A.: Anomalie elettroencefalografiche del sonno negli stati comatosi prolongati posttraumatici. Clin. neuropsichiat. **3**, 25–32 (1966).
Bricolo, A.: Semeotica clinico-strumentale dei quari evolutivi del coma traumatico. In: Gli stati di coscienza, Lugarsi. Pazzaglia, M. (ed.). Bologna: Gaggi, 1971, pp. 291–316.
Bricolo, A., Dalle Ore, G.: Prime esperienze nel trattamento con L-dopa degli stam comatosi posttraumatici. Sist. nerv. **22**, 175–180 (1970).
Bricolo, A., Dolce, G.: Evolutioni cliniche del coma posttraumatico grave, Minerva neurochir. **13**, 61–68 (1969).
Bricolo, A., Formenton, A.: Considerazioni sul trattamento del coma traumatico: nuove prospettive terapeutiche. Fracastoro **64**, 157–172 (1971).
Bricolo, A., Gentilomo, A., Rosadini, G., Rossi, G.F.: Coma posttraumatico prolongato e suoi particolari aspetti poligrafici. Sist. nerv. **4**, 209–216 (1967).
Bricolo, A., Gentilomo, A., Rosadini, G., Rossi, G.F.: Acinetic mutism following craniocerebral trauma. Physiopathological considerations based on sleep-studies. Acta neurochir. (Wien) **17**, 68–77 (1968a).
Bricolo, A., Gentilomo, A., Rosadini, G., Rossi, G.F.: Longlasting posttraumatic unconsciousness. Acta neurol. scand. **44**, 512–532 (1968b).
Bricolo, A., Mazza, C., Sdarretta, G., Turella, G.: Effetti della l-dopa sui fusi da sonno nei parkinsoniani. Riv. sper. Freniat. **94**, 416–424 (1970a).

Bricolo, A., Turella, G., Mazza, C., Buffat, M.R., Gross'-Lercher, J.S.: Modificationi del sonno notturno in parkinsoniani trattati con l–dopa. Sist. nerv. **22**, 181–190 (1970b).
Bricolo, A., Formenton, A., Turella, G., Dalle Ore, G.: Clinical and EEG effects of mechanical hyperventilation in acute traumatic coma. Comunicat. Internat. CBF Symposium Roma–Siena, pp. 28–31, Oct. 1971; Europ. Neurol. **8**, 219–224 (1972).
Brierley, J.B., Adams, J.H., Graham, D.J., Simpson, J.A.: Neocortical death after cardiac arrest. Lancet **1971 I**, 560–565.
Brierley, J.B., Cooper, J.E.: Cerebral complications of hypotensive anesthesia in a healthy adult. J. Neurol. Neurosurg. Psychiat. **25**, 24–30 (1962).
Bright, R.: Observations of jaundice. Guy's Hosp. Rep. **1**, 604–637 (1836).
Brock, M., Schürmann, K., Hadjidimos, A.: Cerebral blood flow and cerebral death. Acta neurochir. (Wien) **20**, 195–209 (1969).
Brodal, A.: The Reticular Formation of the Brain Stem. Anatomical Aspects and Functional Correlations. Edinburgh–London: Oliver and Boyd, 1957, pp. 87–160.
Brodersen, P.: Critical levels of blood flow and oxygen utilization in the brain. Contribution to IInd International Symposium on Nuclear Medicine, Karlovy Vary, May 11–14, 1971. Acta neurol. scand. **51**, 423–424 (1972).
Brown, G.W., Brown, M.L.: Cardiovascular responses to experimental cerebral concussion in the monkey. Arch. Neurol. Psychiat. (Chicago) **71**, 701–713 (1954).
Bruck, J., Gerstenbrand, F.: Funktionelle Dezerebration unter dem Bild eines apallischen Syndroms bei hochdosierter Majeptil-Behandlung. 82nd Wandertagung d. SW-Dtsch. Neurol.-Psychiat. Baden-Baden, June 1966. Nervenarzt **38**, 459–464 (1967).
Buchthal, F., Rosenfalck, A.: Evoked action potentials and conduction velocity in human sensory nerves. Brain Res. **3**, 321–336 (1966).
Büchner, F.: Die Pathologie der zellulären und geweblichen Oxydationen. In: Hypodosen, Vol. IV/2. Berlin–Göttingen–Heidelberg: Springer, 1957, p. 569.
Bürger-Prinz, H., Kaila, M.: Über die Struktur des amnestischen Symptomenkomplexes. Z. ges. Neurol. Psychiat. **124**, 553–595 (1930).
Butenuth, J.: Spinale Mechanismen in einem Fall von Hirntod nach Cyanidintoxikation. Dtsch. Z. Nervenheilk. **197**, 225–284 (1970).
Cadilhac, J., Kassabgui, M.E., Passonant, P.: La réorganisation du sommeil nocturne après les comas posttraumatiques. Rev. neurol. **115**, 529 (1966).
Cairns, H.: Disturbances of consciousness with lesions of the brain-stem and diencephalon. Brain **75**, 109–146 (1952).
Cairns, H., Oldfield, R.C., Pennybacker, J.B., Whitteridge, D.: Akinetic mutism with an epidermoid cyst of the 3rd ventricle. Brain **64**, 273–290 (1941).
Carr, J.A.: Spontaneous ulnar nerve paresis. Brit. med. J. **5058**, 1415 (1957).
Chatrian, G.E., White, L.E., Daly, D.: Electronencephalography pattern resembling those of sleep in certain comatose states after injuries to the head. Electroenceph. clin. Neurophysiol. **15**, 272–280 (1963).
Chaumont, P., Patte, D., Sejournant, P., Antoine, B.: Etude de la vitesse de conduction motrice chez des malades en état de déplétion potassique cronique, avant pendant et après des épreuves de charge en potassium. Rev. neurol. **110**, 318 (1964).
Chavany, J.A., Carrere, J., Perrin, J., Pochard, M.: Sur une variété d'encéphalopathie posttraumatique. Presse méd. **63**, 1840–1842 (1955).
Chomsky, N.: Language and Mind. New York: Harcourt, Brace and World, 1968.
Chopra, J.S., Hurwitz, L.J.: Internodal length of sural nerve fibers in chronic vascular disease. J. Neurol. Neurosurg. Psychiat. **30**, 207 (1967).
Ciganek, L.: The EEG response (evoked potential) to light stimulus in man. Electroenceph. clin. Neurophysiol. **13**, 165–172 (1961).
Ciganek, L.: A comparative study of visual, auditory and somatosensory EEG response in man. Exp. Brain Res. **4**, 118–125 (1967).
Cobb, W.A., Dawson, G.D.: The latency and form in man of the occipital potential evoked by light flashes. J. Physiol. (Lond.) **152**, 108–121 (1960).
Coirault, R., Deligne, P.: L'ANP 235. Agressologie **1**, 113–116 (1960).
Conomy, J.P., Swash, U.: Reversible decerebrate and decorticate postures in hepatic coma. New Engl. J. Med. **278**, 876–879 (1968).
Conrad, K., Delbrügge, M.: Ein remittierter Fall von Panencephalitis subakuta (Pette). Z. ges. Neurol. Psychiat. **169**, 580–583 (1940).
Corcoran, A.C., Page, H., Taylor, R.D.: Lithium poisoning from the use of salt. Substitutes J. Amer. med. Ass. **139**, 685–688 (1949).

Corletto, F., Gentilomo, A., Rosadini, G., Rossi, G.F., Zattoni, J.: Corrélation entre niveau de conscience, EEG et potentiels évoquée chez l'homme. Rev. neurol. **115**, 5–14 (1966).
Costello, F.V., Brown, A.: Myositis ossificans complicating anterior poliomyelitis. J. Bone Jt Surg. **33-B**, 594–597 (1951).
Cowie, J., Lambie, A.T., Robson, J.S.: The influence of extracorporal dialysis of the acidbase composition of blood and cerebrospinal fluid. Clin. Sci. **23**, 379 (1962).
Cravioto, H., Silbermann, J., Feigin, J.: A clinical and pathological study of akinetic mutism. Neurology (Minneap.) **10**, 10–21 (1960).
Creutzfeldt, W., Frerichs, H.: Hypoglykaemia factitia, eine differentialdiagnostisch wichtige Form des Hyperinsulinismus. Dtsch. med. Wschr. **94**, 813–818 (1969).
Crompton, M.R.: Brain stem lesions due to closed head injury. Lancet **1971 I**, 669–673.
Crompton, M.R., Teare, R.D., Bowen, D.A.L.: Prolonged coma after head injury. Lancet **1966 I**, 938–940.
Curri, S.B., Drago, G., Modiano, C., Gonzata, P.: Distribuzione dei fosfolipidi nell'encefalo traumatizzato. Nota II: Determinazioni cromatografiche dell'endefalo umano. Osped. ital. Chir. **10**, 635–652 (1964).
Dagnino, D., Favale, E., Loeb, C., Manfredi, M.: Sensory transmission in the geniculate straite system of the cat during nocturnal sleep arousal. J. Neurophysiol. **28**, 443–456 (1965).
Dahlström, A., Fuxe, K.: Evidence for the existence of monoamines containing neurons in the central nervous system. Acta physiol. scand. **62**, Suppl. 232, 1–55 (1964).
Damansky, M.: Heterotropic ossification in paraplegia. A clinical study. J. Bone Jt Surg. **43-B**, 286 (1961).
Dechaume, J.P., Girard, P.F., Tommasi, M., Trillet, M.: Documents anatomiques concernant les encéphalopaties posttraumatiques (comas prolongés et "morts du cerveau" post-traumatiques). Proc. IV. Internat. Congr. Neurophath., Vol. III, Stuttgart: Thieme, 1967, pp. 238–242.
Degkwitz, R., Luxemburger, O.: Das terminale extrapyramidale Insuffizienz- bzw. Defektsyndrom infolge chronischer Anwendung von Neuroleptika. Nervenarzt **36**, 173–175 (1965).
Déjérine, Mme., Ceillier, M.A.: Trois cas d'ostéomes-ossifications périostés juxta-musculairés et interfasciculairés, chez des paraplégiques par lésion traumatique de la moelle épinière. Rev. neurol. **33**, 159–172 (1918).
Déjérine, Mme., Ceillier, M.A., Déjérine, Y.: Para-ostéoarthropathies des paraleugiques lésions médullaires: Etude anatomique et histologique. Rev. neurol. **35**, 399–407 (1919).
Delay, J., Deniker, P.: Méthodes chémothérapeutiques en psychiatrie. Les nouveaux médicaments psychotropes. Paris: Masson, 1961.
Delay, J., Deniker, P., Greene, A., Mordret, M.: Le syndrome excitomoteur provoqué par les médicaments neuroleptiques. Presse méd. **65**, 1771 (1957).
Delay, J., Deniker, P., Ropert, R., Beek, H., Barande, R., Enrienet, M.: Syndromes neurologiques expérimentaux et thérapeutique psychiatrique. Effects neurologiques d'un nouveau neuroleptique majeur, le 7843 R.P. Press méd. **69**, 123 (1959).
Delay, J., Thuillier, J., Pichot, P., Lamperiere, T., Brion, M.S.: Premiers résultats en clinique psychiatrique du parachlorophénoxy acétate de diméthylam inoéthyle (ANP 235). Ann. med. Psychol. **118**, 133–140 (1960).
Denber, H.C.B., Tursus, C.D., Seemann, M.V.: The therapeutic community: nine years after. Psychiat. Quart. **42**, 531–538 (1968).
Denny-Brown, D.: The Cerebral Control of Movement. Liverpool Univ., 1966.
Deucher, F., Widmer, A.: Zollinger-Ellison-Syndrom. Ther.Umsch. **27**, 233–235 (1970).
Dietze, R.A., Dörffel, E.W., Schoeppner, H.: Apallisches Syndrom als Durchgangssyndrom bei Bestrahlung eines Ponstumors im Kindesalter. Rat. biol. Ther. **9**, 423–430 (1968).
Dolce, G., Fromm, H.: Sleep EEG-investigations in the apallic syndrome. Excerpta med. Int. Congr. Ser. **139**, 104 (1967).
Dolce, G., Fromm, H.: Beeinflussung des visuell evozierten Reaktionspotentials (VRP) durch Veränderung der spezifischen und unspezifischen Afferenzen der Area striata. Z. EEG-EMG **1**, 100–108 (1972a).
Dolce, G., Fromm, H.: An experimental model of the apallic syndrome. Scand. J. Rehabil. Med. **4**, 39–43 (1972b).

Dolce, G., Kaemmerer, E.: Contributo anatomo-clinico alla conoscenza della sindrome apallica. Sist. nerv. **18**, 142–151 (1966).
Dolce, G., Kaemmerer, E.: Contributo anatomico-clinico ed elettroencefalografico alla conoscenza della sindrome apallica. Studio dell'evolutione dell'EEG da sonno in 5 casi. Sist. nerv. **1**, 12–23 (1967).
Dubois, E.F.: Why are fever temperatures over 106° F rare? Amer. J. med. Sci. **217**, 361–368 (1949).
Duensing, F.: Das Elektroenzephalogramm bei Störungen der Bewußtseinslage. Arch. Psychiat. Nervenkr. **183**, 71–115 (1949).
Dumont, S., Dell, P.: Facilitation réticulaire des méchanismes visuels corticaux. Eléctro-encephal. clin. Neurophysiol. **12**, 769–796 (1960).
Dustman, R.E., Beck, E.C.: The effects of maturation and aging of the waveform of the visually evoked potentials. Electroenceph. clin. Neurophysiol. **26**, 2–11 (1969).
Dyck, P.: Experimental hypertrophic neuropathy. Pathogenesis of onion-bulb formations produced by repeated tourniquet applications. Arch. Neurol. **21**, 73 (1969).
Eames, R.A., Lange, L.S.: Clinical and pathological study of ischaemic neuropathy. J. Neurol. Neurosurg. Psychiat. **30**, 215 (1967).
Ebe, M., Nikami, T.: Cortical evoked potentials due to photic stimulation during sleep in man. Tohoku J. exp. Med. **77**, 383–389 (1962).
Eicke, W.J.: Beitrag zur Substantia nigra. Arch. Psychiat. Nervenkr. **115**, 549–565 (1943).
Eik-Nes, K.B., Clark, D.L.: Diurnal variation of plasma 17-hydroxycoxycorticosteroids in subjects suffering severe brain damage. J. clin. Endocr. **18**, 764 (1958).
Engel, G.L., Romano, J., Ferris, E.B., Webb, J.P., Stevens, G.D.: Simple method of determining frequency spectrum in encephalogram observations on effects of physiologic variations in dextrose, oxygen, posture and acid-base balance on normal electroencephalogram. Arch. Neurol. Psychiat. (Chicago) **51**, 134–146 (1944).
Engerth, G., Winkler, W.: Über das Auftreten von Automatoren bei Urämie. Dtsch. Z. Nervenheilk. **132**, 102–113 (1933).
Erbslöh, F.: Die Hirnveränderungen bei Herzstillstand. In: Spezielle Pathologische Anatomie und Histologie, Vol. XIII/2. Berlin–Göttingen–Heidelberg: Springer, 1958, pp. 1330–1337.
Erbslöh, F., Abel, M., Vinken, P.J., Bruyn, G.W.: Deficiency neuropathies. In: Handbook of Clinical Neurology, Vol. VII. Amsterdam: North-Holland Publ. Co.; New York: Elsevier, 1970, pp. 558–663.
Erickson, T.C.: Neurogenic hyperthermia. Brain **62**, 172–190 (1939).
Evans, E.B., Smith, J.R.: Bone and joint changes following burns. A roentgenographic study – preliminary report. J. Bone Jt Surg. **41-A**, 785–799 (1959).
Evans, J., Ishii, S., Tsuji, H.: Brain oedema: some clinical and experimental correlation. In: Proc. Workshop, Brain Oedema. Internat. Congr. Ser. **94**, Amsterdam: Excerpta Med. Found., 1965, Vol. 99.
Evans, W.: An encephalographic ratio for stimating ventricular enlargement and cerebral atrophy. Arch. Neurol. Psychiat. (Chicago) **47**, 931–937 (1942).
Evarts, E.V., Fleming, T.C.: Recovery cycle of visual cortex of the awake and sleeping cat. Amer. J. Physiol. **199**, 375–376 (1960).
Facon, E., Steriade, M., Wertheim, N.: Hypersomnie prolongée engendrée par des lésions bilatérales du systemeactivateur médiale et le syndrome thrombotique de la bifurcation du tronc basilaire. Rev. neurol. **98**, 117–133 (1958).
Falck, B., Hillarp, N.A., Thieme, G., Torp, A.: Fluorescence of catacholamines and related compounds condensed with formaldehyde. J. Histochem. Cytochem. **10**, 348–354 (1962).
Fau, R.: Etude EEG des dégrés de la vigilance au cours d'un coma traumatique très prolongé. Rev. neurol. **94**, 818–834 (1956).
Fazekas, J.F., Alman, R.W.: Coma. Springfield/Ill.: Charles C. Thomas, 1962.
Fazekas, J.F., Bessman, A.N.: Coma mechanism. Amer. J. Med. **15**, 804–812 (1953).
Felix, K.: Presented at 3rd Colloquium der Gesellschaft für physiol. Chemie, Mosbach/Baden, 1952: Die Chemie und der Stoffwechsel des Nervengewebes. Berlin–Göttingen–Heidelberg: Springer 1952.
Fischgold, H., Mathis, P.: Obnubilations comas et stupeurs. Études électroencéphaliques. EEG clin. Neurophysiol., Suppl. II, Paris: Masson, 1959.
Fishman, R.A., Raskin, N.H.: Experimental uraemic encephalopathy. Arch. Neurol. **17**, 10–21 (1967).

Flügel, F.: Erfahrungen mit Megaphen in der psychiatrischen und neurologischen Klinik. Verh. dtsch. Ges. inn. Med. **60**, 135–140 (1954).
Folz, E.L., Ward, A.A., Jr.: Communicating hydrocephalus from subarachnoid bleeding. J. Neurosurg. **13**, 546–566 (1956).
Freeman, R.B., Sheff, M.F., Maher, J.F., Schreiner, G.E.: The blood-cerebro spinal fluid barrier in uraemia. Ann. intern. Med. **56**, 233–240 (1962).
Freiberg, J.A.: Para-artic calcification and ossification following acute anterior poliomyelitis in an adult. J. Bone Jt Surg. **34-A**, 339–348 (1952).
French, J.D.: Brain lesions associated with prolonged unconsciousness. Arch. Neurol. Psychiat. (Chicago) **68**, 727–740 (1952).
French, J.D., Magoun, H.W.: Effects of chronic lesions in central cephalic brain stem of monkeys. AMA Arch. Neurol. Psychiat. **68**, 591–604 (1952).
Frerichs, F.T.: Clinical Treatise on Diseases of the Liver. London: New Sydenham Society, 1860.
Frowein, R.A.: Behandlung der Streckstarre in akutem Stadium nach Kopfverletzungen. Zbl. Chir. **83**, 918–919 (1958).
Frowein, R.A.: Beurteilung und Behandlung der Störungen lebenswichtiger Funktionen im akuten Stadium schwerer Schädel-Hirn-Verletzungen. Acta neurochir. (Wien) **2**, 468–495 (1961).
Frowein, R.A.: Zentrale Atemstörungen bei Schädel-Hirn-Verletzungen und bei Hirntumoren. Berlin–Göttingen–Heidelberg: Springer, 1963.
Frowein, R.A., Haar, K.A.D., Terhaag, D., Kinzel, W., Wieck, H.H.: Arbeitsfähigkeit und Abbausyndrome nach Hirntraumen mit andauernder Bewußtlosigkeit. 100 klinische und 38 testpsychologische Untersuchungen bei Erwachsenen und Kindern. Mschr. Unfallheilk. **71**, 233–249 (1968).
Fruehan, A., Frawley, T.: Current status of anabolic steroids. J. Amer. med. Ass. **184**, 527–531 (1963).
Fuchsig, P.: Zur Klinik und Pathologie der narbigen Trachealstenosen nach Rezidivoperationen. Langenbecks Arch. klin. Chir. **295**, 145 (1960).
Fulton, J.F.: Physiologie des Nervensystems. Stuttgart: Thieme, 1952.
Gamper, E.: Bau und Leistung eines menschlichen Mittelhirnwesens (Arhinencephalie mit Encephalocele), zugleich ein Beitrag zur Teratologie und Fasersystematik. Z. ges. Neurol. Psychiat. **102**, 154–235 (1926); 2. klin. Teil: Z. ges. Neurol. Psychiat. **104**, 49–120 (1926).
Garcia-Austt, E.: Influence of the states of awareness upon sensory evoked potentials. Electroencephal. clin. Neurophysiol. Suppl. **24**, 76–89 (1963).
Gastaut, H.: The brain stem and cerebral electrogenesis in relation to consciousness. In: Brain Mechanism and Consciousness. Oxford: Blackwell, 1954.
Gastaut, H.: A transcranial chronographic and topographic study of cerebral potentials evoked by photostimulation in man. In: Progress in Brain Research, Brain Mechanism, Moruzzi, G. et al. (eds.), Vol. I. Amsterdam: Elsevier, 1963, pp. 374–394.
Gemsenjager, E.: Über einen atypischen Fall von Hirnschädigung nach stumpfer Gewalteinwirkung auf den Schädel. Psychiat. Neurol. **139**, 416–428 (1960).
Genovesi, U., Moruzzi, G., Palestini, M., Rossi, G.F., Zanchetti, A.: EEG and behavioural patterns following lesions of the mesencephalic reticular formation in chronic cats with implanted electrodes. Int. physiol. Sci. Congr. **20**, 335–336 (1956).
Gentilomo, A., Rivano, C., Rosadini, G.: Studio electroclinico longhitudinale del coma cerebrale evolvente verso la sindrome apallica. Rass. Arch. Chir. **4**, 116–132 (1966).
Geraud, J., Bes, A., Rascol, A., Delpla, M., Marc-Vergnes, J.P.: Exploration du débit sanguin cérébral par la méthode au Krypton 85. Presse méd. **73**, 1473–1475 (1965).
Geraud, J., Bes, A., Rascol, A., Delpla, M., Marc-Vergnes, J.P.: Application de la méthode au Krypton 85. Pharmacologie de la circulation cérébrale. Presse méd. **73**, 1577–1582 (1965).
Gerhard, D., Jr.: Cited by Mumenthaler, M., Schliack, H. (1965).
Gerhard, L., Brölsch, C.H.: Veränderungen am basalen Schläfenlappen und Gyrus hippocampus bei Schädelhirntrauma. Acta neuropath. (Berl.) **15**, 20–35 (1970).
German, W.J., Page, W.R., Nims, L.: Cerebral blood flow and cerebral oxygen consumption in experimental intracranial injury. Trans. Amer. neurol. Ass. **72**, 86–88 (1947).
Gerstenbrand, F.: Das traumatische apallische Syndrom. Vienna–New York: Springer 1967.
Gerstenbrand, F.: Neurologische Rehabilitation traumatischer Hirnschäden. Wien. med. Wschr. **118**, 782–786 (1968a).

Gerstenbrand, F.: Rehabilitation of the head-injured. In: The Late Effects of Head Injury. Walker, A.E., Caveness, W.F., Critchley, Mc D. (eds.). Springfield/Ill.: Charles C. Thomas, 1968b, pp. 340–350.
Gerstenbrand, F.: The course of restitution of brain injury in the early and late stages and the rehabilitation measures. Scand. J. Rehabil. Med. **4** (in press).
Gerstenbrand, F., Galanti, T.: Die Bedeutung der Ernährung für die Prognose des apallischen Syndroms. In: Parenterale Ernährung. Hartmann, G., Berger, H. (eds.). Bern: Huber, 1972.
Gerstenbrand, F., Helmer, F., Wolner, H.: Das akute Hirnstamm-Syndrom als Komplikation nach Herzoperationen. Bruns Beitr. klin. Chir. **216**, 210–222 (1968).
Gerstenbrand, F., Hoff, H.: Rehabilitation bei organischer Hirnschädigung, psychiatrische Aspekte. Wien med. Wschr. **118**, 754–757 (1968).
Gerstenbrand, F., Hoff, H., Prosenz, P.: Therapeutische Erfahrungen mit Lucidril bei neuro-psychiatrischen Krankheitsbildern. Wien med.Wschr. **113**, 539–543 (1963a).
Gerstenbrand, F., Jellinger, K., Pateisky, K.: Zur Rehabilitation des apallischen Syndroms nach schwerem gedecktem Schädel-Hirn-Trauma. Wien. Z. Nervenheilk. **21**, 177–185 (1963b).
Gerstenbrand, F., Kaufmann, F., Krenn, J., Zacherl, H.: Sekundärschäden peripherer Nerven bei langdauernden Comazuständen. Wiederbeleb. Organers. Intensivmed. **8**, 57 (1971).
Gerstenbrand, F., Liehe-Kreutzner, M., Bruha, W.:Periartikuläre Ossifikationen beim traumatischen apallischen Syndrom. Zur Klinik, Pathogenese und Therapie. Arch. orthop. Unfall-Chir. **67**, 173 (1970a).
Gerstenbrand, F., Lücking, C.H.: Die akuten traumatischen Hirnstammschäden. Arch. Psychiat. Nervenkr. **213**, 264–281 (1970).
Gerstenbrand, F., Lücking, C.H., Peters, G., Rothemund, E.: Cerebellar symptoms as sequels of traumatic lesions of upper brain atem and cerebellum. Int. J. Neurol. **7**, 271–282 (1970b).
Gerstenbrand, F., Machacek, F.: Traumatisch bedingter Uvula-Nystagmus. Wien Z. Nervenheilk. **26**, 293–303 (1968).
Gerstenbrand, F., Schnack, H., Wewalka, F.: Zur neurologischen Symptomatologie des Coma hepaticum. Verh. dtsch. Ges. inn. Med. **75**, 754–757 (1969).
Gerstenbrand, F., Schultes, H.: Die therapeutische Gemeinschaft in der Rehabilitation Hirnverletzter. In: Kongreßbericht 2. Donau-Symposium für Neurologie. Gerstenbrand, F. (ed.). Vienna: Verl. Wien. med. Akad., 1971, pp. 21–24.
Gilliatt, R.W., Thomas, P.K.: Peripheral nerve conduction with ulnar lesions at the elbow. J. Neurol. Neurosurg. Psychiat. **23**, 312 (1960).
Girard, P.F., Tommassi, M., Trillet, M.: Un nouvel aspect anatomique des encéphalopathies alcooliques: la démyélinisation centrale du pont. Lyon méd. **52**, 1195–1200 (1959).
Girard, P.F., Tommassi, M., Trillet, M.: Les lésions anatomiques de l'encéphalopathie posttraumatiques. (Comas prolongés et "morts du cerveau"). Acta neuropath. (Berl.) **2**, 313–327 (1963).
Girke, W., Mauruschat, W., Kanowski, S.: Kombinationen von amentiellen und aphasischen Störungen unter Psychopharmakotherapie. Arch. Psych. Nervenheil. (in press).
Goldstein, K.: Beobachtungen über die Veränderungen des Gesamtverhaltens bei Gehirnerschütterung. Mschr. Psychiat. Neurol. **68**, 217–242 (1928).
Goodman, L., Gilman, N.: The Pharmacological Basis of Therapeutics. London–New York: MacMillan, 1970, p. 1794.
Gordon, E., Rossanda, N.: The importance of the cerebral spinal fluid acid-base status in the treatment of unconscious patients with brain lesions. Acta anesth. scand. **12**, 51–58 (1968).
Gosztonyi, G., Mattyus, Merrei, F.T.: Über Gehirnveränderungen bei lange überlebenden Hirnverletzungen. In: Proc. VIII. Internat. Congr. Neurol., Vol. I. Vienna, 1965, pp. 375–379.
Gottschlick, J.: Die Leistungen des Nervensystems. Jena: VEB G. Fischer, 1955.
Gottstein, U.: Zirkulation, Sauerstoff- und Glukosestoffwechsel des Gehirns bei den Encephalopathien. Verh. dtsch. Ges. inn. Med. **72**, 185–198 (1966).
Graham, D.J., Adams, J.H.: Ischaemic brain damage in fatal head injuries. In: Brain Hypoxia. Brieley, J.B., Meldrum, B.S. (eds.). London: Heinemann, 1971, pp. 31–40.
Grahmann, H., Hauss, K., Lehmann, H.J.: Progrediente Blockierung corticaler Funktio-

nen bei der adulten Form der metachromatischen Leukodystrophie. Dtsch. Z. Nervenheilk. **195**, 64–78 (1969).
Grahmann, H., Reimer, F.: Psychopharmakotoxische Encephalopathie. Int. Pharmacopsychiat. **1**, 126–128 (1968).
Grčević, N.: In: Diskussion, Round-table-Gespräch, Die Morphologie des apallischen Syndroms. 11. Wiss. Tg. Verein Dtsch. Neuroanat. Neuropath., Göttingen, 1964.
Grčević, N., Jacob, H.: Some observations on pathology and correlative neuroanatomy of cerebral trauma. In: Proc. VIIIth Internat. Congr. Neurol. Vienna, 1965, Vol. I, pp. 369–373.
Griesel, W.: Hauttemperaturmessungen und Diagnose des zentralen Fiebers. Dtsch. Z. Nervenheilk. **148**, 159–170 (1939).
Gross, H., Rupprecht, A., Seitelberger, F.: Anatomische Befunde bei Spättod nach Lachgasnarkose. Wien. Z. Nervenheilk. **10**, 397–405 (1955).
Grosse-Brockhoff, F.: Pathologische Physiologie. Berlin–Heidelberg–New York: Springer, 1969.
Grotjahn, M.: Klinik und Bedeutung akinetischer Zustände nach Luftfüllung des 3. Ventrikels. Mschr. Psychiat. Neurol. **93**, 121–139 (1936).
Grüner, J.E.: Les lésions histologiques des séquelles des traumatismes craniens. In: Proc. VIIIth Internat. Congr. Neurol., Vienna, 1965, Vol. I, pp. 1–9.
Grünthal, E.: Über eine ungewöhnliche Schädigung der Großhirnrinde durch Insulin. Mschr. Psychiat. Neurol. **104**, 301–311 (1941).
Haase, H.J.: Über Vorkommen und Deutung des psychomotorischen Parkinson–Syndroms bei Megaphen-, bzw. Largactil-Dauerbehandlung. Nervenarzt **25**, 486–492 (1954).
Haberland, C.: Clinico-pathological data on late residual of cerebral anoxia with report of a case of cardiac arrest. Excerpta med. Int. Congr. Ser. **39**, 58–59 (1961).
Hakim, S., Adams, R.D.: The special clinical problems of symptomatic hydrocephalus with normal cerebrospinal fluid pressure. J. neurol. Sci. **2**, 307–327 (1965).
Hardy, A.G., Dickson, P.W.: Pathological ossification in traumatic paraplegia. J. Bone Jt Surg. **45**, 76–87 (1963).
Harner, R.N., Dorman, R.N.: Mechanism of electroencephalographic and behavioral changes produced by parenteral L-dopa. Electroenceph. clin. Neurophysiol. **27**, 672 (1969).
Hartcroft, U.S., Wrenshall, G.A.: Correlation of β-cell granulation with extractable insulin of the pancreas. Diabetes **4**, 1 (1955).
Hartmann, K., Hippius, H.: Extrapyramidal-motorische Begleiteffekte der neuroleptischen Therapie und ihrer Behandlung. Ärztl. Wschr. 307-312 (1959).
Hassler, R.: Funktionelle Neuroanatomie und Psychiatrie. In: Psychiatrie der Gegenwart. Kisker, K.P., Meyer, J.E., Müller, M., Strömgren, E. (eds.), Vol. I/A. Berlin–Heidelberg–New York: Springer, 1967, pp. 151–285.
Hassler, R.: Stereotaktische Stimulation. Presented at Conf. „Das apallische Syndrom". April 1970, Verona, Italy.
Hassler, R., Dalle Ore, G., Bricolo, A., Dieckmann, G., Dolce, G.: EEG and clinical arousal induced by bilateral long term stimulation of pallidal systems in traumatic coma. Electroenceph. clin. Neurophysiol. **27**, 689 (1969a).
Hassler, R., Dalle Ore, G., Dieckmann, G., Bricolo, A., Dolce, G.: Behavioral and EEG arousal induced by stimulations of unspecific projection system in a patient with post-traumatic apallic syndrome. Electroenceph. clin. Neurophysiol. **27**, 306–310 (1969b).
Heiss, W.D., Gerstenbrand, F., Prosenz, P., Krenn, J.: The prognostic value of cerebral blood flow measurement in patients with apallic syndrome. J. neurol. Sci. **16**, 372–382 (1972a).
Heiss, W.D., Prosenz, P., Roszuczky, A.: Technical considerations in the use of a gamma-camera 1600 channel analyzer system for the measurement of regular cerebral blood flow. J. Nucl. Med. **13**, 534–543 (1972b).
Heiss, W.D., Prosenz, P., Roszuczky, A., Tschabitscher, H.: Die Verwendung von Gamma-Kamera und Vielkanalspeichern zur Messung der gesamten und regionalen Hirndurchblutung. J. Nucl. Med. **7**, 297–318 (1968).
Hellbronner, K.: Über die Beziehung zwischen Demenz und Aphasie. Arch. Psychiat. Nervenkr. **33**, 366–392 (1900).
Helmchen, H.: Delirante Abläufe unter psychiatrischer Pharmakotherapie. Arch. Psychiat. Nervenkr. **202**, 395–411 (1961).

Helmchen, H., Hippius, H.: Unerwartete neurologische Begleiterscheinungen der Pharmakotherapie von Psychosen. In: Neurolepsie und Schizophrenie. Kran, H., Heinrich, K. (eds.). Stuttgart: Thieme, 1962, pp. 77–87.
Helmchen, H., Hippius, H.: Psychische Nebenwirkungen der psychiatrischen Pharmakotherapie. In: Begleitwirkungen und Mißerfolge der psychiatrischen Pharmakotherapie. Kranz, H., Heinrich, K. (eds.). Stuttgart: Thieme, 1964, pp. 29–40.
Helmchen, H., Künkel, H.: Die prognostische Bedeutung elektroencephalographischer Veränderungen unter psychiatrischer Pharmakotherapie. Arzneimittel-Forsch. **14**, 595–596 (1964).
Hermann, E.: Niezwykly zespol pourazowy: livedo racemosa universalis u osobnika z objawami piramido-pozapiramidowymi i zaburzeniam i psychicznyni. Warszawskie Czasopismo Lekarskie **14**, 83–86; **6**, 107–109 (1937).
Hermann, E., Sulat, H.: Un syndrome particulier post-traumatique vasomoteur: Livédo racémosa universalis, symptômes disséminés pyramidaux et extrapyramidaux et trouble psychiques. Rev. neurol. **101**, 731–740 (1959).
Hermann, K.: Posttraumatic Dysarthria. In: Proc. VIIIth Internat. Congr. Neurol. Vienna, 1965, Vol. I, pp. 135–137.
Hess, R.: Sleep and sleep disturbances in the electroencephalogram. In: Progress in Brain Research, Sleep Mechanism. Akert, K. (ed.), Vol. XVIII. Amsterdam: Elsevier, 1965, p. 247.
Himwich, H.E.: Biochemical and neurophysiological action of psychoactive drugs. In: Drug Behavior. Uhr, L., Miller, J.P. (eds.). New York–London: Wiley, 1960.
Hinreich, H.E.: Brain Metabolism and Cerebral Disorders. Baltimore: Williams and Wilkins, 1951.
Hoagland, H., Himwich, H.E., Campbell, E., Fazenkas, G.F., Hadidian, Z.: Effects of hypoglycemia and phenobarbital sodium on electrical activity of cerebral cortex and hypothalamus (dogs). J. Neurophysiol. **2**, 276–288 (1939).
Hobson, Y.A.: The effects of chronic brain stem lesions on cortical and muscular activity during sleep and waking in the cat. Electroenceph. clin. Neurophysiol. **19**, 41–62 (1965).
Hodes, R., Larrabee, M.G., German, W.: The human electromyogram in response to nerve stimulation and the conduction velocity of motor axons. Arch. Neurol. Psychiat. (Chicago) **60**, 340 (1948).
Hoff, F., Jellinger, K.: Neurological problems of brain edema. In: Brain Edema. Klatzo, I., Seitelberger, F. (eds.). Vienna–New York: Springer, 1967.
Höpker, W.: Die Wirkung des Glukosemangels auf das Gehirn. Leipzig: Thieme, 1954.
Hogage, W.: Tracheostomie, ein sorgfältig abzuwägender Eingriff. Dissertation, Vienna, 1960.
Holdorff, B., Cervos-Navarro, J.: Die Pathologie der inneren ponto-mesenzephalen Venen. Radiologie **2**, 465–471 (1971).
Holländer, H.: Histochemische Untersuchungen von Markabbauprodukten bei der protrahierten Form der posttraumatischen Enzephalopathie. Arch. Psychiat. Z. ges. Neurol. **206**, 161–164 (1964).
Hook, O.: Comments on rehabilitation of the brain injured. In: The Late Effects of Head Injury. Walker, A.E., Caveness, W.F., McCritchley, D. (eds.). Springfield/Ill.: Charles C. Thomas, 1969, pp. 398–407.
Hooker, D.: The Prenatal Origin of Behaviour. Univ. of Kansas Press, 1952.
Hornet, T., Petrescu, A.: Accidents cérébraux après syncope cardiaque. Excerpta med. Int. Congr. Ser. **39**, 59–60 (1961).
Hornykiewicz, O.: Metabolism of brain dopamine in human parkinsonism; neurochemical and clinical aspects. In: Proc. Symp. Parkinson's Disease Information and Research Center. Vol. II. Newlett, N.Y.: Raven Press, 1966, pp. 171–185.
Hotovy, R., Enekel, H.J., Gillissen, J., Jahn, U., Krafta, G., Müller-Calgan, H., Mührmann, P., Sommer, S., Strulla, R.: Zur Pharmakologie von Pyrithioxin. Arzneimittel-Forsch. **14**, 26(1964).
Hubach, H., Poeck, K.: Erkennung, Behandlung und Prognose der traumatischen Dezerebation. Dtsch. med. Wschr. **89**, 556–563 (1964).
Huguenard, P., Roujas, F.: Etudes cliniques de l'émulsion lipidique "Lipiphysan" 15p 100. Ann. Anesth. franç. **9**, 479–486 (1968).
Huhn, B., Jakob, H.: Traumatische Hirnstammläsionen mit vieljähriger Überlebensdauer. Nervenarzt **41**, 326–334 (1970).

Husler, J., Spatz, H.: Die Keuchhusteneklampsie. Z. Kinderheilk. **38**, 428–465 (1924).
Infuso, L.: Apallic syndrome in the metabolic diseases. This volume.
Infuso, L., Cortellaro, M., Bianchi-Porco, G.: Semeiotica e clinica dei disturbi neuropsichici nei comi metabolici. Roma: Pozzi, 1967.
Ingvar, D.H., Brun, A.: Das komplette apallische Syndrom. Arch. Psychiat. Nervenheilk. **215**, 219–239 (1972).
Ingvar, D.H., Haggendahl, E., Nilsson, N.J., Sourander, P., Wickborn, J., Lassen, N.A.: Cerebral circulation and metabolism in comatose patient. Arch. Neurol. **11**, 13–21 (1964).
Ingvar, D.H., Sourander, P.: Destruction of the reticular core of the brain stem. Arch. Neurol. **23**, 1–8 (1970).
Irving, J., Le Brun, H.: Myositis ossificans in hemiplegia. J. Bone Jt Surg. **36-B**, 440 (1954).
Ishii, S., Tsuji, H., Evans, J.: Lipid metabolism in cerebral injruy. Trans Amer. neurol. Ass. **91**, 136–139 (1966).
Ivanoff, V.J.: Ein Fall der schweren Schädel-Hirnverletzung mit langdauerndem Koma und Genesung (in Russian). Vop. Nejrohir. **5**, 55–56 (1962).
Iwanow, C.D.: On the clinical significance of quinine oxidase in the serum. Z. ges. inn. Med. **16**, 787–791 (1961).
Jackson, J.H.: Cited by Pentschew, A.: Endogene (hormonale) Vergiftungen. Insulin. Hdb. spez. path. Anat. Hist., Vol. XIII/28. Berlin–Göttingen–Heidelberg: Springer, 1958, pp. 2372–2893.
Jackson, J.H.: Selected Writings of John Hughlings Jackson. In: Taylor, J. (ed.), Vol. II. New York: Basic Books, 1958.
Jakob, H.: Zur Neuropathologie comatöser Zustandsbilder. Med. Welt **3**, 119–122 (1964).
Jaspers, K.: Allgemeine Psychopathologie. Für Studierende, Ärzte und Psychologen. 7th ed. Berlin–Göttingen–Heidelberg: Springer, 1959.
Jeannopoulos, C.L., Leventen, E.O.: Unusual bilateral pre-articular ossification of the elbows. J. Bone Jt Surg. **43-A**, 876–880 (1961).
Jefferson, G.: The natur of concusion. Brit. med. J. **1944 I**, 1–5.
Jefferson, M.: Altered consciousness associated with brain stem lesions. Brain **75**, 55–67 (1952).
Jellinger, K.: Protrahierte Formen der posttraumatischen Enzephalopathie. Beitr. gerichtl. Med. **23**, 65–118 (1965a).
Jellinger, K.: Protrahierte Form der posttraumatischen Enzephalopathie. In: Proc. 8th Internat. Congr. Neurol. Vienna, 1965, Vol. I, pp. 405–408.
Jellinger, K.: Zur Pathogenese und klinischen Bedeutung von Hirnstammläsionen bei protrahierter posttraumatischer Enzephalopathie. In: Cong. Nat. Soc. Neurol. Psychiat. Hurig, Budapest, 1966.
Jellinger, K.: Häufigkeit und Pathogenese zentraler Hirnläsionen nach stumpfer Gewalteinwirkung auf den Schädel. Wien. Z. Nervenheilk. **25**, 223–249 (1967).
Jellinger, K.: Protrahierte posttraumatische Enzephalopathien. Wien. med. Wschr. **118**, 747–753 (1968).
Jellinger, K.: Pathologie zentralnervöser Störungen bei internen Erkrankungen. Wien. Z. Nervenheilk. **29**, 1–37 (1971).
Jellinger, K., Gerstenbrand, F., Pateisky, K.: die protrahierte Form der posttraumatischen Enzephalopathie. Nervenarzt **34**, 145–163 (1963).
Jellinger, K., Seitelberger, F.: Protracted posttraumatic encephalopathy. Pathology, pathogenesis and clinical implications. J. neurol. Sci. **10**, 51–94 (1970).
Jochova, D., Simkova, D., Licha, H.: Correlation of electroencephalographic findings with clinical picture in pancreatic islet tumors. Sborn ved. Pr. Lek. Fak. Karlovy Univ. **8**, 75–79 (1965).
Johnson, J.T.H.: Atypical myositis ossificans. J. Bone Jt Surg. **39-A**, 189 (1957).
Jouvet, M.: Recherches sur les structures nerveuses et les mechanismes responsables des différentes phases du sommeil physiologique. Arch. ital. Biol. **100**, 125–206 (1962).
Jouvet, M.: Etude neurologique-clinique des troubles de la conscience. Acta neurochir. (Wien) **12**, 258–269 (1964).
Jouvet, M.: Neurophysiology of states of sleep. Physiol. Rev. **47**, 117–177 (1967).
Jouvet, M.: Coma and other disorders of consciousness. In: Handbook of Clinical Neurology. Vinken, P.J., Bruyn, G.W. (eds.), Vol. III. Amsterdam: Holland Publ. Co., 1969, pp. 62–79.

Jouvet, M., Dechaume, J.: Séméiologie des troubles de la conscience. Rev. gén. Med. **9**, 961–968 (1960).
Jouvet, M., Pellin, B., Monier, D.: Etude polygraphique des différentes phases du sommeil au course des troubles de conscience chronique (comas prolongés). Rev. neurol. **105**, 181–186 (1961).
Jung, R.: Nystagmographie – Zur Physiologie und Pathologie des optisch-vestibulären Systems beim Menschen. In: Hdb. inn. Med. Bergmann, G.v., Frey, W., Schwiegk, H. (eds.), Vol. V/1. Berlin–Göttingen–Heidelberg: Springer, 1953, p. 1925.
Jung, R.: Die Vibrationsempfindung der Wirbelsäule als lokaldiagnostisches Hilfsmittel bei spinalen Krankheitsprozessen. J. nerv. ment. Dis. **116**, 585–595 (1952).
Kaplan, H.A., Hart, I.C., Browder, I.: Hypothermia associated with a mesencephalic lesion. J. Neuropath. exp. Neurol. **11**, 116–136 (1952).
Kassabcui, E.M.: Study of the visual evoked responses during waking and sleeping in the child. Electroenceph. clin. Neurophysiol. **21**, 512 (1966).
Kautzky, R., Buchard, U.: Beitrag zur Kenntnis des postenzephalographischen Fiebers und zentraler Temperatursteigerungen im allgemeinen. Dtsch. Z. Nervenheilk. **164**, 143–156 (1950).
Keller, A.D.: Autonomic discharges elicited by physiological stimuli in midbrain preparations. Amer. J. Physiol. **100**, 576–581 (1932).
Keller, A.D., McClaskey, E.B.: Localization by the brain slicing method of the level or levels of the cephalic brain stem upon which effective heat dissipation is dependent. Amer. J. Physiol. **45**, 181–213 (1964).
Kety, S.S.: The physiology of the human cerebral circulation. Anesthesiology **10**, 610–614 (1949).
Kety, S.S., Schmidt, C.F.: The mitrous oxide method for the qualitative determination of the cerebral blood flow in man. J. clin. Invest. **27**, 476 (1948).
Kieser, Ch.: Schwere akute Äthylalkoholvergiftung mit postcomatöser Hirn- und Myocardschädigung bei einem 2 1/2jähr. Knaben. Schweiz. med. Wschr. **87**, 542–549 (1957).
Kinzel, Ch.: Ein Verfahren zur quantitativen Abschätzung des irreversiblen psychischen Defektsyndroms nach Hirnkontusionen. Diss., Erlangen, 1971.
Kitani, T.: Liver-Insufficiency. Sci. Session Jap. Soc. intern. Med. **57**, 29–54 (1959).
Klawans, H.L.: The pharmacology of parkinsonism (a review). Dis. nerv. Syst. **12**, 805 (1968).
Klintworth, G.K.: Paratentorial grooving of human brain with particular reference to transtentorial herniation and the pathogenesis of secondary brain stem hemorrhages. Amer. J. Path. **53**, 391–408 (1968).
Klüver, H., Bucy, P.C.: "Psychic blindness" and other symptoms following bilateral lobectomy in rhesus monkeys. Amer. J. Physiol. **119**, 352–353 (1937).
Koch, E.: Psychopathologische Verlaufskontrolle der Restitution. Deutung der Symptomatik nach einem apallischen Syndrom. Diss. Kiel, 1969.
Koestler (1967): Cited in Valzelli, L.: Elementi di psicofarmacologia sperimentale e clinica. Milano: Manfredin, 1970.
Kooi, K.A., Bagchi, B.K.: Oberservations on photocally evoked occipital and vertex waves during sleep in man. Ann. N.Y. Acad. Sci. **112**, 270–280 (1964).
Kornhuber, H.: Physiologie und Klinik des zentralvestibulären Systems (Blick- und Stützmotorik). In: Hals-, Nasen-, Ohrenheilkunde. Berendes, J., Link, R., Zöllner, F. (eds), Vol. III/3. Stuttgart: Thieme, 1966, p. 2150.
Kornhuber, H.H.: Zur Bedeutung multisensorischer Integration im Nervensystem. Dtsch. Z. Nervenheilk. **187**, 478–484 (1965a).
Kornhuber, H.H.: Über häufige, aber wenig beachtete Arten von Nystagmus und Schwindel: Paroxysmaler Lageschwindel und lateraler Fixationsnystagmus. Nervenarzt **36**, 361–362 (1965b).
Koufen, H., Consbruck, U.: Die Lithium-Intoxikation. Beobachtungen an 6 Fällen. Nervenarzt **43**, 145–152 (1972).
Kramer, W.: Progressive, posttraumatic encephalopathy during reanimation. Acta neurol. scand. **40**, 249–258 (1964).
Krauland, W.: Die pathologische Anatomie des Schädeltraumas. Wien. klin. Wschr. **75**, 489–492 (1963).
Krauland, W.: Über Hirnschäden durch stumpfe Gewalt. Dtsch. Z. Nervenheilk. **163**, 265–328 (1950).

Krenn, J., Kucher, R., Steinbereithner, K.: Pflege des Patienten. In: Intensivstation, -pflege, -therapie. Kucher, R., Steinbereithner, K. (eds.). Stuttgart: Thieme, 1972.
Krenscher, H.: Die Durchblutung und Sauerstoffaufnahme des Gehirns in Narkose: In: Hydrodynamik, Elektrolyt- und Säure-Basen-Haushalt im Liquor und Nervensystem. Kiehle (ed.). Stuttgart: Thieme, 1962, pp. 144–150.
Kretschmer, E.: Das apallische Syndrom. Z. ges. Neurol. Psychiat. **169**, 576–579 (1940).
Kretschmer, E.: Der Begriff der motorischen Schablonen und ihre Rolle in normalen und pathologischen Lebensvorgängen. Arch. Psychiat. Nervenkr. **190**, 1–3 (1953).
Krieger, D.T., Krieger, H.P.: Circadian variations in 17-OHCS in central nervous system diseases. J. clin. Endocr. **26**, 929 (1966).
Krnijevic, K.: Glutamate and gamma-aminobutricic acid brain. Nature (Lond.) **228**, 119 (1970).
Kroll, F.W. von: Hauttemperaturmessungen bei zentralen Fiberstörungen. Dtsch. Z. Nervenheilk. **135**, 232–245 (1935).
Krupka, H.: Psychopathologische Veränderungen in der Rückbildungsphase nach apallischem Syndrom an Hand eines Falles. Diss. Kiel, 1967.
Kryspin-Exner, K.: Zur Behandlung schizophrener Prozeßpsychosen mit Thiobroperazin. Wien. klin. Wschr. **75**, 157–160 (1963).
Kubicki, S.: Bewertung elektroencephalographischer Bilder bei schweren cerebralen Funktionsstörungen. Verh. dtsch. Ges. inn. Med. **69**, 94–99 (1963).
Kubicki, S.: Nervice przwodu pokarmowego. Wiad. lek. **18**, 1761–1766 (1965a).
Kubicki, S.: Nowe mozliwosci w diagnosticg chorob przewody pokarmowego. Pstepy H.G. Med. Posw. **19**, 1761–1766 (9165b).
Kucher, R., Lechner, G., Pokieser, H., Steinbereithner, K.: Spätschäden der Trachea nach Tracheotomie. Anaesthesist **16**, 157 (1967).
Laborit, H., Weber, B., Oruellas, M.R., Baron, C.: Etude pharmacologique de la dihydroxyacétone. Conséquences thérapeutique. Agressologie **7**, 581–596 (1966).
Laederich, L.J., Bernard-Pichon, J.: Dermite bullo-ulcéreuse et polynévrite par intoxication barbituque. Bull. Soc. méd. Hôp. Paris **49**, 1414 (1935).
Laine, E., Fossati, P., Christiaens, J.L., Lefrevre, J., Racadot, J., Leroy, M.N., Linquette, N.: Les perfusions intravénneuses d'émulsion lipidique en réanimation neurochirurgicale. Lille méd. **11**, 368–373 (1966).
Lapresle, J., Benhamida, M.: The dento-olivari pathway. Arch. Neurol. **22**, 135–143 (1970).
Larrabee, M.G., Garcia Ramos, J., Bulbring, E.: Effects of anesthetics on oxygen-consumption and on synaptic transmission in sympathetic ganglia. J. cell comp. Physiol. **40**, 461–494 (1952).
Lasagna, L., Epstein, L.C.: A comparison of the effects of the orally administered barbiturate salts and barbiturate acids on human psychomotor performance. In: Proc. Internat. Symposium on Amphetamine and Related Compounds. New York: Raven Press, 1969.
Lassen, N.A.: Cerebral blood flow and oxygen consumption in man. Physiol. Rev. **39**, 183–238 (1959).
Lassen, N.A.: The luxury perfusion syndrome and its possible relations to acute metabolic acidosis localized within the brain. Lancet **1966 II**, 1113–1115.
Lassen, N.A., Ingvar, D.H.: Regional cerebral blood flow measurement in man. Arch. Neurol. **9**, 615–622 (1963).
Lassen, G.: Disorders of central temperature regulation. In: Modern Aspects of Neurosurgery. Pia, H.W., Grote, E., Mundinger, F., Gleave, J.R.W. (eds.), Vol. I–II. Amsterdam: Excerpta Medica, 1971, pp. 11–115.
Lausberg, G.: Posttraumatische zentrale Hyperthermie und Hypothermie. Acta chir. **5**, 353–358 (1970a).
Lausberg, G.: Der Verlust der Temperaturregelung beim zentralen Tod – reversibel? Dtsch. med. Wschr. **24**, 1301–1303 (1970b).
Lausberg, G.: Signification des troubles de la thermo-régulation chez les polytraumatisés à lésion cranieue prédominate. Cah. Anesth. **19**, 315–324 (1971b).
Lausberg, G.: Zentrale Störungen der Temperaturregulation. Acta neurochir. (Wien), Suppl. **19**, 1–168 (1972).
Lazarus, S.S., Volk, B.W.: Histochemical and electron microscopic studies of a functioning insulinoma. Lab. Invest. **11**, 1279 (1962).
Le Beau, J., Funck-Brentano, J.L., Castaigne, P.: Le traitement des comas prolongés. Presse méd. **66**, 820–833 (1958).

Le Beau, J., Pradat, P., Thoulmonde, M.: Action de la léeglutamine sur les troubles de la conscience en neurochirurgie. Rev. neurol. **106**, 25–33 (1962).
Lehmann, H.J., Gloeckner, R.J.: Cerebral disconnection in multiple sclerosis. Europ. Neurol. **8**, 257–269 (1972).
Lehmann, H.J., Ule, G.: Subakute Enzephalitisformen unbekannter Ätiologie. Arch. Psychiat. Z. ges. Neurol. **206**, 356–366 (1964).
Lepetit, J.M., Vallat, J.N., Mathieu, S., Radvanji, M.F., Eliet-Flescher, J., Fischgold, H.: Etude du nychtemére dans un état comateux prolongé. Etude électro-clinique. Rev. neurol. **115**, 526–529 (1966).
Lesny, J.: Entwicklungsdiagnostik in der Kinderneurologie. Berlin: VEB Volk und Gesundheit, 1965.
Leson, M.: Contribution à l'étude des comas prolongés. Médical thesis, Paris, 1960.
Levine, M.: Pathophysiologie und Klinik. Hdb. des Diabetes mellitus, Vol. I. Munich: Lehmann. 1969.
Lewin, W.: Preliminary observations on external hydrocephalus after severe head injury. Brit. J. Surg. **55**, 747–751 (1968).
Lhermitte, F., Gautier, J.C., Marteau, R., Chain, F.: Troubles de la conscience et mutisme akinétique. Etude anatomo-clinique d'un ramollissement paramédian, bilatéral du pédoncule cérébrale et du thalamus. Rev. neurol. **109**, 115–131 (1963).
Liberson, M.: Soft tissue calcifications in cord lesions. J. Amer. med. Ass. **152**, 1010 (1953).
Liebaldt, G.: Zur synotischen Darstellung cyto-myelo- und angio-architektonischer Strukturen im Zentralnervensystem. Zbl. allg. Path. **105**, 343–346 (1964).
Liebaldt, G., Descalze, J.: Idiopathische (nicht arteriosklerotische) Verkalkungsvorgänge im ZNS. Dtsch. Z. Nervenheilk. **184**, 388–426 (1963).
Liebaldt, G.P., Scheller, H.: Amnestisches Syndrom und Korsakow-Syndrom-2, auch anatomisch-lokalisatorisch unterscheidbare Syndrome. Nervenarzt **42**, 402–412 (1971).
Liepmann, H.: Über die agnostischen Störungen. Neurol. Zbl. **27**, 609–617 (1968).
Lindenberg, R.: Selective Vulnerability of the Brain in Hypoxaemia. Oxford: Blackwell, 1963, p. 189.
Lindenberg, R.: Die Schädigungsmechanismen der Substantia nigra bei Hirntraumen und das Problem des posttraumatischen Parkinsonismus. Dtsch. Z. Nervenheilk. **185**, 637–663 (1964).
Lindenberg, R.: Trauma of meninges and brain. In: Pathology of the Nervous System. Minckler, J. (ed.), Vol. II. New York: McGraw-Hill, 1971, pp. 1705–1765.
Lindenberg, R., Fischer, R.S., Durlacher, S.H., Lovitt, W.V., Freytag, E.: Lesions of the corpus callosum following blunt mechanical trauma to the head. Amer. J. Path. **31**, 297–310 (1955).
Lindenberg, R., Freytag, E.: The mechanism of cerebral contusions. Arch. Path. (Chicago) **69**, 440–469 (1960).
Lindgren, E.: Encephalography in cerebral atrophy. Acta radiol. (Stockh.) **35**, 277–291 (1951).
Lindsley, D.B., Bowden, J.W., Magoun, H.W.: Effects upon the EEG of acute injury to the brain stem activating system. Electroenceph. clin. Neurophysiol. **1**, 475–486 (1949).
Lindsley, D.B., Schreiner, L.H., Knowles, A.B., Magoun, H.W.: Behavioural and EEG changes following chronic brain stem lesions in cats. Electroenceph. clin. Neurophysiol. **2**, 483–498 (1950).
Loeb, C., Rosadini, G.: Correlazioni anatomeletrichi nella perdita dei conscienza. Neurone (Mantova) **5**, 179–182 (1957).
Loeb, C., Rosadini, G., Poggio, G.F.: Electroencephalograms during coma. Normal and borderline records in 5 patients. Neurology (Minneap.) **9**, 610–618 (1959).
Loew, F., Wüstner, S.: Diagnose, Behandlung und Prognose der traumatischen Haematome des Schädelinneren. Acta neurochir. (Wien), Suppl. **VIII** (1960).
Lorber, J.: Ectopic ossification in tuberculous meningitis. Arch. Dis. Childh. **28**, 98 (1953).
Lorente, De No, R.: Vestibulo-ocular reflex arc. Arch. Neurol. Psychiat. (Chicago) **30**, 245 (1933).
Lorente, De No, R.: Analysis of the activity of the chains of internuncial neurons. J. Neurophysiol. **1**, 207 (1938).
Lorenz, K.: Er redete mit dem Vieh, den Vögeln und den Fischen. Cologne: Kiepenheuer 1961; Deutscher Taschenbuch-Verlag, 1964.

Lücking, C.H.: Das apallische Syndrom. Clinical pathophysiology of the apallic syndrome. This volume.
Lücking, C.H.: Sleep-like patterns and abnormal arousal reactions in brain stem lesions. Electroenceph. clin. Neurophysiol. **28**, 214 (1970).
Lücking, C.H.: Das Elektroenzephalogramm in der Intensivtherapie. In: Intensivstation, -pflege und -therapie. Kucher, R., Steinbereithner, K. (eds.). Stuttgart: Thieme, 1972, pp. 367–375.
Mägi, M.A.: Klinische und elektroenzephalographische Untersuchungen bei langdauernden Komazuständen (insbesondere bei Schädel-Hirn-Verletzungen) (in Russian). Vop. klin. neurol. Psychiat. **5**, 45–48 (1965).
Mägi, M.A.: Dynamics of prolonged comatose states (in Russian). Vop. klin. neurol. Psychiat. **7**, 221–231 (1968).
Magliani, A., Bizzi, E., Apelbaum, J., Zanchet, A.: Ascending afferent mechanism maintaining sham-rage behaviour in the acute thalamic cat. Arch. ital. Biol. **101**, 632–647 (1963).
Magnus, K.: Körperstellungen. Berlin–Göttingen–Heidelberg: Springer, 1924.
Magnus, R., de Kleyn, A.: Die Abhängigkeit des Tonus der Extremitätenmuskeln von der Kopfstellung. Pflügers Arch. ges. Physiol. **145**, 455–548 (1912).
Magnus, R., de Kleyn, A.: Körperstellung, Gleichgewicht und Bewegung bei Säuglingen. Haltung und Stellung bei Säuglingen. In: Handbuch der Physiologie. Bethe, A., Bergmann, V. (eds.). Berlin: Springer, 1930.
Malavaud, A., Voldoir, A., Archard, M.: Trois mois de "drip feeding" chez un comateux traumatique. Afr. franç. chir. **16**, 273–275 (1958).
Mantegazzini, P., Ferrara, G.B.: Azione della 3,4-diossifenilalanina (DOPA), della dopamina e dell'adrenalina sulla miosi da sonno. Arch. ital. Sci. farmacol. **10**, 284 (1960).
Marinesco, G., Radovici, H.: Sur un réflexe cutané nouveau, réflexe palmo-mentonnier. Rev. neurol. **36**, 236–240 (1920).
Mason, J.W.: The central nervous system regulation of ACTH secretion. In: Reticular Formation of the Brain. Jasper, H.H. (ed.). Boston: Little Brown, 1958, p. 663.
Maspes, P.E., Marossero, F.: Cosiderazioni cliniche ed elettraencefalografiche su di un caso di rammollimento ischemico circoscritto ad una parte dei nuclei a proiezione diffusa del talamo. Riv. Pat. nerv. ment. **78**, 21–32 (1957).
Masshoff, W.: Allgemeine und spezielle Pathologie der Vita reducta . Verh. dtsch. Ges. inn Med. **69**, 59–64 (1963a).
Masshoff, W.: Allgemeines zur Vita reducta. Verh. dtsch. Ges. inn. Med. **69**, 12–15 (1963b).
Matsumoto, J., Jouvet, M.: Effects de réserpine, DOPA et 5-HTP sur les deux états de sommeil. C.R. Soc. Biol. (Paris) **158**, 2137 (1964).
Matsumoto, J., Nishisho, T., Sadahiro, T., Myoshi, M.: Influence of fatique on sleep. Nature (Lond.) **218**, 177 (1968).
Mattson, R.H., Lecoq, F.R.: Nerve conduction in volocity in fasting patients. Neurology (Minneap.) **18**, 335–339 (1968).
Mayer, E.Th.: Zentrale Hirnschäden nach Einwirkung stumpfer Gewalt auf den Schädel. Arch. Psychiat. Neurol. **210**, 238–262 (1967).
Mayer, E.Th.: Zur Klinik und Pathologie des traumatischen Mittelhirn- und apallischen Syndroms. Ärztl. Forsch. **22**, 163–172 (1968).
Mayer, E.Th.: Zur Pathologie des traumatischen Mittelhirn- und apallischen Syndroms. Radiologie **9**, 16–22 (1969).
McCormick, W.F., Danneel, C.M.: Central pontine myelinosis. Arch. intern. Med. **119**, 444–478 (1967).
McCougall, J., Wyllie, A.M.: A fatal case of paraldehyde poisoning, with post-mortem findings. J. ment. Sci. **78**, 369–376 (1932).
McGeer, P., McGeer, E., Wada, J.: Central aromatic amine levels and behaviour.
McGeer, P., McGeer, E., Wada, J.: Serotonin and catecholamine levels in various cat brain areas following administration of psychoactive drugs or amine precursors. Arch. Neurol. (Paris) **9**, 81–89 (1963).
McLennan, H., York, D.H.: The action of dopamine on neurons of the caudate nucleus. J. Physiol. (Lond.) **189**, 393 (1967).
McNealy, D.E., Plum, E.: Brain stem disfunction with supratentorial mass lesions. Arch. Neurol. (Paris) **7**, 10–32 (1962).

McNeur, J.C.: Calcification round the hips in paraplegia. (Three cases). Proc. roy. Soc. Med. (Section of Orthopaedics) **47**, 14 (1954).
Meister, A.: Metabolism of glutamine. Physiol. Rev. **36**, 103–127 (1957).
Mertens, H.G.: Die disseminierte Neuropathie im Coma. Zur Differenzierung der sogenannten toxischen Polyneuropathien. Nervenarzt **32**, 71 (1961).
Meyer, J.S., Kondo, A., Nomura, F., Sakamoto, K., Teraura, T.: Cerebral hemodynamics and metabolism following experimental head injury. J. Neurosurg. **32**, 304–319 (1970).
Meyer, R.F., Denny-Brown, D.: Conduction velocity in peripheral nerve during experimental demyelination in the cat. Neurology (Minneap.) **14**, 714 (1964).
Michon, P., Larcon, A., Huriet, C., Streiff, F.: Indications et limites de l'emploi du lucidril en réanimation médicale. Agressologie **2**, 575 (1961).
Mifka, P.: Erworbene Demenz bei traumatischen Einflüssen. Wien. med. Wschr. **116**, 396–397 (1966).
Miller, L.F., O'Neill, C.J.: Myositis ossificans in paraplegies. J. Bone Jt Surg. **31-A**, 283 (1949).
Minauf, M., Schacht, L.: Zentrale Hirnschäden nach Einwirkung stumpfer Gewalt auf den Schädel. II. Mitteilung. Läsionen im Bereich der Stammganglien. Arch. Psychiat. Nervenkr. **208**, 162–176 (1966).
Mingrino, S., Molinari, G., Andrioli, G., Frugoni, P.: Some observations upon vestibular reactions in acute head injury. Excerpta med. Int. Congr. Ser. **110**, 26 (1965).
Mingrino, S., Molinari, G., Babighian, G.: Modificazioni del riflesso vestibulo-oculare nel coma sperimentalmente in dotto. Boll. Soc. ital. Biol. sper. **42**, 1900 (1966).
Minkowski, M.: Neurobiologische Studien am menschlichen Foetus. In: Handbuch der biologischen Arbeitsmethoden. Abderhalden, E. (ed.), Vol. V. Berlin–Vienna: Urban & Schwarzenberg, 1928, pp. 511–618.
Model, W.: Drugs of Choice. 1970–1971. St. Louis: Mosby, 1970, p. 924.
Möllmann, M.: Zerebraler Defektzustand nach verlängertem Coma im Verlauf einer Insulinschockbehandlung. Arch. Psychiat. Nervenkr. **112**, 76–89 (1940).
Mollaret, P., Bertrand, J., Mollaret, H.: Coma dépassé et nécroses nerveuses centrales massives. Rev. neurol. **101**, 116–139 (1959).
Mollaret, P., Goulon, M.: Le coma dépassé. Rev. neurol. **101**, 3–15 (1959).
Monnier, M.: Retinal, cortical and motor responses to photic stimulation in man. Retino-cortical time and opto-motor integration time. J. Neurphysiol. **15**, 469–486 (1952).
Monnier, M., Tissot, R.: Action de la réserpine et de ses médiateurs (5-HTP, sérotonine et DOPA-noradrénalin) sur le comportement et le cerveau du lapin. Helv. physiol. Acta **16**, 255 (1958).
Monnier, M., Willi, H.: Die integrative Tätigkeit des Nervensystems beim normalen Säugling und beim bulbo-spinalen Anencephalus (Rautenhirnwesen). Ann. paediat. (Basel) **169**, 289–308 (1947).
Monnier, M., Willi, H.: Die integrative Tätigkeit des Nervensystems beim meso-rhombo-spinalen Anencephalus (Mittelhirnwesen). 1. Physiologisch-klinischer Teil. Mschr. Psychiat. Neurol. **126**, 239–258 (1953).
Moro, E.: Zur Symptomatik des Mongolismus. Dtsch. med. Wschr. **10**, 536 (1920).
Moruzzi, G.: Active processes in the brain stem during sleeping. The Harvey Lectures Series 58. New York:London: Academic Press, 1963, pp. 233–297.
Moruzzi, G.: The sleep-waking cycle. Ergebn. Physiol. **64**, 1–165 (1972).
Moruzzi, G., Magoun, H.W.: Brain stem reticular formation and activation of the EEG. Electroenceph. clin. Neurophysiol. **1**, 455–473 (1949).
Mucha, H.: Flexibilitas ceria unter neuroleptischer Behandlung. Nervenarzt **37**, 272–274 (1966).
Müller, D.: Das Problem der Funktion und der Form des Achsenorgans. In: Neurologie der Wirbelsäule und des Rückenmarks im Kindesalter. Jena: VEB Fischer, 1964, pp. 47–113.
Müller, D.: Fehldiagnosen infolge Massenverschiebung des Gehirns. In: Die klinische Lokalisation der Hirntumoren. Leonhard, K. (ed.). Leipzig: Barth, 1965.
Müller, D.: Neurologische Untersuchung und Diagnostik im Kindesalter. Vienna-New York: Springer, 1968.
Mumenthaler, M.: Dezerebration nach Kohlenmonoxydvergiftung. Schweiz. Arch. Neurol. Neurochir. Psychiat. **88**, 248–272 (1961).
Mumenthaler, M., Schliack, H.: Läsionen peripherer Nerven, Diagnostik und Therapie. Stuttgart: Thieme, 1965.

Muting, D.: Untersuchungen zur Pathogenese des Coma hepaticum. Med. Welt **19**, 1081–1085 (1962).
Myrianthopoulos, N.C., Kurland, A.A., Kurland, L.T.: Hereditary predisposition in drug-induced Parkinsonism. Arch. Neurol. Psychiat. (Chicago) **6**, 19–23 (1962).
Nagel, W., Gött, H., Colmant, H.J.: Klinik, Elektroenzephalogramm und Anatomie eines Falles von subakuter, sklerosierender Leukoenzephalitis (van Bongaert). Ann. paediat. (Basel) **193**, 193–225 (1959).
Nakayama, T., Hardy, J.D.: Unit responses in the rabbit's brain stem to changes in brain and cutaneous temperature. J. appl. Physiol. **27**, 848–857 (1969).
Narabayashi, H.: Athetosis or the spastic state of cerebral palsy. In: 1st Internat. Symp. Stereoencephalotomy, Philadelphia. Confin. neurol. (Basel) **22**, 364–367 (1962).
Neuhaus, G.: Pathophysiologie und Klinik von Erkrankungen bei Patienten unter den Bedingungen der Vita reducta. Verh. dtsch. Ges. inn. Med. **69**, 16–39 (1963).
Nevin, N.C.: Neuropathological changes in the white matter following head injury. J. Neuropath. exp. Neurol. **26**, 77–84 (1967).
Nyström, S.: A case decortication following a severe head injury. Acta psychiat. scand. **35**, 101–112 (1960).
Ojemann, R.G., Fisher, C.M., Adams, R.D., Sweet, W.H., New, P.F.: Further experience with the syndrome of "normal pressure" hydrocephalus. J. Neurosurg. **31**, 279–294 (1969).
Olsen, C.W.: Lesions of peripheral nerves developing during coma. J. Amer. med. Ass. **160**, 39 (1956).
Olszewski, J., Baxter, D.: Cytoarchitecture of the Human Brain Stem. Basel–New York: Karger, 1954.
Opitz, E.: Energieumsatz des Gehirns in situ unter aeroben und anaeroben Bedingungen. In: Die Chemie und der Stoffwechsel des Nervengewebes. 3rd Mosbacher Kolloquium, Berlin–Göttingen–Heidelberg: Springer, 1952.
Oppenheimer, D.R.: Microscopic lesions in the brain following head injury. J. Neurol. Psychiat. Neurosurg. **31**, 229–306 (1968).
Orth, D.W., Island, D.P., Liddle, G.W.: Experimental alterations of the circadian rhythm in plasma cortisol concentration in man. J. clin. Endocr. **27**, 549 (1967).
Orthner, H.: Neuroanatomische Gesichtspunkte der Schlaf-Wach-Regelung. In: Der Schlaf. Jovanović, U. (ed.). Munich: Ambr. Bart, 1969, pp. 69–84.
Osetowska, E.: La leuco-encéphalopathie oedémateuse posttramatique. J. neurol. Sci. **1**, 458–466 (1964).
Otteni, J., Gauthier-Lafaye, P.: Indikationen und Komplikationen bei Tracheotomie und Dauerintubation. Anästhesist **19**, 291–295 (1969).
Owen, O.E., Morgan, A.P., Kemp, H.G., Sullivan, G.M., Herrera, M.G., Cahill, G.F.: Brain metabolism during fasting. J. clin. Invest. **46**, 1589–1595 (1967).
Parsons-Smith, B.G., Summerskill, W.H.J., Dawson, A.M., Sherlock, S.: The electroencephalograph in liver disease. Lancet **273**, 867–871 (1957).
Passonean, J., Lowry, O.H.: Phosphofructokinase and the control of the citric acid circle. Biochem. biophys. Res. Commun. **13**, 372 (1963).
Patton, H.D.: Higher control of autonomic outflows. The hypothalamus. In: Medical Physiology and Biophysics. Ruch, T.C., Fulton, J.F. (eds.). Philadelphia–London: Saunders, 1960, pp. 234–248.
Peiper, A.: Die Eigenart der kindlichen Hirntätigkeit. Leipzig: VEB Thieme, 1949.
Pelage, S., D'Escrivain, Leger, Jonier: A propos du réveil spectaculaire de deux comas traumatiques par le Lucidril. Observations cliniques et EEG. Congr. Psych. Neurol. de Langue Franç., Lille, 1960.
Penin, H.: Über den diagnostischen Wert des Hirnstrombildes bei der hepaportalen Enzephalopathie. Fortschr. Neurol. Psychiat. **35**, 173–234 (1967).
Pentschew, A.: Endogene (hormonale) Vergiftungen. Insulin. In: Hdb. spez. path. Anat. u. Hist. Scholz, W.(ed.), Vol. XIII/2B. Berlin–Göttingen–Heidelberg: Springer, 1958, pp. 2372–2893.
Perria, L., Rivano, C., Rosadini, G., Sannita, W.: Il tratamente con escina nell'edema cerebrale. Rass. clin.-sci. Ist. biochim. ital. **45**, 320–323 (1969).
Peters, G.: Spezielle Pathologie der Krankheiten des zentralen und peripheren Nervensystems. Stuttgart: Thieme, 1951, pp. 220–258.
Peters, G.: Die gedeckten Hirn- und Rückenmarksverletzungen. In: Hdb. spez. path. Anat. u. Hist. Scholz, W. (ed.), Vol. XIII/3. Berlin–Göttingen–Heidelberg: Springer, 1955, pp. 118–136.

Peters, G.: Morphologische Forschung in der Neurologie und Psychiatrie. Nervenarzt **37**, 429 (1966).
Peters, G.: Pathologische Anatomie der Verletzungen des Gehirns und seiner Häute. In: Neuro-Traumatologie. Kessel, F.K., Guttmann, L., Maurer, G. (eds.), Vol. I. Munich–Berlin–Vienna: Urban & Schwarzenberg, 1969, pp. 31–91.
Peters, G.: Neuropathology of the traumatic apallic syndrome. This volume.
Peters, U.H.: Psychopathology of the apallic syndrome. This volume.
Pfeiffer, C.C., Jenny, E.H., Gallagher, W., Smith, R.P., Bevan, W., Jr., Killam, K.F., Killam, E.K., Blackmore, W.: Stimulant effect of 2-dimethylaminoethanol. Possible precursor of brain acetylcholine. Science **126**, 610 (1957).
Pia, H.W.: Die Schädigung des Hirnstamms bei den raumfordernden Prozessen. Ein Beitrag zur Pathogenese, Klinik und Behandlung der Massenverschiebungen des Gehirns. Acta neurochir. (Wien), Suppl. **IV**, 1525–1531 (1957).
Pilleri, G.: Orale Entstellung nach Art des Klüver-Bucy-Syndroms nach hirnatrophischen Prozessen. Schweiz. Arch. Neurol. Psychiat. **87**, 286–298 (1961a).
Pilleri, G.: Über das chronologische Auftreten von motorischen Schablonen des Oralsinnes, deren ontogenetische Bedeutung und klinisch-anatomische Zusammenhänge bei atrophisierenden Hirnerkrankungen. Schweiz. Arch. Neurol. Psychiat. **88**, 273–298 (1961b).
Pilleri, G., Poeck, K.: Arterhaltende und soziale Instinktbewegungen als neurologische Symptome beim Menschen. Psychiat. Neurol. **147**, 193–238 (1964).
Plum, F.: The CSF in hepatic encephalopathy. Exp. Biol. Med. **4**, 34–41 (1971).
Plum, F., Posner, J.B.: Diagnosis of Stupor and Coma. Philadelphia: F.A. Davis, 1966.
Poeck, K., Hubach, H.: Rhythmische orale Automatismen bei Dezerebrationszuständen. Dtsch. Z. Nervenheilk. **185**, 37–52 (1963).
Pötzl, O.: Die optisch-agnostischen Störungen. Leipzig–Vienna: Deuticke, 1928.
Polli, E.E.: Pathogenetic problems and classification of neuropsychic disturbances. Exp. Biol. Med. **4**, 1–14 (1971).
Pompeiano, O., Brodal, A.: Experimental demonstration of a somaticotropic origin of rubro-spinal fibers in the cat. J. comp. Neurol. **108**, 225–251 (1957).
Posner, J.B., Plum, F.: Spinal fluid pH and neurologic symptoms in acidosis. New Engl. J. Med. **277**, 605 (1967).
Prechtl., H.F.R.: Die Entwicklung und Eigenart frühkindlicher Bewegungsweisen. Klin. Wschr. **34**, 281–284 (1956).
Prill, A.: Die neurologische Symptomatologie der Niereninsuffizienz. In: Schriftenreihe Neurologie, Vol. II. Berlin–Heidelberg–New York: Springer, 1969.
Quadbeck, G., Landmann, H.R., Sachsse, W., Schmidt, I.: Der Einfluß von Pyrithiaxin auf die Blut-Hirnschranke. Med. exp. **7**, 144 (1962).
Quadbeck, G., Sachsse, W.: Beeinflussung der Blut-Hirnschranke durch Neuroleptika im Dauerversuch. Arch. Psychiat. Nervenkr. **201**, 580–592 (1961).
Quatember, R., Sluga, W., Tschabitscher, H.: Die Bedeutung der Teamarbeit in der Wiederherstellungstherapie neurologischer Krankheitsbilder. Wien. klin. Wschr. **73**, 174–177 (1961).
Rabe, W., Möller, W.D., Völker, B.: Immunsuppressive Therapie bei der subakuten sklerosierenden Panenzephalitis. Nervenarzt **42**, 603–605 (1971).
Rademaker, G.G.J.: Das Stehen. Statische Reaktionen, Gleichgewichtsreaktionen und Muskeltonus unter besonderer Berücksichtigung ihres Verhaltens bei kleinhirnlosen Tieren. Berlin–Göttingen–Heidelberg: Springer, 1931.
Reichardt, M.: Hirnstamm und Seelisches. Fortschr. Neurol. Psychiat. **16**, 81–105 (1944).
Reis, D., Moorhead, D., Merlino, N.: DOPA-induced excitement in the cat. Arch. Neurol. (Paris) **22**, 31–39 (1970).
Reissigl, H.: Praxis der Flüssigkeitstherapie. Munich–Berlin: Urban & Schwarzenberg, 1965.
Reulen, H.J., Medzihradsky, F., Enzenbach, F., Marguth, F., Brendel, W.: Electrolytes, fluids and energy metabolism in human cerebral edema. Arch. Neurol. (Paris) **21**, 517–525 (1969).
Reymond, J.C., Fau, R.: Coma traumatique exceptionnellement prolongé. Trépanation au troisième mois. Guérison avec un minimum de séquelles. Mém. Acad. Chir. **82**, 39–42 (1956).
Richardson, J.C., Chambers, R.A., Heywood, P.M.: Encephalopathy of anoxia and hypoglycemia. Arch. Neurol. (Paris) **1**, 178–190 (1959).

Riecker, G.: Enzephalopathien als Folge von Elektrolytstörungen. Verh. dtsch. Ges. inn. Med. **72**, 125–141 (1967).
Rioch, D.Mc.K.: Discussion in: Brain Mechanism and Consciousness. Delafresnaje, J.F. (ed.). Springfield/Ill.: Charles C. Thomas, 1954, pp. 133–134.
Riser, M., Geraud, J., Gayral, L.: Les troubles nerveux au cours du traitment par les neuroleptiques et par les nouveaux sédatifs tranquillisants. Médical **59**, 93–101 (1958).
Rix, D.: Experimentelle Untersuchungen über die klinischen Erscheinungsformen der Bewußtseinstrübung und der Bewußtlosigkeit. Diss., Cologne, 1967.
Roberts, E.: Diskussionsbemerkungen in: Exp. Biol. Med. **4**, 31 (1971).
Rodbell, J.: Wirkung des Insulins auf die Zellmembran. In: Hdb. des Diabetes Mellitus. Pathophysiologie und Klinik. Pfeiffer, E.F. (ed.), Vol. I. Munich: J.F. Lehmanns, 1969.
Roger, A., Rossi, G.F., Zirnondoli, A.: Le rôle des nervs craniens dans le maintien de l'état vigile de la préparation "encéphale isolé". Electroenceph. clin. Neurophysiol. **8**, 1–13 (1956).
Rondot, P., Ben Hamida, M.: Myoclonies du volle et myoclonies squeletiques. Etude clinique et anatomique. Rev. neurol. **120**, 59–83 (1968).
Rosadini, G., Gentilomo, A.: Quadri EEG di sonnonella sindrome apallica. Riv. Neurol. **37**, 469–476 (1967).
Rosenblath, W.: Über einen bemerkenswerten Fall von Hirnerschütterung (aus dem Landeskrankenhaus Cassel). Dtsch. Arch. klin. Med. **64**, 406-424 (1899).
Rossi, G.F.: Electroencefalogramma e comportamento dopo lesioni chroniche della sostanza reticolare e delle vie della sensibilita specifica. In: Atti del Congr. di Parma, November 1957, pp. 131–151.
Rossi, G.F.: Sleep.inducing mechanism in the brain stem. Electroenceph. Neurophysiol. Suppl. **24**, 113–132.
Rossi, G.F.: L'influence du tronc cérébrale sur le niveau de conscience et sur l'activité électrique cérébrale. Journée du tronc cérébrale, Marseille (in press).
Rossi, G.F.: Nuove considerazioni sui meccanismi fisiopatologici delle variazioni di conscienza. Minerva neurochir. **6**, 129–141 (1962).
Rossi, G.F.: Discussion at Conf. on the Appallic Syndrome, Verona, Italy. April 1970.
Rossi, G.F., Zanchetti, A.: The brain stem reticular formation. Anatomy and physiology. Arch. ital. Biol. **95**, 199–433 (1957).
Rowbotham, G.F.: Acute Injuries of the Head. Edinburgh: Livingstone, 1945.
Salmon, J.H.: Surgical treatment of severe post-traumatic encephalopathy. Surg. Gynec. Obstet. **133**, 634–636 (1971).
Sauter, R.: Zustand nach apallischem Syndrom: Psychopathologische Untersuchungen. Proc. 8th Internat. Congr. Neurol. Vienna, 1965, Vol. I, pp. 121–124.
Sayk, J.: Über die kortikalen und subkortikalen Funktionsstörungen in Folge Herzstillstand im Vergleich zum neuropathologischen Befund. Arch. Psychiat. Nervenkr. **201**, 565–579 (1961).
Schacht, L., Minauf, M.: Zentrale Hirnschäden nach Einwirkung stumpfer Gewalt auf den Schädel. 1. Mitteilung: Balkenläsionen. Arch. Psychiat. Nervenkr. **207**, 416–427 (1965).
Schaltenbrandt, G.: Normale Bewegungs- und Lagereaktionen bei Kindern. Dtsch. Z. Nervenheilk. **87**, 24–59 (1925).
Schenker, S., McCandless, Brophy, E., Lewis, M.S.: Studies of the intercerebral toxicity of ammonia. J. clin. Invest. **46**, 838–848 (1967).
Scherzer, E.: Die Störungen des Gleichgewichtssystems nach Unfällen. Vienna: Verlag der Wiener med. Akademie, 1968.
Schewe, G., Adebahr, A.: Sekundärschäden am Gehirn bei Schädeltrauma. Z. Rechtsmed. **67**, 129–146 (1970).
Schliack, H.: Neurologische Differentialdiagnose und Prognose in der vita reducta. Verh. dtsch. Ges. inn. Med. **69**, 84–93 (1963).
Schliack, H., Kubicki, S.: Neurologische und elektroenzephalographische Differentialdiagnose und Prognose in der vita reducta. Zbl. Neurochir. **24**, 242–249 (1964).
Schmidt, C.G.: Gehirn und Nerven. In: Hdb. der physiolog. Chemie II, Der Stoffwechsel. Berlin–Göttingen–Heidelberg: Springer, 1956.
Schneider, H.: Der Hirntod. Begriffsgeschichte und Pathogenese. Nervenarzt **41**, 381–387 (1970).
Schneider, K.: Klinische Psychopathologie, 8th ed. Stuttgart: Thieme, 1967.

Scholz, W., Boellaard, J.W., Hager, H.: The morphologic pattern of oxygen deficiency in the human brain. Final report US AF Contract. **AF 61**, 514–945 (1959).
Schou, M.: Lithium als Psychopharmakon. Fortschr. Neurol. Psychiat. **37**, 349–383 (1969).
Schrappe, O.: Die psychopathologischen Gemeinsamkeiten und Unterschiede von Hypoglykämie und Alkoholrausch. Stuttgart: Schattauer, 1968.
Schrappe, O.: Die forensisch-psychiatrische Bedeutung der Hypoglykämie. Verh. dtsch. Ges. inn. Med. **75**, 966–969 (1969).
Scott, H.R.: Rapid staining of beta granules in pancreatic islets. Stain Techn. **27**, 267 (1952).
Seiler, N.R.: Der Stoffwechsel im ZNS. Stuttgart: Thieme, 1966.
Seitelberger, F., Gross, H.: Zur organischen Hirnschädigung des Alkoholkranken. In: Klinik und Therapie des Alkoholismus. Krypsin-Exner, K., Oltenau, T. (eds.). Vienna: Verh. Wien. Med. Akad., 1969, pp. 109–138.
Seitelberger, F., Jonasch, G.: Zentrale pontine Myelinolyse nach Schädeltrauma. Dtsch. Z. Nervenheilk. **197**, 28–41 (1970).
Selbach, H.: Über die vegetative Dynamik in der psychiatrischen Pharmakotherapie. Dtsch. med. Wschr. **12**, 511–517 (1961).
Shalit, M.N., Beller, A.J., Feinsod, M., Drapkin, A.J., Cotev, S.: The blood flow oxygen consumption of the dying brain. Neurology (Minneap.) **20**, 740–748 (1970).
Shalit, M.N., Reinmuth, O.M., Shimojyo, S., Scheinberg, P.: Carbon dioxide and cerebral circulation control. The effect of brain stem lesions. Arch. Neurol. (Paris) **17**, 342–353 (1967).
Shepherd, M., Lader, M., Rodnight, R.: Clinical Psychopharmacology. London: English Univ. Press, 1968.
Sherlock, S.: Altered consciousness in liver failure. Presented at 1st Congr. Internat. Neurol. (Brussels) **7**, 115–134 (1957).
Sherlock, S.: Pathogenesis and management hepatic coma. Amer. J. Med. **24**, 805–813 (1958).
Sherlock, S.: Hepatic coma. Ann. Rev. Med. **11**, 47–58 (1960).
Sherlock, S., Summerskill, G., White, L.P., Hear, E.A.: Portal-system encephalopathy. Neurological complications of liver disease. Lancet **1954**, 453–457.
Sherrington, C.S.: Decerebrate rigidity and reflex coordination of movements. J. Physiol. (Lond.) **22**, 319–328 (1898).
Sherrington, C.S.: The Integrative Action of the Nervous System. 2nd ed. New Haven: Yale, 1947.
Shinton, N.: The cobolamines. Practitioner **196**, 859–867 (1966).
Sieker, H.O., Hickam, J.B.: Carbon dioxide intoxication. Medicine **35**, 389–423 (1956).
Sieracki, J., Marshall, R.B., Horn, R.C.: Tumors of the pancreatic islets. Cancer (Philad.) **13**, 347 (1960).
Silverman, D.: Retrospective study of EEG in coma. Electroenceph. clin. Neurophysiol. **15**, 486–503 (1963).
Simpson, J.A.: Conduction velocity of peripheral nerves in human metabolic disorders. Electroenceph. clin. Neurophysiol. **10**, 357–394 (1958).
Skultety, F.M.: Clinical and experimental aspects of akinetic mutism. Arch. Neurol. **17**, 1–14 (1968).
Sluga, E.: Polyneuropathien. Typen und Differenzierung. Ergebnisse bioptischer Untersuchungen. Berlin–Heidelberg–New York: Springer, 1974.
Smith, A.L., Satterth-Waite, L.S., Sokoloff, L.: Induction of brain D-β-hydroxybutyrate-dehydrogenase activity by fasting. Science **163**, 79–81 (1969).
Sohn, D., Levine, S.: Hypertrophy of the olives: a report on 43 cases. Progr. Neuropath. **1**, 202–217 (1971).
Sokoleff, L.: Neurophysiology and neurochemistry of coma. Exp. Biol. Med. **4**, 15–33 (1971).
Spandri, P., Ambrosio, G., Binda, F., Meo, A., Mingrino, S., Grandesso, R.: Il comportamento dell'asse diencefalo ipofisosurrenalico nel coma da trauma cranico. Minerva med. giul. **15**, I (1968).
Sprague, J.M.: The effects of chronic brain stem lesions on wakefullness and sleep and behaviour. In: Sleep and Altered States of Consciousness. Proc. Ass. Res. nerv. ment. Dis. **45**, 148–188, 591 (1967).
Sprague, J.M., Chambers, W.W.: Regulation of posture in intact and decerebrate cat: Cerebellum, reticular, formation, vestibular nuclei. J. Neurophysiol. **16**, 451–463 (1953).

Sprague, J.M., Levitt, M., Rosbon, K., Liu, C.N., Stellar, E., Chambers, W.W.: Neuroanatomical and behavioural analysis of the syndromes resulting from midbrain lemniscal and reticular lesions in the cat. Arch. ital. Biol. **101**, 225 (1963).
Sprofkin, B.E.: Peroneal paralysis – a hazard of weight reduction. Arch. intern. Med. **102**, 82 (1958).
Staal, A.: General discussion on pressure neuropathies. In: Handbook of Clinical Neurology. Vinken, P.J., Bruyn, G.W. (eds.). New York–Amsterdam: Elsevier, North-Holland Publ. Co., 1970, p. 276.
Steegmann, A.T.: Anoxic encephalopathy and the cerebral circulation with reference to cardiovascular and respiratory disease. VIIth Congr. Neurol. 1961, pp. 197–228.
Stefanelli, N.: Prognose und Lebenserwartung der Leberzirrhose nach dem Auftreten eines Coma hepaticum. Wien. klin. Wschr. **74**, 228–290 (1962).
Steinbrecher, W.: Kurzer Grundriß der klinischen Elektromyographie. Franfurt/M.: Wander, 1962.
Steriade, M., Demetrescu, M.: Unspecific systems of inhibition and facilitation of potentials evoked by intermittent light. J. Neurophysiol. **23**, 602–617 (1960).
Stöckel, O., Beduin, D.: Spätkomplikationen nach Tracheotomie. Ergebnisse und Schlußfolgerungen aus einer katamnestischen Untersuchung. Langenbecks Arch. klin. Chir. **323**, 18 (1968).
Störring, G.E.: Über personale Eingleisigkeit als hirnorganische Erscheinung. Top. Probl. Psychiat. Neurol. **2**, 168–174 (1965).
Störring, G.E., Hauss, K., Ule, G.: Zur topischen Diagnostik des amnestischen Symptomenkomplexes. Psychiat. Neurol. **143**, 161–177 (1962).
Stössel, K.: Zur Klinik enzephalopathischer Zustände nach schweren gedeckten Hirntraumen. Dtsch. Gesundh.-Wes. **21**, 2140–2146 (1966).
Strauss, H.: Strangulationsfolgen und Hirnstamm. Z. Neurol. Psychiat. **131**, 363–374 (1931).
Street, D.M.: Paraarticular bone formation. In: Proc. 7th Ann. Clin. Paraplegia Conf. U.S. Veterans Admin., 1958, p. 31.
Strich, S.J.: Diffuse degeneration of the cerebral white matter in severe dementia following head injury. J. Neurol. Neurosurg. Psychiat. **19**, 163–185 (1956).
Strich, S.J.: Shearing of nerve fibres as a cause of brain damage due to head injury. A pathological study of twenty cases. Lancet **1961 I**, 443–448.
Strich, S.J.: The pathology of brain damage due to blunt head injuries. In: The Late Effect of Head Injury. Walker, A.F., Caveness, W.F., Critchley (eds.). Springfield/Ill.: Charles C. Thomas, 1969, pp. 501–524.
Struck, G.: Morphologische Befunde bei Dezerebrationszuständen mit rhythmischen oralen Automatismen. Dtsch. Z. Nervenheilk. **185**, 53–66 (1963).
Summerskill, W.H.G., Davidson, E.A., Sherlock, S., Steiner, R.E.: The neuropsychiatric syndrome associated with hepatic cirrhosis and an extensive portal collateral circulation. Quart. J. Med. **25**, 245–266 (1956).
Susuki, H., Taira, N.: Effect of reticular stimulation upon synaptic transmission in the cat's lateral geniculate body. Jap. J. Physiol. **11**, 641–655 (1961).
Sutter, J.M., Bardenal, C., Pheline, C., Coundray, J.P.: La catatonie posttraumatique. Ses rapports avec les "états de décérébration" et les comas prolongés". Rev. neurol. **101**, 524–535 (1959).
Swanson, A.G., Iseri, O.A.: Acute encephalopathy due to water intoxication. New Engl. J. Med. **258**, 831–834 (1958).
Szentagothai, J.: The elementary vestibulo-ocular reflex. J. Neurophysiol. **13**, 395 (1950).
Taylor, A.R., Bell, T.K.: Slowing of cerebral circulation after concussional head injury. Lancet **1966 II**, 178–180.
Terzian, H., Dalle Ore, G.: Syndrome of Klüve and Bucy, reproduced in man by bilateral removal of the temporal lobes. Neurology (Minneap.) **5**, 373–381 (1955).
Thomas, P.K., Fullerton, P.M.: Nerve fibre size in carpal-tunnel syndrome. J. Neurol. Neurosurg. Psychiat. **26**, 520 (1963).
Thuillier, J., Rumpf, P., Thullier, G.: Propriétés pharmacologiques de l'acide p. chlorphénoxytacétique (235 ANP). C.R. Soc. Biol. **153**, 1914 (1959).
Tönnies, J.F.: Drehstuhl mit unterschwelliger Anlaufsbeschleunigung. Z. Hals-, Nas.- u. Ohrenheilk. **30**, 353 (1932).
Tönnies, J.F.: Die Ableitungen bioelektrischer Effekte vom uneröffneten Schädel. Physikalische Behandlung des Problems. J. Psychol. Neurol. **15**, 154–171 (1933).

Tönnis, D.: Zur Entstehung von Drucklähmung an den unteren Extremitäten. Fortschr. Neurol. Psychiat. **26**, 483 (1958).
Tönnis, W., Frowein, R.A., Loew, F., Grote, W., Hemmer, R., Klug, W., Finkemeyer, H.: Organisation der Behandlung schwerer Schädel-Hirnverletzungen. Arbeit und Gesundheit, H. 79. Stuttgart: Thieme, 1968.
Tomlinson, B.E., Walton, J.N., Rebeiz, J.J.: The effect of ageing and of cachexia upon skeletal muscle. A histopathological study. J. neurol. Sci. **9**, 321 (1969).
Torelli, L.: La dihydroxyacétone dans la traitement de l'oedeme cérébral. Agressiologie **10**, 177–181 (1969).
Trillet, M.: A propos des encéphalopathies post-traumatiques. Comas prolongés et morts du cerveau post-traumatiques. Doctoral thesis. Faculty of Medicine and Pharmacy, Lyon, **239** (1949).
Trillet, M.: L'encéphalopathie posttraumatique: Comas prolongés et "morts du cerveau". J. Med. Lyon **987**, 631–655; **988**, 705–761; **992**, 1037–1083 (1961).
Tyler, H.R.: Neurologic disorders in renal failure. Amer. J. Med. **44**, 734–748 (1968).
Tyler, H.R.: Neurology disorders seen in the uremic patients. Arch. intern. Med. **126**, 781 (1970).
Tzonos, T., Muke, R.: Die Einwirkung von eilecithinemulgierter Sojabohnenölemulsion (Intralipid) auf das experimentell erzeugte Hirnödem. Acta neurochir. (Wien) **20**, 249–262 (1969).
Ule, G.: Hirnbefunde bei hochgradiger posttraumatischer „Demenz". Verh. dtsch. Ges. Path. **43**, 178 (1959).
Ule, G., Döhner, W., Bues, E.: Ausgedehnte Hemisphärenmarkschädigung nach gedecktem Hirntrauma mit apallischem Syndrom und partieller Spätrehabilitation. Arch. Psychiat. Nervenkr. **202**, 155–176 (1961).
Ule, G., Laux, W., Lehmann, H.J.: Anoetischer Symptomenkomplex und apallisches Syndrom bei der diffusen Form der Multiplen Sklerose. Top. Probl. Psychiat. Neurol. **2**, 168–174 (1965).
Umbach, W., Riechert, T.: Bewußtseinsstörungen unter dem Bild akinetischer-mutistischer Verhaltensweisen nach stereotaktischen Ausschaltungen in den Stammganglien. Arch. Psychiat. Nervenkr. **204**, 96–112 (1963).
Unterharnscheidt, F., Sellier, K.: Pathomorphologie der gedeckten Schädel-Hirnverletzungen. Excerpta med. Internat. Concr. Ser. **93**, 62–73 (1965).
Urhbrand, L., Faurbye, A.: Reversible and irreversible dyskinesia after treatment with perphenazine, chlorpromazine, reserpine and electroconvulsive therapy. Psychopharmacologia (Berl.) **1**, 408–418 (1960).
Valzelli, L.: Elementi di psicopharmacologia sperimentale e clinica. Milan: Manfredi, 1970.
Vanzulli, A.: Evoked responses in man. I. Photic responses. Acta neurol. lat.-amer. **6**, 219–231 (1960).
Verner, J.V., Morrison, A.B.: Islet cell tumor and a syndrome of refractory diarrhea and hypokalemia. Amer. J. Med. **25**, 374 (1958).
Victor, M., Adams, R.D.: In: Principles of Internal Medicine. Harrison, T.R. (ed.). New York: McGraw-Hill, 1962, p. 1400.
Vigouroux, R., Naquet, R., Baurand, C., Choux, M., Salomon, G., Khalil, R.: Evolution électro-radio-clinique de comas graves prolongés post-traumatiques. Rev. neurol. **110**, 72–81 (1964).
Villablanca, J.: Behavioural and poligraphic study of "sleep" and "wakefullness" in chronic decerebrate cats. Electroenceph. clin. Neurophysiol. **21**, 526–577 (1964).
Vincent, C., David, M., Thiebaut, E.: Le cone de pression remporal dans les tumeurs des Hémisphères cérébraux. Symptomatologie, sa gravité, les traitements qu'il convient de lui opposer. Rev. neurol. **65**, 536 (1936).
Vitale, A.: Mutismo acinetico in un caso di lesione circonscrita monoaterale della regione pallido-talamica con attività elettroencefalographica di tipo "cerveau isolé". Minerva neurochir. **8**, 45–52 (1964).
Vuia, O., Rothemund, E.: L:hypertrophie de l'olive bulbaire dans le syndrome apallique post-traumatique. Rev. neurol. **125**, 373–386 (1971).
Waelsch, H.J.: Metabolism of glutamic acid and glutamine. In: Neurochemistry, the Chemical Dynamics of the Brain and Nerve. Springfield/Ill.: Charles C. Thomas, 1955, pp. 173–203.
Walsh, J.T., Cordeau, J.P.: Responsiveness in the visual system during various phases of sleep and waking. Exp. Neurol. **11**, 90–103 (1965).

Weber, W.C., Jung, R.: Über die epileptische Aura. Z..ges. Neurol. Psychiatr. **170**, 211–265 (1940).
Weinberger, L.M., Gibbon, M.H., Gibbon, J.H.: Temporary arrest of the circulation of the CNS. Arch. Neurol. Psychiat. (Chicago) **43**, 615–634 (1940).
Weingarten, K., Seitelberger, F.: Über die subakute sklerosierende Leukoenzephalitis. Wien. Z. Nervenheilk. **6**, 65–90 (1953).
Weinstein, E.: Ophthalmoplegia with reserve of bells phenomenon occurring in a diabetic patient. Arch. Neurol. (Paris) **58** (1947).
Weiss, B., Laties, V.G.: Enhancement of human performance by caffeine and the amphetamines. Pharmacol. Rev. **14**, 1–36 (1962).
Weitzmann, E.D., Schaumburgh, H., Fischbein, W.: Plasma 17-OHCS levels during sleep in man. J. clin. Endocr. **26**, 121 (1966).
Welch, B.L., Graded effect of social simulation upon d-amphetamine toxicity agressiveness and heart and adrenal weight. J. Pharmacol. exp. Ther. **151**, 331 (1966).
Wertheimer, P., Allegre, G.: Note sur les camas traumatiques prolongés. Rev. neurol. **89**, 509–511 (1953).
Wesmann, W., Eggert, H., Kirschstein, H.: Zur Pathogenese und Therapie des Hirnödems. Verh. anat. Ges. Jena: G. Fischer, 1970, p. 126.
Wewalka, F.: Neurologische Komplikationen von Leberkrankheiten. Wien. Z. Nervenheilk. **29**, 95–106 (1971).
Wieck, H.H.: Zur Klinik der sogenannten symptomatischen Psychosen. Dtsch. med. Wschr. **61**, 1345–1349 (1956).
Wieck, H.H.: Funktionspsychosenbegriff und klinische Bedeutung. Med. Welt **18** (N.S.), 1807–1811 (1967a).
Wieck, H.H.: Lehrbuch der Psychiatrie. Stuttgart: Schattauer, 1967b).
Wieck, H.H., Brilmayer, H., Picka, N.: Durchgangssyndrome infolge von Vergiftungen mit Barbituraten. Fortschr. Neurol. Psychiat. **30**, 304–324 (1962).
Wieck, H.H., Stäcker, K.: Zur Dynamik des „amnestischen Durchgangs-Syndroms". Arch. Psychiat. Neurol. (Chicago) **205**, 479–512 (1964).
Wieser, S.: Der Abbau der oralen Leistungen. Ein Beitrag zum Problem der Evolution und Dissolution nervöser Leistungen. Ann. Univ. Saraviensis **5**, 211–269 (1957a).
Wieser, S.: Schlüsselreize raumorientierender Zuwendungsreaktionen. Arch. Psychiat. Nervenkr. **195**, 373–382 (1957b).
Wilhelm, A.: Neues über Druckschäden des Nervus ulnaris und Nervus radialis. Handchirurgie **2**, 143 (1970).
Wilson, S.A.K.: On decerebrate rigidity in man and the occurrence of tonic fits. Brain **43**, 220–268 (1920).
Woltman, H.W.: Pressure neuritis. Amer. J. med. Sci. **179**, 528 (1930).
Woods, J.W.: Behaviour of chronic decerebrate rats. J. Neurophysiol. **27**, 635–645 (1964).
Wyatt, R., Chase, T., Scott, J., Snyder, F., Engeeman, K.: Effect of L-DOPA on sleep in man. Nature (Lond.) **228**, 999–1001 (1970).
Yasuda, M., Namba, H.: Documentazione sul Nicholin. Takeda Pharm. Lab. (Japan), 1970.
Zanchetti, A.: Specificity of the reticular activating system. In: Brain Mechanism. Progress in Brain Res., Vol. I. Amsterdam, 1963, pp. 454–461.
Zander, E.: Die posttraumatische Hydrozephalie und ihre Behandlungsmöglichkeiten. Schweiz. med. Wschr. **99**, 1624–1629 (1969).
Ziegler, D.K., Zosa, A., Zileli, T.: Hypertensive Encephalopathy. Neurol. (Paris) **12**, 472–478 (1965).
Zülch, K.J.: Störungen des intrakraniellen Druckes. In: Handbuch der Neurochirurgie. Olivecrona, H., Tönnis, W. (eds.), Vol. I. Berlin–Göttingen–Heidelberg: Springer, 1955.
Zuppinger, K., Rossi, E.: Kindliche Hypoglykämien. Pädiat. Prax. **6**, 1903–1923 (1967).
Zysno, E., Darv, F., Rechenmiller, H.E., Nieth, H.: EEG-Untersuchungen bei urämischen Enzephalopathien unter intermittierender Peritonealdialyse. Verh. dtsch. Ges. inn. Med. **72**, 227–229 (1966).

Subject Index

Monographien aus dem Gesamtgebiete der Psychiatrie

Herausgeber: H. Hippius, Berlin; W. Janzarik, Heidelberg; C. Müller, Prilly, Schweiz

Band 1
K. Hartmann / **Theoretische und empirische Beiträge zur Verwahrlosungsforschung**
2., neubearbeitete und erweiterte Auflage, 16 Abbildungen, 34 Tabellen. XII, 180 Seiten. 1977. ISBN 3-540-07925-4

Band 2
P. Matussek / **Die Konzentrationslagerhaft und ihre Folgen**
Mit R. Grigat, H. Haiböck, G. Halbach, R. Kemmler, D. Mantell, A. Triebel, M. Vardy, G. Wedel. 19 Abbildungen, 73 Tabellen. X, 272 Seiten. 1971. ISBN 3-540-05214-3

Band 3
A.E. Adams / **Informationstheorie und Psychopathologie des Gedächtnisses**
12 Abbildungen. IX, 124 Seiten, 1971. ISBN 3-540-05215-1

Band 4
G. Nissen / **Depressive Syndrome im Kindes- und Jugendalter**
Beitrag zur Symptomatologie, Genese und Prognose.
11 Abbildungen, 51 Tabellen, IX. 174 Seiten. 1971. ISBN 3-540-05493-6

Band 5
A. Moser / **Die langfristige Entwicklung Oligophrener**
Mit einem Vorwort von Chr. Müller.
4 Abbildungen, 30 Tabellen. X, 102 Seiten. 1971. ISBN 3-540-05599-1

Band 6
H. Feldmann / **Hypochondrie**
Leibbezogenheit – Risikoverhalten – Entwicklungsdynamik.
36 Abbildungen, 5 Tabellen. VI, 118 Seiten. 1972. ISBN 3-540-05753-6

Band 7
S. Meyer-Osterkamp, R. Cohen / **Zur Größenkonstanz bei Schizophrenen**
Eine experimentalpsychologische Untersuchung. Mit einem einführenden Geleitwort von H. Heimann.
5 Abbildungen. VII, 91 Seiten. 1973. ISBN 3-540-06147-9

Band 8
K. Diebold / **Die erblichen myoklonisch-epileptisch-dementiellen Kernsyndrome**
Progressive Myoklonusepilepsien – Dyssynergia cerebellaris myoclonica – myoklonische Varianten der drei nachinfantilen Formen der amaurotischen Idiotie.
31 Abbildungen, IX, 254 Seiten. 1973. ISBN 3-540-06117-7

Band 9
C. Eggers / **Verlaufsweisen kindlicher und präpuberaler Schizophrenien**
3 Abbildungen, IX, 250 Seiten. 1973. ISBN 3-540-06163-0

Band 10
M. Schrenk / **Über den Umgang mit Geisteskranken**
Die Entwicklung der psychiatrischen Therapie vom 'moralischen Regime' in England und Frankreich zu den 'psychischen Kurmethoden' in Deutschland.
20 Abbildungen. X, 194 Seiten, 1973. ISBN 3-540-06267-X

Band 11
H. Schepank / **Erb- und Umweltfaktoren bei Neurosen**
Tiefenpsychologische Untersuchungen an 50 Zwillingspaaren. Unter Mitarbeit von P.E. Becker, A. Heigl-Evers, C.O. Köhler, H. Schepank, G. Wagner.
1 Abbildung, 82 Tabellen. VIII, 227 Seiten. 1974. ISBN 3-540-06647-0

Band 12
L. Ciompi, C. Müller / **Lebensweg und Alter der Schizophrenen**
Eine katamnestische Langzeitstudie bis ins Senium
27 Fallbeispiele, 23 Abbildungen, 48 Tabellen. IX, 242 Seiten. 1976. ISBN 3-540-07567-4

Band 13
L. Süllwold / **Symptome schizophrener Erkrankungen**
Uncharakteristische Basisstörungen.
15 Tabellen. VIII, 112 Seiten, 1977. ISBN 3-540-08203-4

Springer-Verlag Berlin Heidelberg New York

MIX
Papier aus verantwortungsvollen Quellen
Paper from responsible sources
FSC® C105338
FSC
www.fsc.org

If you have any concerns about our products,
you can contact us on
ProductSafety@springernature.com

In case Publisher is established outside the EU,
the EU authorized representative is:
Springer Nature Customer Service Center GmbH
Europaplatz 3, 69115 Heidelberg, Germany

Printed by Libri Plureos GmbH
in Hamburg, Germany